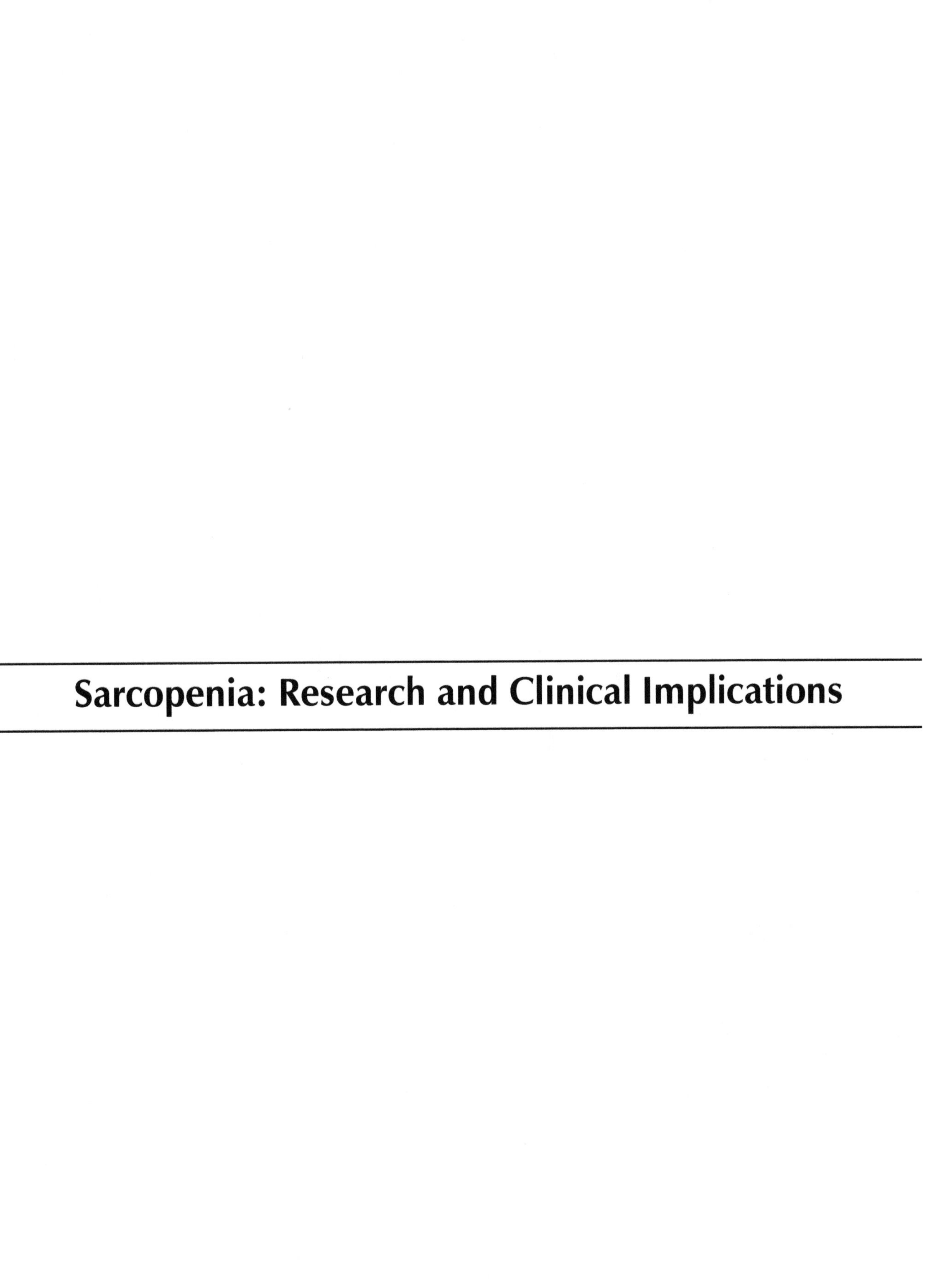

Sarcopenia: Research and Clinical Implications

Sarcopenia: Research and Clinical Implications

Editor: Jonathan Davidson

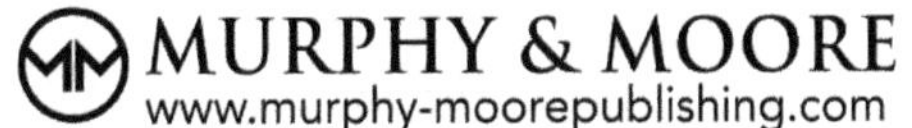

www.murphy-moorepublishing.com

MURPHY & MOORE

Cataloging-in-Publication Data

Sarcopenia : research and clinical implications / edited by Jonathan Davidson.
p. cm.
Includes bibliographical references and index.
ISBN 978-1-63987-777-5
1. Muscles--Diseases. 2. Aging--Physiological aspects. 3. Musculoskeletal diseases in old age.
4. Musculoskeletal system--Diseases. 5. Muscle strength. I. Davidson, Jonathan.
RC925.53 .S27 2023
618.976 7--dc23

Murphy & Moore Publishing
1 Rockefeller Plaza,
New York City,
NY 10020, USA

ISBN 978-1-63987-777-5

Contents

Preface

Every book is a source of knowledge and this one is no exception. The idea that led to the conceptualization of this book was the fact that the world is advancing rapidly; which makes it crucial to document the progress in every field. I am aware that a lot of data is already available, yet, there is a lot more to learn. Hence, I accepted the responsibility of editing this book and contributing my knowledge to the community.

Sarcopenia refers to a type of muscle loss which occurs due to aging or immobility. It is characterized by a progressive loss of skeletal muscle strength, mass and quality, which is dependent on factors such as nutrition, exercise level and co-morbidities. Sarcopenia is a component of the frailty syndrome and can result in decreased quality of life as well as incapacity, falls and fractures. It has become a crucial subject in geriatric medicine and represents a growing area of research. Inactivity is a major risk factor of sarcopenia and regular exercise can significantly decrease the muscle loss. The most beneficial form of exercise is resistance training, which is designed for enhancing the muscle stamina and strength by using resistance weights and bands. This book aims to shed light on some of the unexplored aspects of sarcopenia and the clinical implications of the researches conducted on it. Most of the topics introduced herein cover new techniques for clinical diagnosis and treatment of sarcopenia. The book is appropriate for students seeking detailed information on this disease as well as for experts.

While editing this book, I had multiple visions for it. Then I finally narrowed down to make every chapter a sole standing text explaining a particular topic, so that they can be used independently. However, the umbrella subject sinews them into a common theme. This makes the book a unique platform of knowledge.

I would like to give the major credit of this book to the experts from every corner of the world, who took the time to share their expertise with us. Also, I owe the completion of this book to the never-ending support of my family, who supported me throughout the project.

Editor

1

Melatonin as a Potential Agent in the Treatment of Sarcopenia

Ana Coto-Montes [1,2,*], Jose A. Boga [2,3], Dun X. Tan [2] and Russel J. Reiter [2]

1 Department of Morphology and Cellular Biology, Medicine Faculty, University of Oviedo, Julian Claveria, s/n, Oviedo 33006, Spain
2 Department of Cellular and Structural Biology, UTHSCSA, San Antonio, TX 78229, USA; joseantonio.boga@sespa.es (J.A.B.); tan@uthscsa.edu (D.X.T.); reiter@uthscsa.edu (R.J.R.)
3 Service of Microbiology, Hospital Universitario Central de Asturias, Avenida de Roma, s/n, Oviedo 33011, Spain
* Correspondence: acoto@uniovi.es

Academic Editor: Charles J. Malemud

Abstract: Considering the increased speed at which the world population is aging, sarcopenia could become an epidemic in this century. This condition currently has no means of prevention or treatment. Melatonin is a highly effective and ubiquitously acting antioxidant and free radical scavenger that is normally produced in all organisms. This molecule has been implicated in a huge number of biological processes, from anticonvulsant properties in children to protective effects on the lung in chronic obstructive pulmonary disease. In this review, we summarize the data which suggest that melatonin may be beneficial in attenuating, reducing or preventing each of the symptoms that characterize sarcopenia. The findings are not limited to sarcopenia, but also apply to osteoporosis-related sarcopenia and to age-related neuromuscular junction dysfunction. Since melatonin has a high safety profile and is drastically reduced in advanced age, its potential utility in the treatment of sarcopenic patients and related dysfunctions should be considered.

Keywords: melatonin; sarcopenia; frailty; skeletal muscle; aging

---

1. Introduction

Worldwide estimates predict 2 billion people will be over 65 years old by 2050 [1]. Thus, an increasingly significant percentage of the population demands remedies and treatments for the deleterious processes that age induces. The scientific community is currently at a loss when it comes to meeting these requirements. Aging is a multifactorial process that provokes slow and persistent functional decline. This gradual physiological deterioration becomes disabling for a high percentage of the elderly population, where it impairs quality of life and increases the demands on primary caregivers and healthcare providers. Of all the degenerative processes, the development of limitations in mobility is one of the most common, leading to a reduced capacity for daily living activities, disability and loss of independence. Slow walking speed, together with unintentional weight loss, self-reported exhaustion, weakness (grip strength) and low physical activity, are the criteria that characterize frailty status. This aging phenotype has been described in detail by Fried et al. [2]. This state of frailty also is characterized by a reduced capacity to respond to demands caused by diminishing functional reserve; this puts the individual in a special risk category when facing minor stressors and is associated with poor outcomes (disability, hospitalization and death) [3,4].

In older adults, mobility limitations have been defined as the self-reported inability to walk a mile, climb stairs or perform heavy housework [5]. This impaired mobility is very often associated with a well-established factor of age-related decline in muscle mass designated as sarcopenia [6].

Sarcopenia, however, not only refers to muscle mass deterioration; numerous other factors are involved in the reduction in muscle quality associated with aging. These include derangement of skeletal myocytes, vascular dysfunction, reduced aerobic capacity, fat infiltration and a decline in bone mineral density [6,7].

The high number of individuals affected by this syndrome or at least by some sarcopenia-related features has caused sarcopenia to reach epidemic proportions. Moreover, there is no effective cure currently available for this condition and likewise no known treatments, even palliative, are available. The need to develop interventions to prevent or treat sarcopenia has been repeatedly claimed in the literature [8–10]. In the current brief review, we summarize previous data suggesting that melatonin mayto limit the development of several of the derangements associated with sarcopenia. Melatonin has a variety of beneficial effects that may slow the development or reduce the severity of the deleterious processes which inevitably lead to sarcopenia in aging population. To date, the evidence for melatonin's efficacy relative to reducing sarcopenia has not been systematically summarized.

2. Sarcopenia Syndrome

Sarcopenia is a term derived from the Greek words *sarx* (flesh) and *penia* (loss) that was introduced by Rosenberg [11] and was used to classically describe the decline in muscle mass among older people [7,12]. Currently, sarcopenia is a well-documented condition associated with the impaired mobility that occurs with aging [13]. There is increasingly evidence, however, that not only the decline in muscle mass is responsible for sarcopenia, but also a failure in muscle strength or power (referred to as dynapenia) is commonly associated with sarcopenia [6,14,15]. Both sarcopenia and dynapenia typically increase with advancing age, but there are individuals in whom there is a discrepancy between changes in muscle mass and muscle strength, mainly related to occupational physical activity in their midlife [6]. Such activity appears to delay sarcopenia development, while dynapenia is a more constant factor that compromises wellbeing at old ages [15]. To take into account this discrepancy, a new term (i.e., muscle quality) is being increasingly used, referring to the force generating capacity per unit cross-sectional area [6,16,17]. Muscle quality is negatively affected by several processes.

Sarcopenia and energetic imbalance are characteristics of the physiological framework that explain frailty and its consequences [18]. Walston and Fried suggest that there is some feedback between these components, the so-called frailty cycle. This cycle stems from the physiological changes associated with aging, which results in an imbalance between anabolism and catabolism. This state embraces multiple systems and cellular pathways implicated in age-dependent muscle degeneration (reviewed by [7,14]). Thus, sarcopenic muscle exhibits several cellular dysfunctions which result from oxidative stress, mainly due to mitochondrial dysfunction and a reduction of radical scavenging capability. Also included is a reduction in cellular turnover with a significant decrease in the number of satellite cells, alterations in proteolytic activities including those of the proteasome, autophagic dysregulation and even changes in apoptosis. These cellular derangements are associated or are even part of the more general perturbations also involved in sarcopenia development. These include a decrease in sex hormones [19] and an elevated pro-inflammatory state [20]. Eventually, sarcopenia is related to adipocyte infiltration with increases in both intra- and inter-muscular adipose tissue which significantly contributes to the decline in muscle quality [21]. Additional contributing factors include osteoporosis due to close relationship between muscle and bone, which are a single functional unit [7] and a decline in neurophysiological activity. This relates to the fact that age-related changes in the neuromuscular junction (NMJ) play a key role in musculoskeletal impairment, preceding or following the decline in muscle mass [22].

Collectively, the described alterations are embodied in the term sarcopenia and all are well-established risk factors for the major negative health-related conditions and events that characterize aging, including frailty, disability, institutionalization and mortality [23]. The development of preventive and therapeutic strategies against sarcopenia is considered an urgent need by health professionals. Based on what is known about the actions of melatonin, we propose that this molecule may have the potential to counteract sarcopenic damage or, moreover, may prevent some of the alterations associated with muscle quality loss. Additionally, we cited the published literature that shows the efficacious and beneficial effects of melatonin against the features which constitute the multi-pathology called sarcopenia.

3. Why Melatonin?

Melatonin, also known as *N*-acetyl-5-methoxytryptamine, is a derivative of tryptophan, an essential amino acid [24]. It is produced by the pineal gland in a circadian manner with maximal production during the night. It is involved in synchronization of circadian rhythms in physiological functions including sleep timing, blood pressure, seasonal reproduction and many others [25–29]. There is also evidence that all other cells produce melatonin [30,31], continually throughout the day, mainly as an antioxidant and free radical scavenger [32–35]. Melatonin is present in all biological fluids including cerebrospinal fluid, saliva, bile, synovial fluid, amniotic fluid, and breast milk [36,37]; and perhaps in mitochondria and chloroplasts where it may have the capacity to synthesize and metabolize melatonin itself [31,38]. This molecule has important protective capabilities, mainly based on its high potency as a free radical scavenger, low toxicity and solubility in both aqueous and organic media [30,39].

Pineal production and plasma melatonin levels progressively drop during aging [40–42] to the extent that in advanced age its levels are almost null. The loss of melatonin during aging may have great importance in the general deterioration that the elderly experience. Several investigations have reported a general improvement in life quality due to melatonin supplementation in older adults [43–45]. Moreover, numerous articles relate the age-associated decline in melatonin levels with the development of several diseases [46–48].

Melatonin is undoubtedly more than a zeitgeber and an antioxidant molecule since it seems to be essential at the cellular level as a physiological regulator of homeostasis. Its therapeutic applications are numerous, from pediatric [49–51] to geriatric diseases [52–54]; this includes cancer [55,56], sleep disturbances [57,58] and neurodegenerative diseases [59,60].

Several clinical trials with melatonin supplementation as a treatment have been successfully performed [61]. These melatonin treatments have often had positive outcomes in different pathologies: reducing cardiac morbidity [62], controlling adverse effects of chemotherapy [63] and alleviating bipolar disorders [64] among others. Also, melatonin has been used as a treatment with significant success in Duchenne muscular dystrophy [65] where it reduced the muscle degenerative process. Based on previous knowledge about the role of melatonin and sarcopenia (as summarized below), it is likely that melatonin may be effective in treating this condition.

4. Cellular Impact of Sarcopenia

Sarcopenia is a highly burdensome geriatric syndrome. The heterogeneity of its clinical correlates and the complexity of its pathogenesis make the development of effective preventive and therapeutic measures difficult. In this section we describe the numerous changes that occur at the cellular level in sarcopenic muscle [66].

4.1. Increase in Oxidative Stress and Mitochondrial Alterations

Aging is characterized by an increase in oxidative stress which is exacerbated during sarcopenia development. The relationship of oxidative stress to sarcopenia has been experimentally defined [67,68]. Considering this, theoretically at least, the addition of an antioxidant should produce beneficial effects in this condition. However, not all reactive species are harmful. Certainly, it is well-established that some reactive oxygen species (ROS), reactive nitrogen species (RNS), and a basal level of oxidative stress are essential for cell survival [69]. Oxidant generation, within a hormetic range, is essential for intracellular signaling [70] and optimal force production [71]. Thus, very highly efficient antioxidants may paradoxically be harmful unless their effects on the redox balance are closely titrated [72].

However, melatonin seems not to be a typical radical scavenger and many publications show that melatonin also regulates cellular homeostasis [37] and could even promote the generation of free radicals when necessary [34]. For example, we have shown that when high oxidative stress is necessary for adequate organ development, daily melatonin injections initially induce a reduction of oxidative stress but, subsequently, when the melatonin injections are continued, free radical generation is restored [73]. The collective findings indicate that melatonin is able to reduce free radical concentrations but maintain them inside homeostatic limits and, moreover, melatonin's action as a free radical scavenger and as antioxidant are context specific as described by Proietti and colleagues [74].

The rise in oxidative stress in sarcopenia is mainly a result of mitochondrial dysfunction. Any derangements in skeletal myocyte mitochondrial function are recognized as major factors that contribute to age-dependent muscle degeneration [67]. In this regard, it is noteworthy that slow walking speed has been adopted as a criterion for defining sarcopenia [75]; this is likely due to a mitochondrial bioenergetic decline during muscle aging [76]. Melatonin and its metabolites are powerful antioxidants protecting the electron transport chain and mitochondrial DNA from oxidative damage more efficiently than other conventional antioxidants [77]. This protection of the respiratory chain allows melatonin to increase ATP production in mitochondria [78].

4.2. Cellular Vacuolization: Alterations in Autophagy

The process of vacuolization is currently poorly understood. According to Henics and Wheatley [79], vacuolization is simply the state of being with vacuoles; this implies a continual process of becoming progressively more vacuolated. This occurs in most cell types spontaneously or via a wide range of inductive stimuli. Vacuoles can be formed from several organelle types of the endosomal/lysosomal compartment and is generally considered a degenerative process. The involvement of autophagosomes in vacuole formation is widely accepted [80]. Also, some agents impair autophagy, inducing blockage, which results in vacuole accumulation [81]. Strongly supporting this hypothesis, several articles show functional defects in autophagy as a characteristic of sarcopenic muscle [7,82]; this has been occasionally accompanied by perinuclear accumulation of autophagic vacuoles [83].

Melatonin, in its role as a homeostasis stabilizer, has been shown to induce [84] or reduce [85] autophagy. In relation to muscle, melatonin is highly versatile molecule and either induces autophagy [86] or inhibits it [87], depending on pathological processes involved, since oxidative stress has a close relationship with autophagy. For example, melatonin induces autophagy in myoblast cells collaborating in myogenic differentiation (MyoD) degradation [88] but it inhibits autophagy in muscles from carbon tetrachloride-treated mice by reducing oxidative stress-induced damage [89].

4.3. Protein Degradation Deterioration

Sarcopenia is a syndrome where the cell's catabolic machinery has collapsed or has become misregulated [90]. The accumulation of lipofuscin granules in an increasing number of lysosomes of sarcopenic muscles is an example of impaired lysosomal degradative capacity [91]. In this process, only a small amount of lysosomal enzymes remains available for degradative pathways [67]; this significantly contributes to the reduction in the degenerative capacity of these organelles. On the other hand, higher levels of myostatin, a transforming growth factor-β (TGF-β) family member, induce muscle wasting by activating proteasomal-mediated catabolism of intracellular proteins [92]. In addition, defects in protein synthesis has been detected in muscles of sarcopenic patients [93]

Melatonin reduces endoplasmic reticulum stress in skeletal muscle by increasing the expression of several proteins as well as mRNA levels [89]; this improves protein synthesis. Likewise, melatonin is an important regulator of proteasome [94] and lysosomal mechanisms [88], thereby enhancing cell quality.

4.4. Decrease in Satellite Cells and Increase in Apoptosis

Satellite cells in skeletal muscle are quiescent mono-nucleated myogenic cells, located between the sarcolemma and basement membrane of terminally-differentiated muscle fibres [95]. The life-long maintenance of muscle tissue involves satellite cells, since under homeostatic conditions satellite cells are activated by stimuli such as physical trauma or growth signals [96]. Sarcopenia increases the susceptibility to muscle injury [97] and the reduced muscle mass contributes to falls [98]; in these situations satellite cell activation would be essential for improving regeneration of these old muscles. However, satellite cells are drastically reduced in sarcopenia increasing the negative consequences of sarcopenic muscle [99] and/or its funcionality [100]. Unfortunately, these changes are sarcopenic characteristics [7].

Melatonin also increases satellite cells following muscle injury in rats [101] by reducing the apoptotic processes via modulation of signaling pathways which causes significant muscle regeneration in these animals. Antiapoptotic actions of melatonin have been described in many tissues and in a variety of normal cell types [102,103]. However, melatonin's role in apoptosis can differ among normal and cancer cells, since several publications have shown melatonin's capability to destroy cancer cells by triggering apoptosis [104–106]. In contrast, in normal skeletal muscle, some authors have described in detail how melatonin prevents apoptosis and limits the oxidative stress that causes mitochondria permeability transition and subsequent death [107]. Melatonin, for example, attenuates apoptotic processes during ischemia/reperfusion in skeletal muscle [108]. Considering these findings, melatonin has been proven to significantly reduce or, even, counteract several pathophysiological processes specifically associated with sarcopenia [7].

4.5. Chronic Low Inflammation

There are other processes, some of them being a result of the changes described above, which are common to different pathologies and are part of the sarcopenic complex. Melatonin may also counteract or reduce those pathologies. One example is the systemic subacute inflammation which is a predominant characteristic of the aging process [109]. This low grade inflammation has been implicated in the development of a number of chronic diseases [110] and is associated with sarcopenia development as well [67,111]. The damaging agents in this process are notably interleukin 6 (IL-6), C-reactive protein (CRP) and tumor necrosis factor α (TNF-α) [112,113]. Recent evidence has documented a role for melatonin in reducing inflammation in muscle cells, acting specifically against these cytokines in rats [114] and also in humans [115]. The anti-inflammatory actions of melatonin are well-documented in numerous organs [116].

4.6. Endocrine Signaling

Studies on the nature and magnitude of age-related perturbations in circulating hormones as well as the responsiveness of target tissues are major features of sarcopenia research [82]. A number of hormone levels change during sarcopenia, including myokines and adipokines, due to the crosstalk between muscle and adipose tissue [117,118]. Also, alterations in the renin–angiotensin system promote muscular inflammation, mitochondrial dysfunction, and apoptosis [119]; insulin resistance leads to perturbed metabolism and misrouted signaling [120]. Also, reductions in testosterone and dehydroepiandrosterone contribute to muscle loss or weakness [121], while growth hormone (GH) and insulin-like growth factor 1 (IGF-1) decrease, which is deleterious to the physical function of skeletal muscle with age [122].

Hormonal supplementation in the older adults has been used to restore endocrine signaling. This procedure is controversial and disappointing results in sarcopenic individuals have been obtained [67]. As a result, great disparities between recommendations from scientific societies related to aging and elderly patients in general have been mentioned [121]. Consequently, hormonal supplementation seems not to be a desirable option. As an example, special attention should be paid regarding GH where long-time supplementation as an anti-aging strategy has caused a number of severe side effects associated with this treatment, and the Growth Hormone Research Society has warned against the use of GH or its secretagogues [123].

With regard to supplementation with melatonin, firstly, no significant adverse effects have been reported with its use at any concentration or at any treatment time. Also, melatonin, as an effective testosterone substitute, has been shown to prevent muscular atrophy in rats induced by castration through the IGF-1 axis [124]. Moreover, melatonin reduces adipogenesis in obese mice [85], collaborates in insulin resistance attenuation in *Caenorhabditis elegans* [125] and has a regulatory role in autocrine and paracrine responses in muscle and adipose tissue [126]. Additionally, melatonin has been shown to be more effective than GH in recovering physiological functions in smooth muscle from old rats [127].

4.7. Vascular Aging

Aging of the vascular system significantly hinders the uptake of oxygen and nutrients by muscle cells; this is closely related to sarcopenia development. Thus, aged skeletal muscle shows reduced blood flow capacity [128] together with extensive damage to endothelium-dependent vasodilation. Both processes promote mitochondrial destruction in muscle cells due to a reduction in microvascular oxygenation [129]; this in turn, induces ATP failure, increases ROS generation that also affects blood vessel integrity. Thus, a vicious cycle involving oxidant production and vascular and muscular damage ensues [67].

In contrast, a long-term treatment with melatonin has vasculoprotective properties [130]; for example, it restores vascular dysfunction in a model of accelerated aging (i.e., the senescence accelerated mouse-prone 8 (SAMP8)). Moreover, melatonin improves endothelial damage and causes important improvements in vessel cytoarchitecture in aged animals [131]. Finally, benefits in delaying age-related cellular damage in the cardiovascular system have been observed in aged rats supplemented with caffeic acid phenethyl ester and melatonin [132].

Age-related damage of skeletal muscle cannot be studied as an isolated entity because to its close relation with bone and the involvement of neuromuscular junctions. Unrepaired damage to one of these two systems renders treatments for improving sarcopenia useless. It is essential that melatonin's capability of restoring the integrity of the musculoskeletal system and neuromuscular junctions also be considered in any attempts to reduce sarcopenia.

5. Sarcopenia and Osteoporosis

As mentioned above, bone and muscle are closely interrelated. Thus, when aging affects one of these two tissues, the functionality of the other is likewise compromised [66]. Thus, as muscle quality deteriorates during aging, also bone becomes weakened when it develops osteoporosis.

Osteoporosis literally means "porous bone". It is a consequence of a reduction in bone mineral density which significantly increases fracture risk, which is the most serious complication of osteoporosis [133]. Muscle force has an important influence on essential bone properties such as mass, size, shape, and, even, architecture [134]. Thus, in elderly sarcopenic patients when the muscle strain falls below a given threshold, bone remodeling activates a so-called disuse mode, which results in less bone formation and greater bone resorption [66]. The reliance of muscle health on bone and vice versa is so interrelated that several researchers consider it one syndrome, with terms including sarco-osteopenia, sarco-osteoporosis, or dysmobility syndrome to distinguish disorders which are prone to a high risk of fractures [66,135,136].

Oxidative stress and autophagic alterations have been implicated in the development of osteoporosis [137], which could account for the beneficial effects of melatonin in this disease [138]. A recent published clinical trial has provided evidence related to the ability of melatonin to improve bone mineral density in humans [139], thereby protecting them against fractures. The ability of melatonin to protect against osteroporosis would also provide benefits in terms of limiting sarcopenia, since elevated bone strength is usually associated with greater muscular tone.

6. Neuromuscular Junction

The NMJ is the site at which efferent neurons communicate with muscle fibers. They function in the transmission of signals from the motor neuron to the skeletal muscle fibers to ensure precise control of skeletal muscle contraction and therefore voluntary movement. When the function of the motor neuron terminal is lost, the muscular fiber innervated by this neuron loses its contact to the nervous system and becomes incapable of generating volitional muscle contractions [22]. Although aging is usually associated with a reduction in NMJ function, the mechanisms involved are not well understood. Some lines of evidence point to the changes being causally related to the decline in muscle mass and function as observed in sarcopenia; however, which occurs first, sarcopenia or a reduction in the function of the NMJ, remains unknown [22].

Once again, oxidative stress seems to be implicated in NMJ impairment together with mitochondrial dysfunction and inflammation being prominent features [140]. Thus, melatonin, due to its potent antioxidant activities could be a key player in resolving or preventing this deregulation. In fact, published reports using different animals show that melatonin reverses age-related neuromuscular transmission dysfunction [141] and improves, at the same time, muscle physiology [142].

While still limited, the scientific evidence is consistent in terms of suggesting that melatonin significantly improves aged muscle as well as other cellular alterations characteristic of sarcopenia. Melatonin's action also applies to the pathophysiological processes associated to sarcopenia including muscle dysfunction that is closely interlinked to sarcopenia. Finally, it is necessary to remember that melatonin levels are gradually lost throughout life [41], being almost undetectable in the elderly; this could easily facilitate sarcopenia development. In light of these findings, it is reasonable to assume that maintaining normal endogenous levels of melatonin or administering it as an exogenous supplement may alleviate age-related muscular decline and the development of sarcopenia.

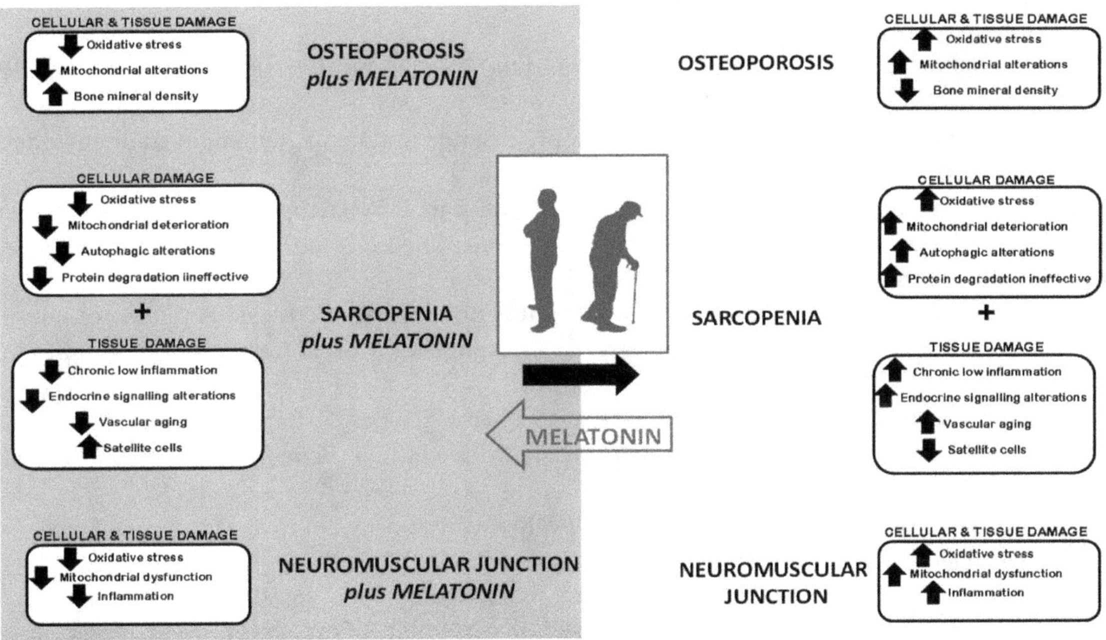

Figure 1. Schematic overview of the potential beneficial effects of melatonin in osteoporosis, sarcopenia and disruption of the neuromuscular junction.

7. Conclusions

Sarcopenia is a highly burdensome geriatric syndrome. It is commonly associated with osteroporosis and neuromuscular dysfunction. Currently, no effective treatment for this degenerative process has been identified. Melatonin has a high safety profile and no serious toxicity related to melatonin usage has been reported. Here, we summarized the scientific evidence that melatonin prevents and counteracts mitochondrial impairments, reduces oxidative stress and autophagic alterations in muscle cells, increases the number of satellite cells and limits sarcopenic changes in skeletal muscle. Likewise, melatonin lowers chronic low inflammation levels and reduces vascular aging, all of which are usually present in sarcopenic muscle. Similarly, melatonin improves the endocrine signaling which deteriorates in aged individuals. As a consequence, melatonin may be useful to prevent or treat sarcopenia-associated diseases including osteoporosis and neuromuscular dysfunction (Figure 1). Collectively, the published data suggest that melatonin may be a useful aid in slowing age-related muscle deterioration (i.e., sarcopenia as well as its associated conditions). If so, stronger muscles could translate into fewer falls and bone fractures in the older population, which are factors that normally seriously compromise aged individuals' health.

Acknowledgments: Ana Coto-Montes and Jose A. Boga are members of the INPROTEOLYS and INEUROPA network. Ana Coto-Montes and Jose A. Boga are team-leaders from the cellular Response to Oxidative Stress (cROS) research group within the Campus of International Excellence (University of Oviedo). This study and stays of Ana Coto-Montes and Jose A. Boga were supported by the "Salvador de Madariaga" Programme from the Ministerio de Educacion, Cultura y Deportes, FISS-13-RD12/0043/0030, FISS-11-01381 and FISS-14-PI13/02741 (Instituto de Salud Carlos III), GRUPIN14-071 (Plan de Ciencia, Tecnología e Innovación (PCTI) del Principado de Asturias), and Fondo Europeo de Desarrollo Regional (FEDER) funds.

Author Contributions: All authors have equally contributed to the development of this review.

References

1. United Nations, Department of Economic and Social Affairs, Population Division. *World Population Ageing*; United Nations: New York, NY, USA, 2015; ST/ESA/SER.A/390.
2. Fried, L.P.; Tangen, C.M.; Walston, J.; Newman, A.B.; Hirsch, C.; Gottdiener, J.; Seeman, T.; Tracy, R.; Kop, W.J.; Burke, G.; et al. Frailty in older adults: Evidence for a phenotype. *J. Gerontol. A Biol. Sci. Med. Sci.* **2001**, *56*, M146–M156. [CrossRef] [PubMed]
3. Campbell, A.J.; Buchner, D.M. Unstable disability and the fluctuations of frailty. *Age Ageing* **1997**, *26*, 315–318. [CrossRef] [PubMed]
4. Rockwood, K.; Hogan, D.B.; MacKnight, C. Conceptualisation and measurement of frailty in elderly people. *Drugs Aging* **2000**, *17*, 295–302. [CrossRef] [PubMed]
5. Dufour, A.B.; Hannan, M.T.; Murabito, J.M.; Kiel, D.P.; McLean, R.R. Sarcopenia definitions considering body size and fat mass are associated with mobility limitations: The Framingham Study. *J. Gerontol. A Biol. Sci. Med. Sci.* **2013**, *68*, 168–174. [CrossRef] [PubMed]
6. McGregor, R.A.; Cameron-Smith, D.; Poppitt, S.D. It is not just muscle mass: A review of muscle quality, composition and metabolism during ageing as determinants of muscle function and mobility in later life. *Longev. Healthspan* **2014**, *3*, 9. [CrossRef] [PubMed]
7. Tarantino, U.; Piccirilli, E.; Fantini, M.; Baldi, J.; Gasbarra, E.; Bei, R. Sarcopenia and fragility fractures: Molecular and clinical evidence of the bone-muscle interaction. *J. Bone Jt. Surg. Am.* **2015**, *97*, 429–437. [CrossRef] [PubMed]
8. Brass, E.P.; Sietsema, K.E. Considerations in the development of drugs to treat sarcopenia. *J. Am. Geriatr. Soc.* **2011**, *59*, 530–535. [CrossRef] [PubMed]
9. Chumlea, W.C.; Cesari, M.; Evans, W.J.; Ferrucci, L.; Fielding, R.A.; Pahor, M.; Studenski, S.; Vellas, B.; International Working Group on Sarcopenia Task Force Members. Sarcopenia: Designing phase IIB trials. *J. Nutr. Health Aging* **2011**, *15*, 450–455. [CrossRef] [PubMed]
10. Matthews, G.D.; Huang, C.L.; Sun, L.; Zaidi, M. Translational musculoskeletal science: Is sarcopenia the next clinical target after osteoporosis? *Ann. N. Y. Acad. Sci.* **2011**, *1237*, 95–105. [CrossRef] [PubMed]
11. Rosenberg, I.H. Summary comments: Epidemiological and methodological problems in determining nutritional status of older persons. *Ann. Intern. Med.* **1989**, *50*, 1231–1233.
12. Rosenberg, I.H. Sarcopenia: Origins and clinical relevance. *J. Nutr.* **1997**, *127*, 990S–991S. [CrossRef] [PubMed]
13. Nair, K.S. Aging muscle. *Am. J. Clin. Nutr.* **2005**, *81*, 953–963. [PubMed]

14. Kalinkovich, A.; Livshits, G. Sarcopenia: The search for emerging biomarkers. *Ageing Res. Rev.* **2015**, *22*, 58–71. [CrossRef] [PubMed]
15. Mitchell, W.K.; Williams, J.; Atherton, P.; Larvin, M.; Lund, J.; Narici, M. Sarcopenia, dynapenia, and the impact of advancing age on human skeletal muscle size and strength; a quantitative review. *Front. Physiol.* **2012**, *3*, 260. [CrossRef] [PubMed]
16. Barbat-Artigas, S.; Rolland, Y.; Zamboni, M.; Aubertin-Leheudre, M. How to assess functional status: A new muscle quality index. *J. Nutr. Health Aging* **2012**, *16*, 67–77. [CrossRef] [PubMed]
17. Beavers, K.M.; Beavers, D.P.; Houston, D.K.; Harris, T.B.; Hue, T.F.; Koster, A.; Newman, A.B.; Simonsick, E.M.; Studenski, S.A.; Nicklas, B.J.; et al. Associations between body composition and gait-speed decline: Results from the Health, Aging, and Body Composition Study. *Am. J. Clin. Nutr.* **2013**, *97*, 552–560. [CrossRef] [PubMed]
18. Walston, J.; Fried, L.P. Frailty and the older man. *Med. Clin. N. Am.* **1999**, *83*, 1173–1194. [CrossRef]
19. Iannuzzi-Sucich, M.; Prestwood, K.M.; Kenny, A.M. Prevalence of sarcopenia and predictors of skeletal muscle mass in healthy, older men and women. *J. Gerontol. A Biol. Sci. Med. Sci.* **2002**, *57*, M772–M777. [CrossRef] [PubMed]
20. Leng, Y.; Ahmadi-Abhari, S.; Wainwright, N.W.; Cappuccio, F.P.; Surtees, P.G.; Luben, R.; Brayne, C.; Khaw, K.T. Daytime napping, sleep duration and serum C reactive protein: A population-based cohort study. *BMJ Open* **2014**, *11*, e006071. [CrossRef] [PubMed]
21. Miljkovic, N.; Lim, J.-Y.; Miljkovic, I.; Frontera, W.-R. Aging of skeletal muscle fibers. *Ann. Rehabil. Med.* **2015**, *39*, 155–162. [CrossRef] [PubMed]
22. Gonzalez-Freire, M.; de Cabo, R.; Studenski, S.A.; Ferrucci, L. The neuromuscular junction: Aging at the crossroad between nerves and muscle. *Front. Aging Neurosci.* **2014**, *6*, 208. [CrossRef] [PubMed]
23. Visser, M.; Schaap, L.A. Consequences of sarcopenia. *Clin. Geriatr. Med.* **2011**, *27*, 387–399. [CrossRef] [PubMed]
24. Stehle, J.; Reuss, S.; Riemann, R.; Seidel, A.; Vollrath, L. The role of arginine-vasopressin for pineal melatonin synthesis in the rat: Involvement of vasopressinergic receptors. *Neurosci. Lett.* **1991**, *123*, 131–134. [CrossRef]
25. Dawson, D.; Encel, N. Melatonin and sleep in humans. *J. Pineal Res.* **1993**, *15*, 1–12. [CrossRef] [PubMed]
26. Reiter, R.J.; Tan, D.X.; Korkmaz, A. The circadian melatonin rhythm and its modulation: Possible impact on hypertension. *J. Hypertens. Suppl.* **2009**, *27*, S17–S20. [CrossRef] [PubMed]
27. Calvo, J.R.; González-Yanes, C.; Maldonado, M.D. The role of melatonin in the cells of the innate immunity: A review. *J. Pineal Res.* **2013**, *55*, 103–120. [CrossRef] [PubMed]
28. Reiter, R.J.; Tamura, H.; Tan, D.X.; Xu, X.Y. Melatonin and the circadian system: Contributions to successful female reproduction. *Fertil. Steril.* **2014**, *102*, 321–328. [CrossRef] [PubMed]
29. Pechanova, O.; Paulis, L.; Simko, F. Peripheral and central effects of melatonin on blood pressure regulation. *Int. J. Mol. Sci.* **2014**, *15*, 17920–17937. [CrossRef] [PubMed]
30. Venegas, C.; García, J.A.; Escames, G.; Ortiz, F.; López, A.; Doerrier, C.; García-Corzo, L.; López, L.C.; Reiter, R.J.; Acuña-Castroviejo, D. Extrapineal melatonin: Analysis of its subcellular distribution and daily fluctuations. *J. Pineal Res.* **2012**, *52*, 217–227. [CrossRef] [PubMed]
31. Tan, D.X. Mitochondria and chloroplasts as the original sites of melatonin synthesis: A hypothesis related to melatonin's primary function and evolution in eukaryotes. *J. Pineal Res.* **2013**, *54*, 127–138. [CrossRef] [PubMed]
32. Hardeland, R.; Tan, D.X.; Reiter, R.J. Kynuramine, metabolites of melatonin and other indoles: The resurrection of an almost forgotten class of biogenic amines. *J. Pineal Res.* **2009**, *47*, 109–126. [CrossRef] [PubMed]
33. Tan, D.X.; Manchester, L.C.; Terron, M.P.; Flores, L.J.; Reiter, R.J. One molecule, many derivatives: A never-ending interaction of melatonin with reactive oxygen and nitrogen species? *J. Pineal Res.* **2007**, *42*, 28–42. [CrossRef] [PubMed]
34. Zhang, H.M.; Zhang, Y. Melatonin: A well-documented antioxidant with conditional pro-oxidant actions. *J. Pineal Res.* **2014**, *57*, 131–146. [CrossRef] [PubMed]
35. Galano, A.; Medina, M.E.; Tan, D.X.; Reiter, R.J. Melatonin and its metabolites as copper chelating agents and their role in inhibiting oxidative stress: A physicochemical analysis. *J. Pineal Res.* **2015**, *58*, 107–116. [CrossRef] [PubMed]

36. Reiter, R.J.; Tan, D.X.; Rosales-Corral, S.; Manchester, L.C. The universal nature, unequal distribution and antioxidant functions of melatonin and its derivatives. *Mini Rev. Med. Chem.* **2013**, *13*, 373–384. [CrossRef] [PubMed]
37. Acuña-Castroviejo, D.; Escames, G.; Venegas, C.; Díaz-Casado, M.E.; Lima-Cabello, E.; López, L.C.; Rosales-Corral, S.; Tan, D.X.; Reiter, R.J. Extrapineal melatonin: Sources, regulation, and potential functions. *Cell. Mol. Life Sci.* **2014**, *71*, 2997–3025. [CrossRef] [PubMed]
38. Manchester, L.C.; Coto-Montes, A.; Boga, J.A.; Andersen, L.P.H.; Zhou, Z.; Galano, A.; Vriend, J.; Tan, D.X.; Reiter, R.J. An ancient molecule that makes oxygen metabolically tolerable. *J. Pineal Res.* **2015**, *59*, 403–419. [CrossRef] [PubMed]
39. Tan, D.X.; Korkmaz, A.; Reiter, R.J.; Manchester, L.C. Ebola virus disease: Potential use of melatonin as a treatment. *J. Pineal Res.* **2014**, *57*, 381–384. [CrossRef] [PubMed]
40. Reiter, R.J.; Richardson, B.A.; Johnson, L.Y.; Ferguson, B.N.; Dinh, D.T. Pineal melatonin rhythm: Reduction in aging Syrian hamsters. *Science* **1980**, *210*, 1372–1373. [CrossRef] [PubMed]
41. Reiter, R.J.; Craft, C.M.; Johnson, J.E., Jr.; King, T.S.; Richardson, B.A.; Vaughan, G.M.; Vaughan, M.K. Age-associated reduction in nocturnal pineal melatonin levels in female rats. *Endocrinology* **1981**, *109*, 1295–1297. [CrossRef] [PubMed]
42. Iguichi, H.; Kato, K.I.; Ibayashi, H. Age-dependent reduction in serum melatonin concentrations in healthy human subjects. *J. Clin. Endocrinol. Metab.* **1982**, *55*, 27–29. [CrossRef] [PubMed]
43. Caballero, B.; Vega-Naredo, I.; Sierra, V.; Huidobro-Fernández, C.; Soria-Valles, C.; de Gonzalo-Calvo, D.; Tolivia, D.; Gutierrez-Cuesta, J.; Pallas, M.; Camins, A.; et al. Favorable effects of a prolonged treatment with melatonin on the level of oxidative damage and neurodegeneration in senescence-accelerated mice. *J. Pineal Res.* **2008**, *45*, 302–311. [CrossRef] [PubMed]
44. García-Macia, M.; Vega-Naredo, I.; de Gonzalo-Calvo, D.; Rodríguez-González, S.M.; Camello, P.J.; Camello-Almaraz, C.; Martín-Cano, F.E.; Rodríguez-Colunga, M.J.; Pozo, M.J.; Coto-Montes, A.M. Melatonin induces neural SOD2 expression independent of the NF-kappaB pathway and improves the mitochondrial population and function in old mice. *J. Pineal Res.* **2011**, *50*, 54–63. [CrossRef] [PubMed]
45. Rosales-Corral, S.A.; Lopez-Armas, G.; Cruz-Ramos, J.; Melnikov, V.G.; Tan, D.X.; Manchester, L.C.; Munoz, R.; Reiter, R.J. Alterations in lipid levels of mitochondrial membranes induced by Amyloid-β: A protective role of melatonin. *Int. J. Alzheimer's Dis.* **2012**, *2012*, 459806. [CrossRef] [PubMed]
46. Bubenik, G.A.; Konturek, S.J. Melatonin and aging: Prospects for human treatment. *J. Physiol. Pharmacol.* **2011**, *62*, 13–19. [PubMed]
47. Ito, K.; Colley, T.; Mercado, N. Geroprotectors as a novel therapeutic strategy for COPD, an accelerating aging disease. *Int. J. Chronic Obstr. Pulm. Dis.* **2012**, *7*, 641–652. [CrossRef] [PubMed]
48. Hill, S.M.; Cheng, C.; Yuan, L.; Mao, L.; Jockers, R.; Dauchy, B.; Blask, D.E. Age-related decline in melatonin and its MT1 receptor are associated with decreased sensitivity to melatonin and enhanced mammary tumor growth. *Curr. Aging Sci.* **2013**, *6*, 125–133. [CrossRef] [PubMed]
49. Gitto, E.; Pellegrino, S.; Gitto, P.; Barberi, I.; Reiter, R.J. Oxidative stress of the newborn in the pre- and postnatal period and the clinical utility of melatonin. *J. Pineal Res.* **2009**, *46*, 128–139. [CrossRef] [PubMed]
50. Marseglia, L.; Aversa, S.; Barberi, I.; Salpietro, C.D.; Cusumano, E.; Speciale, A.; Saija, A.; Romeo, C.; Trimarchi, G.; Reiter, R.J.; et al. High endogenous melatonin levels in critically ill children: A pilot study. *J. Pediatr.* **2013**, *162*, 357–360. [CrossRef] [PubMed]
51. Schwichtenberg, A.J.; Malow, B.A. Melatonin Treatment in Children with Developmental Disabilities. *Sleep Med. Clin.* **2015**, *10*, 181–187. [CrossRef] [PubMed]
52. Cardinali, D.P.; Vigo, D.E.; Olivar, N.; Vidal, M.F.; Furio, A.M.; Brusco, L.I. Therapeutic application of melatonin in mild cognitive impairment. *Am. J. Neurodegener. Dis.* **2012**, *1*, 280–291. [PubMed]
53. Gallucci, M.; Flores-Obando, R.; Mazzuco, S.; Ongaro, F.; di Giorgi, E.; Boldrini, P.; Durante, E.; Frigato, A.; Albani, D.; Forloni, G.; et al. Melatonin and the Charlson Comorbidity Index (CCI): The Treviso Longeva (Trelong) study. *Int. J. Biol. Markers* **2014**, *29*, e253–e260. [CrossRef] [PubMed]
54. Boga, J.A.; Coto-Montes, A.; Rosales-Corral, S.A.; Tan, D.X.; Reiter, R.J. Beneficial actions of melatonin in the management of viral infections: A new use for this "molecular handyman"? *Rev. Med. Virol.* **2012**, *22*, 323–338. [CrossRef] [PubMed]

55. Hill, S.M.; Belancio, V.P.; Dauchy, R.T.; Xiang, S.; Brimer, S.; Mao, L.; Hauch, A.; Lundberg, P.W.; Summers, W.; Yuan, L.; et al. Melatonin: An inhibitor of breast cancer. *Endocr. Relat. Cancer* **2015**, *22*, R183–R204. [CrossRef] [PubMed]
56. Xin, Z.; Jiang, S.; Jiang, P.; Yan, X.; Fan, C.; Di, S.; Wu, G.; Yang, Y.; Reiter, R.J.; Ji, G. Melatonin as a treatment for gastrointestinal cancer: A review. *J. Pineal Res.* **2015**, *58*, 375–387. [CrossRef] [PubMed]
57. Song, Y.; Dowling, G.A.; Wallhagen, M.I.; Lee, K.A.; Strawbridge, W.J. Sleep in older adults with Alzheimer's disease. *J. Neurosci. Nurs.* **2010**, *42*, 190–198. [CrossRef] [PubMed]
58. Golombek, D.A.; Pandi-Perumal, S.R.; Brown, G.M.; Cardinali, D.P. Some implications of melatonin use in chronopharmacology of insomnia. *Eur. J. Pharmacol.* **2015**, *762*, 42–48. [CrossRef] [PubMed]
59. Rosales-Corral, S.A.; Acuña-Castroviejo, D.; Coto-Montes, A.; Boga, J.A.; Manchester, L.C.; Fuentes-Broto, L.; Korkmaz, A.; Ma, S.; Tan, D.X.; Reiter, R.J. Alzheimer's disease: Pathological mechanisms and the beneficial role of melatonin. *J. Pineal Res.* **2012**, *52*, 167–202. [CrossRef] [PubMed]
60. Miller, E.; Morel, A.; Saso, L.; Saluk, J. Melatonin redox activity. Its potential clinical applications in neurodegenerative disorders. *Curr. Top. Med. Chem.* **2015**, *15*, 163–169. [CrossRef] [PubMed]
61. Sánchez-Barceló, E.J.; Mediavilla, M.D.; Tan, D.X.; Reiter, R.J. Clinical uses of melatonin: Evaluation of human trials. *Curr. Med. Chem.* **2010**, *17*, 2070–2095. [CrossRef] [PubMed]
62. Gögenur, I.; Kücükakin, B.; Panduro Jensen, L.; Reiter, R.J.; Rosenberg, J. Melatonin reduces cardiac morbidity and markers of myocardial ischemia after elective abdominal aortic aneurysm repair: A randomized, placebo-controlled, clinical trial. *J. Pineal Res.* **2014**, *57*, 10–15. [CrossRef] [PubMed]
63. Sookprasert, A.; Johns, N.P.; Phunmanee, A.; Pongthai, P.; Cheawchanwattana, A.; Johns, J.; Konsil, J.; Plaimee, P.; Porasuphatana, S.; Jitpimolmard, S. Melatonin in patients with cancer receiving chemotherapy: A randomized, double-blind, placebo-controlled trial. *Anticancer Res.* **2014**, *34*, 7327–7337. [PubMed]
64. Mostafavi, A.; Solhi, M.; Mohammadi, M.R.; Hamedi, M.; Keshavarzi, M.; Akhondzadeh, S. Melatonin decreases olanzapine induced metabolic side-effects in adolescents with bipolar disorder: A randomized double-blind placebo-controlled trial. *Acta Med. Iran.* **2014**, *52*, 734–739. [PubMed]
65. Chahbouni, M.; Escames, G.; Venegas, C.; Sevilla, B.; García, J.A.; López, L.C.; Muñoz-Hoyos, A.; Molina-Carballo, A.; Acuña-Castroviejo, D. Melatonin treatment normalizes plasma pro-inflammatory cytokines and nitrosative/oxidative stress in patients suffering from Duchenne muscular dystrophy. *J. Pineal Res.* **2010**, *48*, 282–289. [CrossRef] [PubMed]
66. Tarantino, U.; Baldi, J.; Celi, M.; Rao, C.; Liuni, F.M.; Iundusi, R.; Gasbarra, E. Osteoporosis and sarcopenia: The connections. *Aging Clin. Exp. Res.* **2013**, *25*, S93–S95. [CrossRef] [PubMed]
67. Marzetti, E.; Calvani, R.; Cesari, M.; Buford, T.W.; Lorenzi, M.; Behnke, B.J.; Leeuwenburgh, C. Mitochondrial dysfunction and sarcopenia of aging: From signaling pathways to clinical trials. *Int. J. Biochem. Cell Biol.* **2013**, *45*, 2288–2301. [CrossRef] [PubMed]
68. Hepple, R.T. Mitochondrial involvement and impact in aging skeletal muscle. *Front. Aging Neurosci.* **2014**, *6*, 211. [CrossRef] [PubMed]
69. Yan, L.J. Positive oxidative stress in aging and aging-related disease tolerance. *Redox Biol.* **2014**, *2*, 165–169. [CrossRef] [PubMed]
70. Handy, D.E.; Loscalzo, J. Redox regulation of mitochondrial function. *Antioxid. Redox Signal.* **2012**, *16*, 1323–1367. [CrossRef] [PubMed]
71. Reid, M.B.; Khawli, F.A.; Moody, M.R. Reactive oxygen in skeletal muscle. III. Contractility of unfatigued muscle. *J. Appl. Physiol.* **1993**, *75*, 1081–1087. [PubMed]
72. Cerullo, F.; Gambassi, G.; Cesari, M. Rationale for antioxidant supplementation in sarcopenia. *J. Aging Res.* **2012**, *2012*, 316943. [CrossRef] [PubMed]
73. Vega-Naredo, I.; Caballero, B.; Sierra, V.; García-Macia, M.; de Gonzalo-Calvo, D.; Oliveira, P.J.; Rodríguez-Colunga, M.J.; Coto-Montes, A. Melatonin modulates autophagy through a redox-mediated action in female Syrian hamster Harderian gland controlling cell type and gland activity. *J. Pineal Res.* **2012**, *52*, 80–92. [CrossRef] [PubMed]
74. Proietti, S.; Cucina, A.; Dobrowolny, G.; D'Anselmi, F.; Dinicola, S.; Masiello, M.G.; Pasqualato, A.; Palombo, A.; Morini, V.; Reiter, R.J.; et al. Melatonin down-regulates MDM2 gene expression and enhances p53 acetylation in MCF-7 cells. *J. Pineal Res.* **2014**, *57*, 120–129. [CrossRef] [PubMed]

75. Cruz-Jentoft, A.J.; Baeyens, J.P.; Bauer, J.M.; Boirie, Y.; Cederholm, T.; Landi, F.; Martin, F.C.; Michel, J.P.; Rolland, Y.; Schneider, S.M.; et al. Sarcopenia: European consensus on definition and diagnosis: Report of the European Working Group on Sarcopenia in Older People. *Age Ageing* **2010**, *39*, 412–423. [CrossRef] [PubMed]
76. Coen, P.M.; Jubrias, S.A.; Distefano, G.; Amati, F.; Mackey, D.C.; Glynn, N.W.; Manini, T.M.; Wohlgemuth, S.E.; Leeuwenburgh, C.; Cummings, S.R.; et al. Skeletal muscle mitochondrial energetics are associated with maximal aerobic capacity and walking speed in older adults. *J. Gerontol. A Biol. Sci. Med. Sci.* **2013**, *68*, 447–455. [CrossRef] [PubMed]
77. Ramis, M.R.; Esteban, S.; Miralles, A.; Tan, D.X.; Reiter, R.J. Protective effects of melatonin and mitochondria-targeted antioxidants against oxidative stress: A review. *Curr. Med. Chem.* **2015**, *22*, 2690–2711. [CrossRef] [PubMed]
78. Agil, A.; El-Hammadi, M.; Jiménez-Aranda, A.; Tassi, M.; Abdo, W.; Fernández-Vázquez, G.; Reiter, R.J. Melatonin reduces hepatic mitochondrial dysfunction in diabetic obese rats. *J. Pineal Res.* **2015**, *59*, 70–79. [CrossRef] [PubMed]
79. Henics, T.; Wheatley, D.N. Cytoplasmic vacuolation, adaptation and cell death: A view on new perspectives and features. *Biol. Cell* **1999**, *91*, 485–498. [CrossRef]
80. Shubin, A.V.; Demidyuk, I.V.; Lunina, N.A.; Komissarov, A.A.; Roschina, M.P.; Leonova, O.G.; Kostrov, S.V. Protease 3C of hepatitis A virus induces vacuolization of lysosomal/endosomal organelles and caspase-independent cell death. *BMC Cell Biol.* **2015**, *16*, 4. [CrossRef] [PubMed]
81. Vega-Naredo, I.; Caballero, B.; Sierra, V.; Huidobro-Fernández, C.; de Gonzalo-Calvo, D.; García-Macia, M.; Tolivia, D.; Rodríguez-Colunga, M.J.; Coto-Montes, A. Sexual dimorphism of autophagy in Syrian hamster Harderian gland culminates in a holocrine secretion in female glands. *Autophagy* **2009**, *5*, 1004–1017. [CrossRef] [PubMed]
82. Sakuma, K.; Yamaguchi, A. Sarcopenia and age-related endocrine function. *Int. J. Endocrinol.* **2012**, *2012*, 127362. [CrossRef] [PubMed]
83. Sabatelli, P.; Castagnaro, S.; Tagliavini, F.; Chrisam, M.; Sardone, F.; Demay, L.; Richard, P.; Santi, S.; Maraldi, N.M.; Merlini, L.; et al. Aggresome-autophagy involvement in a sarcopenic patient with rigid spine syndrome and a p.C150R Mutation in FHL1 gene. *Front. Aging Neurosci.* **2014**, *6*, 215. [CrossRef] [PubMed]
84. Coto-Montes, A.; Boga, J.A.; Rosales-Corral, S.; Fuentes-Broto, L.; Tan, D.X.; Reiter, R.J. Role of melatonin in the regulation of autophagy and mitophagy: A review. *Mol. Cell. Endocrinol.* **2012**, *361*, 12–23. [CrossRef] [PubMed]
85. De Luxán-Delgado, B.; Caballero, B.; Potes, Y.; Rubio-González, A.; Rodríguez, I.; Gutiérrez-Rodríguez, J.; Solano, J.J.; Coto-Montes, A. Melatonin administration decreases adipogenesis in the liver of ob/ob mice through autophagy modulation. *J. Pineal Res.* **2014**, *56*, 126–133. [CrossRef] [PubMed]
86. Hong, Y.; Won, J.; Lee, Y.; Lee, S.; Park, K.; Chang, K.T.; Hong, Y. Melatonin treatment induces interplay of apoptosis, autophagy, and senescence in human colorectal cancer cells. *J. Pineal Res.* **2014**, *56*, 264–274. [CrossRef] [PubMed]
87. Hong, Y.; Kim, J.H.; Jin, Y.; Lee, S.; Park, K.; Lee, Y.; Chang, K.T.; Hong, Y. Melatonin treatment combined with treadmill exercise accelerates muscular adaptation through early inhibition of CHOP-mediated autophagy in the gastrocnemius of rats with intra-articular collagenase-induced knee laxity. *J. Pineal Res.* **2014**, *56*, 175–188. [CrossRef] [PubMed]
88. Kim, C.H.; Kim, K.H.; Yoo, Y.M. Melatonin-induced autophagy is associated with degradation of MyoD protein in C2C12 myoblast cells. *J. Pineal Res.* **2012**, *53*, 289–297. [CrossRef] [PubMed]
89. San-Miguel, B.; Crespo, I.; Sánchez, D.I.; González-Fernández, B.; Ortiz de Urbina, J.J.; Tuñón, M.J.; González-Gallego, J. Melatonin inhibits autophagy and endoplasmic reticulum stress in mice with carbon tetrachloride-induced fibrosis. *J. Pineal Res.* **2015**, *59*, 151–162. [CrossRef] [PubMed]
90. Brunk, U.T.; Terman, A. The mitochondrial-lysosomal axis theory of aging: Accumulation of damaged mitochondria as a result of imperfect autophagocytosis. *Eur. J. Biochem.* **2002**, *269*, 1996–2002. [CrossRef] [PubMed]
91. Terman, A.; Kurz, T.; Navratil, M.; Arriaga, E.A.; Brunk, U.T. Mitochondrial turnover and aging of longlived postmitotic cells: The mitochondrial-lysosomal axis theory of aging. *Antioxid. Redox Signal.* **2010**, *12*, 503–535. [CrossRef] [PubMed]

92. Sriram, S.; Subramanian, S.; Sathiakumar, D.; Venkatesh, R.; Salerno, M.S.; McFarlane, C.D.; Kambadur, R.; Sharma, M. Modulation of reactive oxygen species in skeletal muscle by myostatin is mediated through NF-κB. *Aging Cell* **2011**, *10*, 931–948. [CrossRef] [PubMed]
93. Sakuma, K.; Aoi, W.; Yamaguchi, A. Current understanding of sarcopenia: Possible candidates modulating muscle mass. *Pflug. Arch.* **2015**, *467*, 213–229. [CrossRef] [PubMed]
94. Vriend, J.; Reiter, R.J. Melatonin as a proteasome inhibitor. Is there any clinical evidence? *Life Sci.* **2014**, *115*, 8–14. [CrossRef] [PubMed]
95. Morgan, J.E.; Partridge, T.A. Muscle satellite cells. *Int. J. Biochem. Cell Biol.* **2003**, *35*, 1151–1156. [CrossRef]
96. Dumont, N.A.; Bentzinger, C.F.; Sincennes, M.C.; Rudnicki, M.A. Satellite cells and skeletal muscle regeneration. *Compr. Physiol.* **2015**, *5*, 1027–1059. [PubMed]
97. Faulkner, J.A.; Brooks, S.V.; Zerba, E. Muscle atrophy and weakness with aging: Contraction-induced injury as an underlying mechanism. *J. Gerontol. A Biol. Sci. Med. Sci.* **1995**, *50*, 124–129. [PubMed]
98. Tinetti, M.E. Where is the vision for fall prevention? *J. Am. Geriatr. Soc.* **2001**, *49*, 676–677. [CrossRef] [PubMed]
99. Alway, S.E.; Myers, M.J.; Mohamed, J.S. Regulation of satellite cell function in sarcopenia. *Front. Aging Neurosci.* **2014**, *6*, 246. [CrossRef] [PubMed]
100. Van der Meer, S.F.; Jaspers, R.T.; Jones, D.A.; Degens, H. Time-course of changes in the myonuclear domain during denervation in young-adult and old rat gastrocnemius muscle. *Muscle Nerve* **2011**, *43*, 212–222. [CrossRef] [PubMed]
101. Stratos, I.; Richter, N.; Rotter, R.; Li, Z.; Zechner, D.; Mittlmeier, T.; Vollmar, B. Melatonin restores muscle regeneration and enhances muscle function after crush injury in rats. *J. Pineal Res.* **2012**, *52*, 62–70. [CrossRef] [PubMed]
102. Li, Z.; Nickkholgh, A.; Yi, X.; Bruns, H.; Gross, M.L.; Hoffmann, K.; Mohr, E.; Zorn, M.; Büchler, M.W.; Schemmer, P. Melatonin protects kidney grafts from ischemia/reperfusion injury through inhibition of NF-kB and apoptosis after experimental kidney transplantation. *J. Pineal Res.* **2009**, *46*, 365–372. [CrossRef] [PubMed]
103. Jou, M.J.; Peng, T.I.; Hsu, L.F.; Jou, S.B.; Reiter, R.J.; Yang, C.M.; Chiao, C.C.; Lin, Y.F.; Chen, C.C. Visualization of melatonin multiple mitochondria levels of protection against mitochondrial Ca(2+) mediated permeability transition and beyond in rat brain astrocytes. *J. Pineal Res.* **2010**, *48*, 20–38. [CrossRef] [PubMed]
104. Tanaka, T.; Yasui, Y.; Tanaka, M.; Tanaka, T.; Oyama, T.; Rahman, K.M. Melatonin suppresses AOM/DSS-induced large bowel oncogenesis in rats. *Chem. Biol. Interact.* **2009**, *177*, 128–136. [CrossRef] [PubMed]
105. Leja-Szpak, A.; Jaworek, J.; Pierzchalski, P.; Reiter, R.J. Melatonin induces pro-apoptotic signaling pathway in human pancreatic carcinoma cells (PANC-1). *J. Pineal Res.* **2010**, *49*, 248–255. [CrossRef] [PubMed]
106. Mao, L.; Cheng, Q.; Guardiola-Lemaître, B.; Schuster-Klein, C.; Dong, C.; Lai, L.; Hill, SM. In vitro and in vivo antitumor activity of melatonin receptor agonists. *J. Pineal Res.* **2010**, *49*, 210–221. [CrossRef] [PubMed]
107. Hibaoui, Y.; Roulet, E.; Ruegg, U.T. Melatonin prevents oxidative stress-mediated mitochondrial permeability transition and death in skeletal muscle cells. *J. Pineal Res.* **2009**, *47*, 238–252. [CrossRef] [PubMed]
108. Wang, W.Z. Melatonin reduces ischemia/reperfusion-induced superoxide generation in arterial wall and cell death in skeletal muscle. *J. Pineal Res.* **2006**, *41*, 255–260. [CrossRef] [PubMed]
109. De Gonzalo-Calvo, D.; Fernández-García, B.; de Luxán-Delgado, B.; Rodríguez-González, S.; García-Macia, M.; Suárez, F.M.; Solano, J.J.; Rodríguez-Colunga, M.J.; Coto-Montes, A. Long-term training induces a healthy inflammatory and endocrine emergent biomarker profile in elderly men. *Age (Dordr)* **2012**, *34*, 761–771. [CrossRef] [PubMed]
110. De Gonzalo-Calvo, D.; Neitzert, K.; Fernández, M.; Vega-Naredo, I.; Caballero, B.; García-Macía, M.; Suárez, F.M.; Rodríguez-Colunga, M.J.; Solano, J.J.; Coto-Montes, A. Differential inflammatory responses in aging and disease: TNF-alpha and IL-6 as possible biomarkers. *Free Radic. Biol Med.* **2010**, *49*, 733–737. [CrossRef] [PubMed]
111. Cesari, M.; Kritchevsky, S.B.; Baumgartner, R.N.; Atkinson, H.H.; Penninx, B.W.; Lenchik, L.; Palla, S.L.; Ambrosius, W.T.; Tracy, R.P.; Pahor, M. Sarcopenia, obesity, and inflammation results from the Trial of Angiotensin Converting Enzyme Inhibition and Novel Cardiovascular Risk Factors study. *Am. J. Clin. Nutr.* **2005**, *82*, 428–434. [PubMed]

112. Ferrucci, L.; Penninx, B.W.; Volpato, S.; Harris, T.B.; Bandeen-Roche, K.; Balfour, J.; Leveille, S.G.; Fried, L.P.; Md, J.M. Change in muscle strength explains accelerated decline of physical function in older women with high interleukin-6 serum levels. *J. Am. Geriatr. Soc.* **2002**, *50*, 1947–1954. [CrossRef] [PubMed]
113. Michaud, M.; Balardy, L.; Moulis, G.; Gaudin, C.; Peyrot, C.; Vellas, B.; Cesari, M.; Nourhashemi, F. Proinflammatory cytokines, aging, and age-related diseases. *J. Am. Med. Dir. Assoc.* **2013**, *14*, 877–882. [CrossRef] [PubMed]
114. Borges, L.S.; Dermargos, A.; da Silva Junior, E.P.; Weimann, E.; Lambertucci, R.H.; Hatanaka, E. Melatonin decreases muscular oxidative stress and inflammation induced by strenuous exercise and stimulates growth factor synthesis. *J. Pineal Res.* **2015**, *58*, 166–172. [CrossRef] [PubMed]
115. Ochoa, J.J.; Díaz-Castro, J.; Kajarabille, N.; García, C.; Guisado, I.M.; de Teresa, C.; Guisado, R. Melatonin supplementation ameliorates oxidative stress and inflammatory signaling induced by strenuous exercise in adult human males. *J. Pineal Res.* **2011**, *51*, 373–380. [CrossRef] [PubMed]
116. Mauriz, J.L.; Collado, P.S.; Veneroso, C.; Reiter, R.J.; González-Gallego, J. A review of the molecular aspects of melatonin's anti-inflammatory actions: Recent insights and new perspectives. *J. Pineal Res.* **2013**, *54*, 1–14. [CrossRef] [PubMed]
117. Iwabu, M.; Yamauchi, T.; Okada-Iwabu, M.; Sato, K.; Nakagawa, T.; Funata, M.; Yamaguchi, M.; Namiki, S.; Nakayama, R.; Tabata, M.; et al. Adiponectin and AdipoR1 regulate PGC-1alpha and mitochondria by Ca^{2+} and AMPK/SIRT1. *Nature* **2010**, *464*, 1313–1319. [CrossRef] [PubMed]
118. Li, L.; Pan, R.; Li, R.; Niemann, B.; Aurich, A.C.; Chen, Y.; Rohrbach, S. Mitochondrial biogenesis and peroxisome proliferator-activated receptor-γ coactivator-1α (PGC-1α) deacetylation by physical activity: Intact adipocytokine signaling is required. *Diabetes* **2011**, *60*, 157–167. [CrossRef] [PubMed]
119. Carter, C.S.; Onder, G.; Kritchevsky, S.B.; Pahor, M. Angiotensin-converting enzyme inhibition intervention in elderly persons: Effects on body composition and physical performance. *J. Gerontol. A Biol. Sci. Med. Sci.* **2005**, *60*, 1437–1446. [CrossRef] [PubMed]
120. Kob, R.; Bollheimer, L.C.; Bertsch, T.; Fellner, C.; Djukic, M.; Sieber, C.C.; Fischer, B.E. Sarcopenic obesity: Molecular clues to a better understanding of its pathogenesis? *Biogerontology* **2015**, *6*, 15–29. [CrossRef] [PubMed]
121. Samaras, N.; Papadopoulou, M.A.; Samaras, D.; Ongaro, F. Off-label use of hormones as an antiaging strategy: A review. *Clin. Interv. Aging* **2014**, *9*, 1175–1186. [CrossRef] [PubMed]
122. Giovannini, S.; Marzetti, E.; Borst, S.E.; Leeuwenburgh, C. Modulation of GH/IGF-1 axis: Potential strategies to counteract sarcopenia in older adults. *Mech. Ageing Dev.* **2008**, *129*, 593–601. [CrossRef] [PubMed]
123. Thorner, M.O. Statement by the Growth Hormone Research Society on the GH/IGF-I axis in extending health span. *J. Gerontol. A Biol. Sci. Med. Sci.* **2009**, *64*, 1039–1044. [CrossRef] [PubMed]
124. Oner, J.; Oner, H.; Sahin, Z.; Demir, R.; Ustünel, I. Melatonin is as effective as testosterone in the prevention of soleus muscle atrophy induced by castration in rats. *Anat. Rec. (Hoboken)* **2008**, *291*, 448–455. [CrossRef] [PubMed]
125. Das, U.N. A defect in the activity of Delta6 and Delta5 desaturases may be a factor predisposing to the development of insulin resistance syndrome. *Prostaglandins Leukot. Essent. Fat. Acids* **2005**, *72*, 343–350. [CrossRef] [PubMed]
126. Luchetti, F.; Canonico, B.; Bartolini, D.; Arcangeletti, M.; Ciffolilli, S.; Murdolo, G.; Piroddi, M.; Papa, S.; Reiter, R.J.; Galli, F. Melatonin regulates mesenchymal stem cell differentiation: A review. *J. Pineal Res.* **2014**, *56*, 382–397. [CrossRef] [PubMed]
127. Pascua, P.; Camello-Almaraz, C.; Camello, P.J.; Martin-Cano, F.E.; Vara, E.; Fernandez-Tresguerres, J.A.; Pozo, M.J. Melatonin, and to a lesser extent growth hormone, restores colonic smooth muscle physiology in old rats. *J. Pineal Res.* **2011**, *51*, 405–415. [CrossRef] [PubMed]
128. De Van, A.E.; Eskurza, I.; Pierce, G.L.; Walker, A.E.; Jablonski, K.L.; Kaplon, R.E.; Seals, D.R. Regular aerobic exercise protects against impaired fasting plasma glucose-associated vascular endothelial dysfunction with aging. *Clin. Sci. (Lond.)* **2013**, *124*, 325–331. [CrossRef] [PubMed]
129. Behnke, B.J.; Padilla, D.J.; Ferreira, L.F.; Delp, M.D.; Musch, T.I.; Poole, D.C. Effects of arterial hypotension on microvascular oxygen exchange in contracting skeletal muscle. *J. Appl. Physiol.* **1985**, *100*, 1019–1026. [CrossRef] [PubMed]

130. Rosei, C.A.; de Ciuceis, C.; Rossini, C.; Porteri, E.; Rezzani, R.; Rodella, L.; Favero, G.; Sarkar, A.; Rosei, E.A.; Rizzoni, D. 7D.10: Effects of melatonin on contractile responses in small arteries of ageing mice. *J. Hypertens.* **2015**, *33* (Suppl. S1), e103. [CrossRef] [PubMed]
131. Rodella, L.F.; Favero, G.; Rossini, C.; Foglio, E.; Bonomini, F.; Reiter, R.J.; Rezzani, R. Aging and vascular dysfunction: Beneficial melatonin effects. *Age (Dordr)* **2013**, *35*, 103–115. [CrossRef] [PubMed]
132. Eşrefoğlu, M.; Gül, M.; Ateş, B.; Erdoğan, A. The effects of caffeic acid phenethyl ester and melatonin on age-related vascular remodeling and cardiac damage. *Fundam. Clin. Pharmacol.* **2011**, *25*, 580–590. [CrossRef] [PubMed]
133. Cummings, S.R.; Melton, L.J. Epidemiology and outcomes of osteoporotic fractures. *Lancet* **2002**, *359*, 1761–1767. [CrossRef]
134. Frost, H.M. Muscle, bone, and the Utah paradigm: A 1999 overview. *Med. Sci. Sports Exerc.* **2000**, *32*, 911–917. [CrossRef] [PubMed]
135. Binkley, N.; Buehring, B. Beyond FRAX: It's time to consider "sarco-osteopenia". *J. Clin. Densitom.* **2009**, *12*, 413–416. [CrossRef] [PubMed]
136. Binkley, N.; Krueger, D.; Buehring, B. What's in a name revisited: Should osteoporosis and sarcopenia be considered components of "dysmobility syndrome?". *Osteoporos. Int.* **2013**, *24*, 2955–2959. [CrossRef] [PubMed]
137. Yang, Y.H.; Li, B.; Zheng, X.F.; Chen, J.W.; Chen, K.; Jiang, S.D.; Jiang, L.S. Oxidative damage to osteoblasts can be alleviated by early autophagy through the endoplasmic reticulum stress pathway-implications for the treatment of osteoporosis. *Free Radic. Biol. Med.* **2014**, *77*, 10–20. [CrossRef] [PubMed]
138. Maria, S.; Witt-Enderby, P.A. Melatonin effects on bone: Potential use for the prevention and treatment for osteopenia, osteoporosis, and periodontal disease and for use in bone-grafting procedures. *J. Pineal Res.* **2014**, *56*, 115–125. [CrossRef] [PubMed]
139. Amstrup, A.K.; Sikjaer, T.; Heickendorff, L.; Mosekilde, L.; Rejnmark, L. Melatonin improves bone mineral density at the femoral neck in postmenopausal women with osteopenia: A randomized controlled trial. *J. Pineal Res.* **2015**, *59*, 221–229. [CrossRef] [PubMed]
140. Peterson, C.M.; Johannsen, D.L.; Ravussin, E. Skeletal muscle mitochondria and aging: A review. *J. Aging Res.* **2012**, *2012*, 194821. [CrossRef] [PubMed]
141. Gomez-Pinilla, P.J.; Camello, P.J.; Pozo, M.J. Melatonin treatment reverts age-related changes in guinea pig gallbladder neuromuscular transmission and contractility. *J. Pharmacol. Exp. Ther.* **2006**, *319*, 847–856. [CrossRef] [PubMed]
142. Gomez-Pinilla, P.J.; Camello, P.J.; Pozo, M.J. Effects of melatonin on gallbladder neuromuscular function in acute cholecystitis. *J. Pharmacol. Exp. Ther.* **2007**, *323*, 138–146. [CrossRef] [PubMed]

2

Efficacy of Nutritional Interventions as Stand-Alone or Synergistic Treatments with Exercise for the Management of Sarcopenia

Sarah Damanti [1,2,†], Domenico Azzolino [1,2,*,†], Carlotta Roncaglione [1], Beatrice Arosio [1,3], Paolo Rossi [1] and Matteo Cesari [1,3]

1 Geriatric Unit, Fondazione IRCCS Ca' Granda Ospedale Maggiore Policlinico, 20122 Milan, Italy
2 Phd Course in Nutritional Sciences, University of Milan, 20122 Milan, Italy
3 Department of Clinical Sciences and Community Health, University of Milan, 20122 Milan, Italy
* Correspondence: domenico.azzolino@policlinico.mi.it
† These authors contributed equally to this work.

Abstract: Sarcopenia is an age-related and accelerated process characterized by a progressive loss of muscle mass and strength/function. It is a multifactorial process associated with several adverse outcomes including falls, frailty, functional decline, hospitalization, and mortality. Hence, sarcopenia represents a major public health problem and has become the focus of intense research. Unfortunately, no pharmacological treatments are yet available to prevent or treat this age-related condition. At present, the only strategies for the management of sarcopenia are mainly based on nutritional and physical exercise interventions. The purpose of this review is, thus, to provide an overview on the role of proteins and other key nutrients, alone or in combination with physical exercise, on muscle parameters.

Keywords: sarcopenia; nutrition; physical exercise; synergism; older people

---

1. Sarcopenia

Muscle mass and strength progressively decline after the age of 40. Then, these age-related changes substantially accelerate after the age of 60, especially in the presence of sedentary behavior and comorbidities [1]. This clinical manifestation of aging is called sarcopenia (from the Ancient Greek σάρξ (sárx, "flesh") + πενῐ́ᾱ (peníā, "poverty"), and has recently been the object of increasing attention from researchers, clinicians, and public health authorities. Its growing relevance is paradigmatically exemplified by the recent inclusion of a specific ICD-10 code for it [2].

Contrary to lean mass decline, there is an increase in fat mass, with aging [3]. Adipose tissue can infiltrate muscles both at macroscopic (between muscle groups) and microscopic level (between and inside myocytes) with a further reduction in muscle mass and quality [4].

Sarcopenia represents an important sanitary problem since it affects 20% of people over 70 and 50% of people over 80 [5]. Moreover, considering the important function of muscle tissue beyond locomotion (e.g., influence on glucose and protein metabolism and on bone density) [6], it is associated with many adverse clinical outcomes (falls, fractures, functional and cognitive decline, cardiac and respiratory disease, reduced quality of life and independence, hospitalization, and mortality) [7–19]. Therefore, an early detection and treatment of this condition is pivotal.

In recent years, many studies have consistently demonstrated that muscle strength declines more rapidly (1.5%–5% year after the age of 50) than muscle mass (1%–2% year after the age of 50) [1,20–27], allowing an earlier identification of muscle impairment. Moreover, muscle strength correlates better than muscle mass with adverse health outcomes [28]. Therefore, in 2009, the European Working Group on Sarcopenia in Older People (EWGSOP) met to elaborate a definition of sarcopenia, which included both the presence of low muscle mass and function [29]. Sarcopenia was defined as a geriatric syndrome characterized by a progressive loss of muscle mass and strength. However, recently this definition has been updated [30] in light of the recognition of the role as disease of sarcopenia and of the scientific advantages, which stress the role of muscle strength as a principal determinant of the condition. Sarcopenia is now defined as a muscle disease, which can be considered probable if reduced muscle strength is detected. The main tools used to assess muscle strength are the hand grip dynamometer [31] or the chair stand test [32,33]. The diagnosis is confirmed in the presence of reduced muscle mass. The main instrument to assess muscle mass used for research purpose is the dual-energy X-ray absorptiometry (DXA). Bioelectrical impedance analysis [34] is another possibility, though less precise and more sensitive to body water content changes. Finally, in selected settings (i.e., oncologic patients), abdominal CT scans [35] performed for other purposes can be employed to estimate body muscle mass. Instead, anthropometric measures (i.e., calf circumference), though easy to assess, are not considered a reliable measure of muscle mass [36].

The severity of the condition can be then graded by measuring muscle performance. The most common used tools are the Short Physical Performance Battery32, the timed 'up and go' test [37], and the 400 m walking test [38].

Several mechanisms concur to the development of sarcopenia, including malnutrition, hormonal changes (i.e., reduction of growth hormone, estrogens, and testosterone), increased production of pro-inflammatory cytokines (also by the adipose tissue infiltrating the muscle [9]), higher muscle protein breakdown, myocytes loss, reduced satellite cell replenishment, loss of α-motor neurons, muscular mitochondrial dysfunction, altered myocyte autophagy, accelerated apoptosis of myonuclei, and impaired satellite cell function. Recently, the role of the fibromodulin has been highlighted, which is an extracellular matrix protein and predominantly controls a wide range of myogenesis-related genes (i.e., myogenin, myosin light chain 2, and transcriptional activity of myostatin) [39,40]. Fibromodulin is an essential part of the myogenic program and its role in the regulation of myoblasts may help in the development of new therapeutic agents (i.e., novel myostatin inhibitors) for the treatment of different muscle atrophies like as sarcopenia [39,40]. Furthermore, insulin resistance reduces the ability to use the available proteins [41]. Insulin resistance in the skeletal muscle results in whole-body metabolic disturbances associated with type 2 diabetes, which are further exacerbated by sarcopenia [42,43]. All these alterations are differently responsible for an imbalance between the anabolic and catabolic process at the muscular level [44]. Nevertheless, this list of pathophysiological pathways has to be considered as non-exhaustive, especially because novel mechanisms are under study and continuously propose novel/complementary possibilities. Pathophysiological mechanisms represent a possible target for therapeutic interventions.

2. Nutritional Interventions

Malnutrition is a state resulting from the lack of intake or uptake of nutritional elements, which alters body composition and body cell mass. Its etiologies can be heterogeneous: Starvation [45], cachexia [46], or simply aging [47]. Malnutrition has serious consequences, thus impairing both physical and mental functions and predisposing to adverse clinical outcomes from diseases [48]. Indeed, reduced intake of specific nutrients compromises the anabolic signal to muscles whereas their altered uptake configures a situation of anabolic resistance. Both conditions contribute to the development of sarcopenia [49].

Recently, the European Society of Clinical Nutrition and Metabolism (ESPEN) has validated the new diagnostic criteria for malnutrition [50]. The diagnosis can be performed if body mass index (BMI) is <18.5 kg/m^2 or if an unintentional weight loss is associated with either a reduced BMI (<20 kg/m^2 in younger or <22 kg/m^2 in older patients) or a low-fat free mass index. Moreover, malnutrition should be screened in all individual who are potentially at risk.

2.1. Proteins and Essential Amino Acids

Dietary proteins stimulate skeletal muscle protein synthesis and inhibit muscle protein breakdown [51–53]. Some observational studies have showed an association between protein intake and muscle mass and strength [54–56].

The effect of protein supplementation has been particularly evident on muscle strength and function [57] rather than on mass. However, protein supplementation alone could not be sufficient in cases of severe catabolism [58].

Older people frequently fail to reach the recommended dietary allowance (RDA) of proteins and calories. First of all, there is a reduction in appetite with aging, the so-called "anorexia of aging" [59,60]. Moreover, eating habits change due to swallowing and/or economic problems. Thus, the consumption of proteins rich nutrients switches in favor of energy-dilute foods (grains, vegetables, and fruits) [61].

Recently, two consensus studies (ESPEN [62] and PROT-AGE study group [41]) have stated that the traditional RDA of proteins for adults of all ages (0.8 g/kg body weight/day [63]) was not sufficient for older people. People aged 65 and older need more proteins to activate the muscle protein synthesis, compared to younger people [41,64]. Actually, older people have to counteract an anabolic resistance underpinned by an increased splanchnic sequestration of amino acids, lower postprandial perfusion of muscles, decreased muscle uptake of dietary amino acids, reduced anabolic signaling for protein synthesis, and an impaired digestive capacity [41,65,66]. Moreover, they require more proteins to offset inflammatory and catabolic conditions associated with chronic and acute diseases [67]. Thus, both the ESPEN and the PROT-AGE group concord in suggesting the assumption of 1–1.2 g proteins/kg body weight/day. A high-protein diet does not damage the kidney in healthy old individuals [68,69], whereas people with a severe kidney disease who do not undergo dialysis should limit their protein intake at about 0.8 g/kg body weight/day [41].

The protein source and amino acid composition are also important: Plant proteins have a lower anabolic effect compared to animal proteins [70], probably because they have a lower content of leucine. Moreover, independently from the amino acid content, proteins could have different absorption kinetics, which could influence their anabolic effect. There is a debate whether slow or fast digested proteins could better influence a muscle synthetic response [71–73]. It seems that fast proteins are more effective in stimulating muscle protein accretion41 even if results should be confirmed in larger trials.

Spread feeding patterns, in which an equal amount of protein is ingested at each meal, seems to optimize the protein synthetic capacity [74]. Nevertheless, some studies have also showed that with pulse feeding (with a main high protein meal), anabolic benefits can be reached [75,76]. Thus, additional trials are needed to establish the optimal timing of protein administration.

Moreover, some proteins are metabolized to short-chain fatty acids (like propionate, butyrate, and acetate) which are used by muscle cells to produce energy [77–80]. Indeed, short-chain fatty acids promote muscle anabolism and display anti-inflammatory proprieties positively, influencing muscle health [81–84].

Essential amino acids (EAAs), in particular leucine, are an important anabolic stimulus, too [85]. The main dietary sources of EEAs are lean meat, dairy products, soybeans, cowpeas, and lentils. The biological pathways on which leucine act are the activation of the mammalian target of rapamycin (mTOR) [86] and the inhibition of the proteasome [87]. However, supplementation with high doses of EEAs (10–15 g) and leucine (at least 3 g) is necessary to overcome anabolic resistance in older people [88].

A recent meta-analysis has confirmed that leucine is able to increase muscle protein synthesis in older people [89] and its consumption has been found to be directly correlated with muscle mass retention in healthy older people [90]. What is more, the supplementation with EAA in older people has been effective in increasing both muscle mass and function [91].

2.2. β-Hydroxy β-Methylbutyrate

ß-hydroxy ß-methylbutyrate (HMB) is one of the metabolites of leucine, which exerts anabolic effects through the activation of the mTOR pathway and the stimulation of the growth hormone/IGF-1 axis [92]. HMB also has anticatabolic effects: It decreases ubiquitin-proteasome expressions [93,94] and attenuates the up-regulation of caspases [95]. Moreover, it increases mitochondrial biogenesis and fat oxidation [96], possibly contributing to the improvement of muscle performance. HMB also favors sarcolemmal integrity via its conversion into hydroxymethylglutaryl-CoA [97]. Therefore, its final effects are induction of myogenic proliferation and differentiation [98]. Only 5% of leucine is usually metabolized to HMB [99] and there is an age-related decline in its concentrations [100]. Thus, there is a rationale for supplementation with HMB in old sarcopenic individuals. HMB is frequently used by athletes to better their physical performance [101]. It has been shown to be effective in improving muscle mass and strength in older adults too. What is more, HMB contributes to the preservation of muscle mass during bed rest, a known wasting condition [102–105].

2.3. Ornithine α-Ketoglutarate

Ornithine α-ketoglutarate (OKG) is a compound formed by ornithine (a non-proteinogenic amino acid) and α-ketoglutarate (a keto acid derived from the deamination of glutamate). It can offset sarcopenia through various mechanisms. OKG is the precursor of many amino acids (glutamate, glutamine, arginine, and proline), and of nitric oxide (NO), which improves hemodynamics in skeletal muscles [106]. Furthermore, it acts as a secretagogue of anabolic hormones like insulin and the growth hormone [106,107]. Therefore, OKG has successfully been used in experimental conditions of hypercatabolism (e.g., malnutrition, cancer cachexia, burn injury, and surgery) to reduce muscle wasting [108–111]. However, its effects have not been investigated yet, in non-malnourished older people.

2.4. Vitamin D

Deficit of vitamin D has been associated with reduced muscle mass and strength in prospective studies [112,113]. Most older people have serum levels of vitamin D below the normal range. The etiology of this deficit is multifactorial: Insufficient dietary intake, inadequate sunshine exposure, altered skin synthesizing capacity, and diminished renal conversion to the active form [114]. Moreover, there is a reduction in the expression of vitamin D receptors on muscle tissue [115,116] with aging.

The effects of vitamin D are mediated by its link with nuclear (VDR) and membrane-bound vitamin D receptors. The former activate the transcription of target genes involved in calcium uptake, phosphate transport, satellite cells proliferation, and terminal differentiation [117] while the latter regulate the release of calcium into the cytosol, respectively. This is pivotal for muscle contraction and induces protein synthesis [118].

Vitamin D supplementation can modulate the expression of VDR [119] with positive effects on muscle performance and strength [120,121]. What is more, it also improves muscle fiber composition and morphology [122]. Curiously, benefits seem to be appreciable only in people with low levels of vitamin D.

Therefore, it is recommended to dose vitamin D in all sarcopenic patients and to prescribe supplements in those who are deficient. Promotion of an adequate sunshine exposure together with the consumption of foods rich in vitamin D (salmon, mackerel, herring, sun-dried mushrooms) should instead be suggested in all older people.

2.5. Creatine Monohydrate

Creatine (Cr) is a compound that can be assumed with food (lean red meat, tuna, and salmon) or can be synthetized endogenously in the liver and kidneys using the amino acids glycine, arginine, and methionine.

Most of the creatine is stored in the skeletal muscles where it is converted into a high-energy metabolite phosphocreatine (PCr) by the enzyme creatine kinase. PCr acts as an energy buffer: At the beginning of muscular contraction, it donates a phosphate group to ADP to form ATP in order to produce energy anaerobically. During rest, the opposite process takes place and the excess of ATP is used to regenerate PCr from Cr [123,124].

Moreover, Cr activates the transcription of genes involved in muscle protein synthesis and satellite cells activation probably mediated by the mTOR pathway [125–127]. In fact, creatine may enhance muscle mass and force probably by increasing the expression of IGF-1 [127,128], which seems to activate the key elements of protein synthesis of the IGF1-IRS1-PI3K-AKT-mTOR pathway [129–131]. Indeed, it is well known that the activation of the IGF1-IRS1-PI3K-AKT-mTOR pathway induces muscle hypertrophy [132,133]. The consequent increase of IGF-1 via Cr is also observable in the significantly increased expression of several myogenic regulatory factors (i.e., Myo-D, Myf-5 and MRF-4) [128], which are responsible for satellite cell activation, proliferation, and differentiation [134]. This positive effect of creatine on muscle is probably only observable together with exercise [135–137]. Just recently, Ferretti et al. [138] demonstrated that during resistance training, Cr monohydrate increases muscle size and performance, suggesting a higher activation of muscle protein synthesis via IGF1-IRS1-PI3K-AKT-mTOR pathway.

Considering that in older people intramuscular Cr levels are reduced [139], the supplementation with Cr could be very beneficial. Indeed, there is evidence that high consumption of creatine can improve muscle mass and functions in older people [140].

2.6. Antioxidants and polyunsaturated fatty acids

Aging is characterized by oxidative stress-induced damages in various organs and systems [141].

In the pathogenesis of sarcopenia, there is an oxidative damage to muscle mitochondria and membranes, which compromises ATP production and increases sarcolemma permeability. Both alterations cause energy deprivation and activate stress pathways, which lead to muscle cell apoptosis [142–145].

The base of this damage is an imbalance between reactive oxygen species production and antioxidant defenses. Supplementation of exogenous antioxidants has been proposed in older people, since it can help the action of endogenous antioxidant enzymatic systems (i.e., superoxide dismutase, glutathione peroxidase)

It is true that high-plasma carotenoids have been associated with a lower risk of developing walking disability and decline in muscle strength in community-dwelling older people [146,147]. Anyway, excessive vitamin C and E supplementation can compromise muscular adaptations to strength training in older people [148]. This is because a limited ROS production is pivotal to promote adaptation to exercise [149]. In fact, it favors force production and mitochondrial biogenesis [150,151]. Excessive antioxidant supplementation in people who are not deficient could therefore compromise the mechanism of adaption to exercise. Thus, the supplementation can have a final negative effect on muscle mass and performance.

Moreover, many antioxidants (like selenium, vitamin A, vitamin C, vitamin E, and β-carotene) can also behave as potent pro-oxidants under some circumstances [152]. This is one more reason why supplementation with antioxidant in people who are not deficient can blunt the beneficial effects of physical exercise [153]. Meta-analyses and systematic reviews have demonstrated an increased mortality in both healthy people and those with various diseases who have been supplemented with antioxidants [154–156]. Considering the possible harms of antioxidant supplementation, its use to prevent or treat sarcopenia should be avoided unless an overt deficit is documented [157]. Instead, promoting the regular consumption of foods naturally rich in antioxidant could be beneficial in older people [158].

Supplementation with polyunsaturated fatty acids (PUFAs), and in particular with omega-3 fatty acids, improves muscle protein anabolism. PUFAs seem to directly act on mTOR signaling [159] and reduce inflammation [160,161]. The main dietary source of PUFAs is fatty fish: Salmon, mackerel, herring, lake trout, sardines, albacore tuna, and their oils. A higher dietary consumption of PUFAs has been associated with a greater fat-free mass [162]. A positive correlation between fatty fish (which is rich in PUFA) and grip strength was found in community-dwelling older people [163] too.

However, many studies on supplementation with PUFAs (with different dosages and for different periods) have produced different but mainly inconsistent results so far [164,165]. Moreover, the risk for potential adverse events associated with long-term supplementation has not been clearly elicited. Therefore, there is insufficient evidence to promote the systematic consumption of PUFAs in sarcopenic individuals.

2.7. Ursolic Acid

Ursolic acid is a compound with anti-inflammatory properties, which is abundant in apple peels, plum, cranberry, blueberry, rosemary, hawthorn, thyme, basil, oregano, and peppermint [166].

In murine models, ursolic acid has displayed anabolic proprieties mediated by the repression of atrophy-associated genes (atrogin-1 and MuRF1), and the induction of trophic genes (PKB/Akt and S6 kinase). Furthermore, it was able to stimulate the insulin/IGF-1 axis producing muscular hypertrophy [167]. However, supplementation in sarcopenic individuals has not been performed yet.

2.8. Nitrate-Rich Foods

Nitrate (NO3–)-rich foods (e.g., celery, cress, chervil, lettuce, red beetroot, spinach, and rocket) have a potential role in the treatment of sarcopenia. Food-derived NO3– is reduced to NO2– by commensal bacteria of the oral cavity [168]. Through several mechanisms, NO2– is then converted to nitric oxide (NO), which is the active mediator of the anti-sarcopenic effects of these compounds. The increase in gastric levels of NO attenuates the aging anorexia by reducing the earlier satiety feeling [59]. Furthermore, by improving the endothelial function, NO improves nutrient supply to muscles [169].

Finally, NO optimizes mitochondrial bioenergetics, by reducing the metabolic cost of exercise [170,171]. Indeed, NO was effective in improving muscular performance in young individuals [172]. On the contrary, short-term supplementation with nitrate-rich foods did not improve muscular performance and strength [173] in older people. Thus, there has been insufficient evidence so far to recommend the supplementation with nitrate-rich foods in sarcopenic individuals.

2.9. Prebiotics, Probiotics, and Symbiotics

Recently, gut microbiota has been proposed as a contributor in the pathogenesis of sarcopenia, so interventions that promote its health can be beneficial. Older people tend to develop an intestinal dysbiosis, which is associated with an increased gut permeability. Alterations of the gut barrier facilitate the passage of endotoxins and other microbial products with inflammatory effects into the blood stream. This contributes to the development of a deleterious state of systemic inflammation [174] contributing to muscle wasting [78,175].

Moreover, the reduction of intestinal mobility, typical of older persons, also alters the species of bacteria colonizing the gut (*Bacteroidetes* and *Firmicutes*) in favor of species with greater proteolytic potential (*Proteobacteria*) [176], consequently influencing the proper utilization of dietary proteins [175]. An enhanced proteolytic capacity and anabolic resistance of the gut microbiota, characteristic of older age, have been reported. These mechanisms are probably mediated by the age-related proinflammatory state [175,177,178].

Furthermore, it has been demonstrated in murine models that intestinal dysbiosis can alter neuromuscular transmission with a consequent promotion of muscle protein catabolism [179].

Thus, the administration of prebiotics, probiotics, and symbiotics, substances that improve microbiota health, has been proposed as a possible treatment for sarcopenia. Prebiotics are specific fermented ingredients that can induce changes in the composition and/or in the activity of the gastrointestinal microflora with a final beneficial effect for the host organism [79,180].

The actually available prebiotics are non-digestible oligosaccharides (i.e., inulin, oligofructose, (trans)galactooligosaccharides). They modulate the metabolism of the intestinal flora and show immunomodulatory properties [180]. Indeed, a study of Buigues [181] demonstrated that 13-week supplementation with prebiotics improved exhaustion and handgrip strength in older people.

Probiotics are instead viable microorganisms that can exert beneficial effects when administered in adequate quantities for reaching the intestine in an active state [182]. Probiotics modulate the intestinal microflora of the host by reducing microbial aberrancies and having an inflammatory effect [180].

The most used probiotics are Bifidobacteri and Lactobacilli [183]. Indeed, in animal studies, the administration of Lactobacillus reuteri, which modulates the transcriptional factor Forkhead Box N1 (FoxN1), was able to prevent cachexia in murine models of cancer [184]. Other probiotics, like *Faecalibacterium prausnitzii*, has anti-inflammatory proprieties [185] and in animal models, can improve the marker of oxidative stress [186].

Finally, symbiotics are a combination of prebiotics and probiotics exerting synergic effects [187].

Proteins, which are a known nutritional treatment for sarcopenia, represent a substrate for gut microbiota too.

Proteins increase microbiota diversity [188] and the number of protein-fermenting bacteria, which increase the bioavailability of dietary amino acids [175,188].

Short-chain fatty acids and secondary biliary salty acids, produced by microbiota, may counteract age-related muscle decline, too, thanks to their positive effects on muscle mitochondria. Moreover, they reduce host inflammation by decreasing TNFα-mediated immune responses and inflammasomes (i.e., NLRP3) [78].

We have to underline that the evidence of the effectiveness of prebiotics, probiotics, and symbiotics comes mainly from animal studies. Therefore, further research targeting specifically sarcopenic individuals is needed to recommend their routinely use.

3. Synergies between Nutritional and Physical Exercise Interventions

Inactivity is one of the main causes of sarcopenia [189] because it determines a resistance to muscle anabolic stimuli [190]. Therefore, the combination of nutritional interventions and physical exercise acts synergically to improve muscle health. Indeed, up to now it has been the most effective strategy for the management of sarcopenia.

The World Health Organization recommends performing at least 150 min/week of moderate-intensity physical activity or at least 75 min/week of vigorous-intensity physical activity or an equivalent combination of the two. An additional benefit can be obtained by increasing the amount of moderate-intensity physical activity to 300 min/week and by performing strengthening activities involving the major muscle groups on two or more days a week. Furthermore, for people with poor mobility, it is suggested to do exercises to enhance balance and prevent falls on three or more days per week [191]. Since sarcopenia involves muscles in the whole-body [7,192,193] it has been recently recommended to perform an holistic training involving all muscle groups [192].

It is interesting to note that when exercise is proposed to older people, they usually show a positive attitude and also enjoy the social component of the activities [194], even in the hospital setting [195].

The maximum effect of exercise is achieved within the first 3 h after training, but it can persist up to 24 h after the bout is over [196].

In particular, resistance training reduces insulin resistance, sensitizes muscles to other anabolic stimuli, and promotes mitochondrial biogenesis [78]. Therefore, resistance training is established to increase the synthesis of myofibrillar proteins in older people [197] with a consequent positive effect on muscle mass, strength, and performance [198–204]. These results are even appreciable at an extremely advanced age (i.e., centenarians) [205–207].

There are also potential indirect effects of exercise on gut microbiota that are noteworthy. By affecting intestinal mobility [208], exercise seems to reduce the dysbiosis, which negatively impacts muscle protein anabolism [209,210].

Here, we revise the major nutritional interventions that showed to have a synergic effect with physical exercise.

3.1. *Protein/Amino Acid and Exercise*

Exercise sensitizes the muscle to the anabolic actions of amino acids [211]. Indeed, the combination of protein/amino acid administration with physical exercise has proved to augment muscle protein anabolism compared to each intervention alone [212]. The synergistic effect is appreciable both in young and older people [213]. The sensitizing effect of exercise to amino-acid anabolic effects is maximal 3 h after the physical effort [211]. Therefore, proteins should be assumed 2–3 h after training [41]. Both resistance [73,197,214] and aerobic exercise [215,216] improve the protein anabolic stimulus. The effect is appreciable even if the intensity of exercise is only moderate [215]. Indeed, a metanalysis of 22 randomized controlled trials have confirmed that the combination of protein supplementation with resistance training has produced a greater increase in fat-free mass, type I and II muscle fiber cross-sectional area, and muscle strength compared to exercise alone [217]. These results have partially been endorsed by a more recent systematic review [218]. This review has included heterogeneous studies in terms of populations, duration, and dose of daily proteins. There have been negative findings in some of the included studies. These were mainly in older participants already with a sufficient protein and caloric intake and in people receiving soy proteins.

In summary, combination of protein/EAAs supplementation should be recommended in people who are deficient in association with physical exercise to prevent and reverse sarcopenia.

3.2. *HMB and Exercise*

The rationale for associating HMB supplementation and exercise is that HMB seems to promote the regenerative capacity of skeletal muscles after high-intensity exercise. Attenuation of markers of skeletal muscle damage after exercise were seen in case of administration of HMB [219]. Moreover, in one study, supplementation with HMB in association with strength training in older people increased more muscle mass and strength compared to exercise alone [220].

HMB effects are mainly appreciable in untrained people undergoing strenuous exercise, but also in trained people performing high physical stress training [95].

Indeed, a recent systematic review [221] has shown that the association of HMB plus resistance training enhances training-induced muscle mass and strength, attenuates markers of muscle damage, and improves markers of aerobic fitness. However, in another systematic review, the additional effect of HMB plus exercise was found only in one out of three randomized controlled trials for muscle mass and no additional effect was demonstrated for muscle strength and performance [218]. These negative findings can be explained by the fact that the suppression of proteolysis mediated by HMB may blunt the adaptation to training [95]. Moreover, a long period of pre-exercise supplementation may be necessary to achieve results [222].

3.3. *Creatinine and Exercise*

Considering the role of creatinine as energy buffer, it appears to be particularly useful in high-intensity exercise. The creatine-phosphocreatine system is highly used during these performances, so it can provide energy at a rapid rate.

The combination of Cr supplementation and resistance training increases IGF-1 at muscular level [127]. In turn, IGF-1 favors protein synthesis by activating the central mediator, PKB/AKT; and, subsequently, mTOR [223]. The final effect is an increase in muscle mass and strength, which can continue until 12 weeks after Cr withdrawal [224]. These results were confirmed both in young [225–228] and older [229–231] adults, though with some conflicting results [229,232–234].

Therefore, the PROT-AGE study group suggests supplementation only in older people who are deficient or at high risk of deficiency [41].

3.4. *Vitamin D and Exercise*

Vitamin D has a pivotal role on muscle tropism and function [235,236]. The effects of its deficiency on muscles are severe (extreme weakness and muscle pain) [236]. Anyway, in a recent review, no additional effect of vitamin D supplementation plus exercise was found for muscle mass and only conflicting results in terms of muscle performance [203]. Moreover, in the study of Bunout et al. [237], people were supplemented with a dose that was below (400 UI/daily) the recommended daily dose (800 UI/daily), while the study of Binder et al. [238] was considered of poor quality. It is reasonable that only individuals who are deficient would display an additional benefit of vitamin D supplementation over exercise. The deficit, causing muscle weakness and pain, would prevent the benefit from exercise training. Supplementation increases vitamin D receptor expression at muscle level with a positive effect in terms of muscle tropism and performance. Therefore, supplementation creates a positive background for the action of exercise in people who are deficient.

3.5. *PUFA and Exercise*

Results on the synergic effect of PUFA supplementation and exercise on muscle mass and performance are conflicting. In one study, the supplementation with PUFAs (fish oil) plus strength training produced great improvements in muscle strength and performance compared to exercise alone [239]. Anyway, another study has found that 12-week supplementation with α linoleic acid combined with resistance training had only marginal effects on muscle mass and strength [240]. A recent narrative review [241] has concluded that the synergic effect of the two interventions on muscle mass are still equivocal and conflicting about muscle function in older people. Therefore, there is insufficient evidence to recommend this intervention in sarcopenic individuals.

3.6. *Practical Application*

It is well known that older adults frequently have health-related problems, which may compromise the capacity to perform exercise tasks. Furthermore, since it has been shown that individual responses to nutrition/exercise interventions may be quite variable, a personalized approach to counteract muscle decline seem to be promising [242]. As mentioned above, resistance training is the most effective type of exercise to counteract and/or reverse sarcopenia. However, various training-related parameters (i.e., frequency, duration, intensity, volume, etc.), specifics for the older person, need to be considered in the implementation of exercise training programs [243].

Resistance training should be supervised both for compliance and safety (especially for those who are frail or sarcopenic) [244,245]. Furthermore, the time of intervention should be of at least three months to obtain significant improvement in muscle parameters (i.e., muscle strength and physical performance) [244] and exercise frequency should be of two or more nonconsecutive sessions per week [41]. An exercise duration of 10 to 15 min per session with eight repetition for each muscle group is considered sufficient to counteract muscle decline in healthy older people [41]. However, in frail and sarcopenic subjects, more time and repetitions may be needed to improve muscle parameters. A high-intensity resistance training (i.e., 80%–95% 1 repetition maximum) is recommended to induce maximum muscle hypertrophy or muscle fiber adaption [246,247]. Some authors reported that high-intensity resistance training is tolerated in older adults [206,248–250]. Unfortunately, this exercise intensity may not be achieved by frail subjects [251]. Nevertheless, lower intensities of exercise training (i.e., from 50% to 75%) may be sufficient to induce strength gains [192,243].

In a recent systematic review, Liao et al. [251] reported that protein supplementation, in addition to muscle strengthening exercise, is effective in promoting gain both in muscle mass and strength and enhancing physical performance in older adults with a high risk of sarcopenia or frailty.

In addition to increasing dietary protein intake to at least 1.2 g protein/kg of BW or providing supplements, it is recommended to supplement proteins or EEAs close after exercise sessions (i.e., 20 g of proteins) [41]. Nutritional status should be assessed before each intervention and the amount of proteins should be individually adjusted with regard to nutritional status, physical activity level, disease status, and tolerance [252].

4. Conclusions

The severe adverse consequences of sarcopenia and their impact on individuals and health systems make the treatment of this condition compelling. Importantly, the complexity of its pathogenesis represents a challenge for its management. Unfortunately, a contemporary pharmacological therapy is not yet available. However, nutritional interventions have shown to produce important beneficial effects on muscle parameters in older adults. Moreover, new dietary components with promising effects are emerging (i.e., gut microbiota manipulation). What is more, promotion of physical exercise according to the WHO guidelines is another efficacious modality considering the beneficial synergisms of nutritional and physical interventions.

In conclusion, sarcopenic individuals should assume 1–1.2 g proteins/kg body weight/day, with high content of EEAs (10–15 g) and leucine (at least 3 g) preferentially 2–3 h after exercise to maximize their anabolic effect. Older individuals who are deficient or at high risk of deficiency of vitamin D, creatinine, and HMB should be integrated.

Personalization of the diet and exercise programs according to patients' needs remain the pivotal step for the treatment of sarcopenia. Moreover, preventive strategies to maximize the peak of muscle mass during the adulthood and reduce midlife muscle mass decline should be promoted configuring a life course approach to this condition, so that muscle function is preserved for as long as possible; and, thus positively affecting quality of life and health span.

Author Contributions: S.D. and D.A. equally contributed to conceptualizing and writing the manuscript. C.R., B.A., P.R., and M.C. edited and revised manuscript. S.D., D.A., C.R., B.A., P.R., and M.C. approved the final version of manuscript.

References

1. Hughes, A.V.; Frontera, W.R.; Roubenoff, R.; Evans, W.J.; Singh, M.A.F. Longitudinal changes in body composition in older men and women: Role of body weight change and physical activity. *Am. J. Clin. Nutr.* **2002**, *76*, 473–481. [CrossRef] [PubMed]
2. Anker, S.D.; Morley, J.E.; Von Haehling, S. Welcome to the ICD-10 code for sarcopenia. *J. Cachex Sarcopenia Muscle* **2016**, *7*, 512–514. [CrossRef] [PubMed]
3. Forbes, G.B. Longitudinal changes in adult fat-free mass: Influence of body weight. *Am. J. Clin. Nutr.* **1999**, *70*, 1025–1031. [CrossRef] [PubMed]
4. Naimo, A.M.; Gu, J.K.; Lilly, C.; Kelley, A.G.; Baker, B.A. Resistance Training Frequency Confers Greater Muscle Quality in Aged Individuals: A Brief Nhanes Report. *JCSM Clin. Rep.* **2018**, *3*, 1–8. [CrossRef]
5. Thomas, D.R. Sarcopenia. *Clin. Geriatr. Med.* **2010**, *26*, 331–346. [CrossRef] [PubMed]
6. Welch, A.A. Nutritional influences on age-related skeletal muscle loss. *Proc. Nutr. Soc.* **2014**, *73*, 16–33. [CrossRef]
7. Cruz-Jentoft, A.J.; Sayer, A.A. Sarcopenia. *Lancet* **2019**, *393*, 2636–2646. [CrossRef]
8. Akune, T.; Muraki, S.; Oka, H.; Tanaka, S.; Kawaguchi, H.; Tokimura, F.; Yoshida, H.; Suzuki, T.; Nakamura, K.; Yoshimura, N. Incidence of certified need of care in the long-term care insurance system and its risk factors in the elderly of Japanese population-based cohorts: The ROAD study. *Geriatr. Gerontol. Int.* **2014**, *14*, 695–701. [CrossRef]
9. Sarcopenia and the Cardiometabolic Syndrome: A Narrative Review—EM|consulte. Available online: https://www.em-consulte.com/en/article/1055336 (accessed on 30 July 2019).

10. Beaudart, C.; Biver, E.; Reginster, J.Y.; Rizzoli, R.; Rolland, Y.; Bautmans, I.; Petermans, J.; Gillain, S.; Buckinx, F.; Dardenne, N.; et al. Validation of the SarQoL®, a specific health-related quality of life questionnaire for Sarcopenia. *J. Cachexia Sarcopenia Muscle* **2017**, *8*, 238. [CrossRef]
11. Bischoff-Ferrari, H.A.; Orav, J.E.; Kanis, J.A.; Rizzoli, R.; Schlogl, M.; Staehelin, H.B.; Willett, W.C.; Dawson-Hughes, B. Comparative performance of current definitions of sarcopenia against the prospective incidence of falls among community-dwelling seniors age 65 and older. *Osteoporos. Int.* **2015**, *26*, 2793–2802. [CrossRef]
12. Bone, E.A.; Hepgul, N.; Kon, S.; Maddocks, M. Sarcopenia and frailty in chronic respiratory disease. *Chronic Respir. Dis.* **2017**, *14*, 85–99. [CrossRef] [PubMed]
13. Chang, K.V.; Hsu, T.H.; Wu, W.T.; Huang, K.C.; Han, D.S. Association Between Sarcopenia and Cognitive Impairment: A Systematic Review and Meta-Analysis. *J. Am. Med Dir. Assoc.* **2016**, *17*, e7–e15. [CrossRef] [PubMed]
14. De Buyser, S.L.; Petrovic, M.; Taes, Y.E.; Toye, K.R.C.; Kaufman, J.-M.; Lapauw, B.; Goemaere, S. Validation of the FNIH sarcopenia criteria and SOF frailty index as predictors of long-term mortality in ambulatory older men. *Age Ageing* **2016**, *45*, 603–608. [CrossRef] [PubMed]
15. dos Santos, L.; Cyrino, E.S.; Antunes, M.; Santos, D.A.; Sardinha, L.B. Sarcopenia and physical independence in older adults: The independent and synergic role of muscle mass and muscle function. *J. Cachexia Sarcopenia Muscle* **2017**, *8*, 245–250. [CrossRef] [PubMed]
16. Malmstrom, T.K.; Miller, D.K.; Simonsick, E.M.; Ferrucci, L.; Morley, J.E. SARC-F: A symptom score to predict persons with sarcopenia at risk for poor functional outcomes. *J. Cachexia Sarcopenia Muscle* **2016**, *7*, 28–36. [CrossRef] [PubMed]
17. Morley, J.E.; Abbatecola, A.M.; Argilés, J.M.; Baracos, V.; Bauer, J.; Bhasin, S.; Cederholm, T.; Coats, A.J.S.; Cummings, S.R.; Evans, W.J.; et al. Sarcopenia with Limited Mobility: An International Consensus. *J. Am. Med Dir. Assoc.* **2011**, *12*, 403–409. [CrossRef]
18. Schaap, L.A.; van Schoor, N.M.; Lips, P.; Visser, M. Associations of Sarcopenia Definitions, and Their Components, With the Incidence of Recurrent Falling and Fractures: The Longitudinal Aging Study Amsterdam. *J. Gerontol. A Biol. Sci. Med. Sci.* **2018**, *73*, 1199–1204. [CrossRef]
19. Steffl, M.; Bohannon, R.W.; Sontakova, L.; Tufano, J.J.; Shiells, K.; Holmerova, I. Relationship between sarcopenia and physical activity in older people: A systematic review and meta-analysis. *Clin. Interv. Aging* **2017**, *12*, 835–845. [CrossRef]
20. Frontera, W.R.; Hughes, V.A.; Fielding, R.A.; Fiatarone, M.A.; Evans, W.J.; Roubenoff, R. Aging of skeletal muscle: A 12-yr longitudinal study. *J. Appl. Physiol.* **2000**, *88*, 1321–1326. [CrossRef]
21. Keller, K.; Engelhardt, M. Strength and muscle mass loss with aging process. Age and strength loss. *Muscles Ligaments Tendons J.* **2013**, *3*, 346–350. [CrossRef]
22. Lauretani, F.; Russo, C.R.; Bandinelli, S.; Bartali, B.; Cavazzini, C.; Di Iorio, A.; Corsi, A.M.; Rantanen, T.; Guralnik, J.M.; Ferrucci, L. Age-associated changes in skeletal muscles and their effect on mobility: An operational diagnosis of sarcopenia. *J. Appl. Physiol.* **2003**, *95*, 1851–1860. [CrossRef] [PubMed]
23. Lexell, J.; Taylor, C.C.; Sjöström, M. What is the cause of the ageing atrophy? Total number, size and proportion of different fiber types studied in whole vastus lateralis muscle from 15 to 83-year-old men. *J. Neurol. Sci.* **1988**, *84*, 275–294. [CrossRef]
24. Newman, A.B.; Kupelian, V.; Visser, M.; Simonsick, E.; Goodpaster, B.; Nevitt, M.; Kritchevsky, S.B.; Tylavsky, F.A.; Rubin, S.M.; Harris, T.B. Sarcopenia: Alternative Definitions and Associations with Lower Extremity Function. *J. Am. Geriatr. Soc.* **2003**, *51*, 1602–1609. [CrossRef] [PubMed]
25. Von Haehling, S.; Morley, J.E.; Anker, S.D. From muscle wasting to sarcopenia and myopenia: Update 2012. *J. Cachex Sarcopenia Muscle* **2012**, *3*, 213–217. [CrossRef] [PubMed]
26. Dhillon, R.J.; Hasni, S. Pathogenesis and Management of Sarcopenia. *Clin. Geriatr. Med.* **2017**, *33*, 17–26. [CrossRef] [PubMed]
27. Tieland, M.; Trouwborst, I.; Clark, B.C. Skeletal muscle performance and ageing. *J. Cachexia Sarcopenia Muscle* **2018**, *9*, 3–19. [CrossRef] [PubMed]
28. Studenski, S.A.; Peters, K.W.; Alley, D.E.; Cawthon, P.M.; McLean, R.R.; Harris, T.B.; Ferrucci, L.; Guralnik, J.M.; Fragala, M.S.; Kenny, A.M.; et al. The FNIH Sarcopenia Project: Rationale, Study Description, Conference Recommendations, and Final Estimates. *J. Gerontol. Ser. A Biol. Sci. Med. Sci.* **2014**, *69*, 547–558. [CrossRef] [PubMed]

29. Cruz-Jentoft, A.J.; Baeyens, J.P.; Bauer, J.M.; Boirie, Y.; Cederholm, T.; Landi, F.; Martin, F.C.; Michel, J.P.; Rolland, Y.; Schneider, S.M.; et al. Sarcopenia: European consensus on definition and diagnosis: Report of the European Working Group on Sarcopenia in Older People. *Age Ageing* **2010**, *39*, 412–423. [CrossRef]
30. Cruz-Jentoft, A.J.; Bahat, G.; Bauer, J.; Boirie, Y.; Bruyère, O.; Cederholm, T.; Cooper, C.; Landi, F.; Rolland, Y.; Sayer, A.A.; et al. Sarcopenia: Revised European consensus on definition and diagnosis. *Age Ageing* **2019**, *48*, 601. [CrossRef]
31. Roberts, H.C.; Denison, H.J.; Martin, H.J.; Patel, H.P.; Syddall, H.; Cooper, C.; Sayer, A.A. A review of the measurement of grip strength in clinical and epidemiological studies: Towards a standardised approach. *Age Ageing* **2011**, *40*, 423–429. [CrossRef]
32. Guralnik, J.M.; Simonsick, E.M.; Ferrucci, L.; Glynn, R.J.; Berkman, L.F.; Blazer, D.G.; Scherr, P.A.; Wallace, R.B. A Short Physical Performance Battery Assessing Lower Extremity Function: Association with Self-Reported Disability and Prediction of Mortality and Nursing Home Admission. *J. Gerontol.* **1994**, *49*, M85–M94. [CrossRef] [PubMed]
33. Jones, C.J.; Rikli, R.E.; Beam, W.C. A 30-s Chair-Stand Test as a Measure of Lower Body Strength in Community-Residing Older Adults. *Res. Q. Exerc. Sport* **1999**, *70*, 113–119. [CrossRef] [PubMed]
34. Sergi, G.; De Rui, M.; Stubbs, B.; Veronese, N.; Manzato, E. Measurement of lean body mass using bioelectrical impedance analysis: A consideration of the pros and cons. *Aging Clin. Exp. Res.* **2017**, *29*, 591–597. [CrossRef] [PubMed]
35. Mitsiopoulos, N.; Baumgartner, R.N.; Heymsfield, S.B.; Lyons, W.; Gallagher, D.; Ross, R. Cadaver validation of skeletal muscle measurement by magnetic resonance imaging and computerized tomography. *J. Appl. Physiol.* **1998**, *85*, 115–122. [CrossRef] [PubMed]
36. Tosato, M.; Marzetti, E.; Cesari, M.; Savera, G.; Miller, R.R.; Bernabei, R.; Landi, F.; Calvani, R. Measurement of muscle mass in sarcopenia: From imaging to biochemical markers. *Aging Clin. Exp. Res.* **2017**, *29*, 19–27. [CrossRef] [PubMed]
37. Iversen, M.D.; Weyh, A.; Akos, R.; Conzelmann, M.; Dick, W.; Bischoff, H.A.; Stähelin, H.B.; Monsch, A.U.; Von Dechend, M.; Theiler, R. Identifying a cut-off point for normal mobility: A comparison of the timed 'up and go' test in community-dwelling and institutionalised elderly women. *Age Ageing* **2003**, *32*, 315–320.
38. Newman, A.B.; Simonsick, E.M.; Naydeck, B.L.; Boudreau, R.M.; Kritchevsky, S.B.; Nevitt, M.C.; Pahor, M.; Satterfield, S.; Brach, J.S.; Studenski, S.A.; et al. Association of Long-Distance Corridor Walk Performance With Mortality, Cardiovascular Disease, Mobility Limitation, and Disability. *JAMA* **2006**, *295*, 2018–2026. [CrossRef] [PubMed]
39. Lee, E.J.; Jan, A.T.; Baig, M.H.; Ashraf, J.M.; Nahm, S.S.; Kim, Y.W.; Park, S.Y.; Choi, I. Fibromodulin: A master regulator of myostatin controlling progression of satellite cells through a myogenic program. *FASEB J.* **2016**, *30*, 2708–2719. [CrossRef]
40. Jan, A.T.; Baig, M.H.; Malik, A.; Choi, I.; Lee, E.J.; Ahmad, K.; Rabbani, G.; Kim, T.; Park, S.Y. Fibromodulin and regulation of the intricate balance between myoblast differentiation to myocytes or adipocyte-like cells. *FASEB J.* **2018**, *32*, 768–781.
41. Bauer, J.; Biolo, G.; Cederholm, T.; Cesari, M.; Cruz-Jentoft, A.J.; Morley, J.E.; Phillips, S.; Sieber, C.; Stehle, P.; Teta, D.; et al. Evidence-Based Recommendations for Optimal Dietary Protein Intake in Older People: A Position Paper From the PROT-AGE Study Group. *J. Am. Med. Dir. Assoc.* **2013**, *14*, 542–559. [CrossRef]
42. Ahmad, K.; Lee, E.J.; Moon, J.S.; Park, S.Y.; Choi, I. Multifaceted Interweaving Between Extracellular Matrix, Insulin Resistance, and Skeletal Muscle. *Cells* **2018**, *7*, 148. [CrossRef] [PubMed]
43. Cleasby, E.M.; Jamieson, P.M.; Atherton, P.J. Insulin resistance and sarcopenia: Mechanistic links between common co-morbidities. *J. Endocrinol.* **2016**, *229*, R67–R81. [CrossRef] [PubMed]
44. Marzetti, E.; Lees, H.A.; Wohlgemuth, S.E.; Leeuwenburgh, C. Sarcopenia of aging: Underlying cellular mechanisms and protection by calorie restriction. *BioFactors* **2009**, *35*, 28–35. [CrossRef] [PubMed]
45. Thomas, D.R. Loss of skeletal muscle mass in aging: Examining the relationship of starvation, sarcopenia and cachexia. *Clin. Nutr.* **2007**, *26*, 389–399. [CrossRef] [PubMed]
46. Haboubi, N. Assessment and management of nutrition in older people and its importance to health. *Clin. Interv. Aging* **2010**, *5*, 207. [CrossRef]
47. Morley, E.J. Anorexia of aging: Physiologic and pathologic. *Am. J. Clin. Nutr.* **1997**, *66*, 760–773. [CrossRef] [PubMed]
48. Sobotka, L. *Basics in Clinical Nutrition*, 5th ed.; Galén: Prague, Czech Republic, 2011.

49. Trouwborst, I.; Verreijen, A.; Memelink, R.; Massanet, P.; Boirie, Y.; Weijs, P.; Tieland, M. Exercise and Nutrition Strategies to Counteract Sarcopenic Obesity. *Nutrients* **2018**, *10*, 605. [CrossRef]
50. Cederholm, T.; Bosaeus, I.; Barazzoni, R.; Bauer, J.; Van Gossum, A.; Klek, S.; Muscaritoli, M.; Nyulasi, I.; Ockenga, J.; Schneider, S.; et al. Diagnostic criteria for malnutrition—An ESPEN Consensus Statement. *Clin. Nutr.* **2015**, *34*, 335–340. [CrossRef]
51. Koopman, R.; Verdijk, L.; Manders, R.J.F.; Gijsen, A.P.; Gorselink, M.; Pijpers, E.; Wagenmakers, A.J.M.; Van Loon, L.J.C. Co-ingestion of protein and leucine stimulates muscle protein synthesis rates to the same extent in young and elderly lean men. *Am. J. Clin. Nutr.* **2006**, *84*, 623–632. [CrossRef]
52. Paddon-Jones, D.; Sheffield-Moore, M.; Katsanos, C.S.; Zhang, X.J.; Wolfe, R.R. Differential stimulation of muscle protein synthesis in elderly humans following isocaloric ingestion of amino acids or whey protein. *Exp. Gerontol.* **2006**, *41*, 215–219. [CrossRef]
53. Paddon-Jones, D.; Sheffield-Moore, M.; Zhang, X.J.; Volpi, E.; Wolf, E.S.; Aarsland, A.; Ferrando, A.A.; Wolfe, R.R. Amino acid ingestion improves muscle protein synthesis in the young and elderly. *Am. J. Physiol. Metab.* **2004**, *286*, 321–328. [CrossRef] [PubMed]
54. Houston, D.K.; Nicklas, B.J.; Ding, J.; Harris, T.B.; Tylavsky, A.F.; Newman, A.B.; Lee, J.S.; Sahyoun, N.R.; Visser, M.; Kritchevsky, S.B.; et al. Dietary protein intake is associated with lean mass change in older, community-dwelling adults: The Health, Aging, and Body Composition (Health ABC) Study. *Am. J. Clin. Nutr.* **2008**, *87*, 150–155. [CrossRef] [PubMed]
55. Isanejad, M.; Mursu, J.; Sirola, J.; Kröger, H.; Rikkonen, T.; Tuppurainen, M.; Erkkilä, A.T. Dietary protein intake is associated with better physical function and muscle strength among elderly women. *Br. J. Nutr.* **2016**, *115*, 1281–1291. [CrossRef] [PubMed]
56. Landi, F.; Calvani, R.; Tosato, M.; Martone, A.M.; Picca, A.; Ortolani, E.; Savera, G.; Salini, S.; Ramaschi, M.; Bernabei, R.; et al. Animal-derived protein consumption is associated with muscle mass and strength in community-dwellers: Results from the Milan Expo survey. *J. Nutr. Health Aging* **2017**, *21*, 1050–1056. [CrossRef] [PubMed]
57. Tieland, M.; Van De Rest, O.; Dirks, M.L.; Van Der Zwaluw, N.; Mensink, M.; Van Loon, L.J.; De Groot, L.C. Protein Supplementation Improves Physical Performance in Frail Elderly People: A Randomized, Double-Blind, Placebo-Controlled Trial. *J. Am. Med. Dir. Assoc.* **2012**, *13*, 720–726. [CrossRef]
58. Trappe, T.A.; Burd, N.A.; Louis, E.S.; Lee, G.A.; Trappe, S.W. Influence of concurrent exercise or nutrition countermeasures on thigh and calf muscle size and function during 60 days of bed rest in women. *Acta Physiol.* **2007**, *191*, 147–159. [CrossRef] [PubMed]
59. Morley, J.E. Anorexia of aging: A true geriatric syndrome. *J. Nutr. Health Aging* **2012**, *16*, 422–425. [CrossRef]
60. Malafarina, V.; Uriz-Otano, F.; Gil-Guerrero, L.; Iniesta, R. The anorexia of ageing: Physiopathology, prevalence, associated comorbidity and mortality. A systematic review. *Maturitas* **2013**, *74*, 293–302. [CrossRef]
61. Drewnowski, A.; Shultz, J.M. Impact of aging on eating behaviors, food choices, nutrition, and health status. *J. Nutr. Health Aging* **2001**, *5*, 75–79.
62. Deutz, N.E.P.; Bauer, J.M.; Barazzoni, R.; Biolo, G.; Boirie, Y.; Bosy-Westphal, A.; Cederholm, T.; Cruz-Jentoft, A.J.; Krznaric, Z.; Nair, K.S.; et al. Protein intake and exercise for optimal muscle function with aging: Recommendations from the ESPEN Expert Group. *Clin. Nutr.* **2014**, *33*, 929–936. [CrossRef]
63. WHO/FAO/UNU. *Protein and Amino Acid Requirements in Human Nutrition*; Report of a Joint WHO/FAO/UNU Expert Consultation; WHO: Geneva, Switzerland, 2007.
64. Gray-Donald, K.; St-Arnaud-McKenzie, D.; Gaudreau, P.; Morais, J.A.; Shatenstein, B.; Payette, H. Protein intake protects against weight loss in healthy community-dwelling older adults. *J. Nutr.* **2014**, *144*, 321–326. [CrossRef] [PubMed]
65. Burd, N.A.; Gorissen, S.H.; Van Loon, L.J. Anabolic Resistance of Muscle Protein Synthesis with Aging. *Exerc. Sport Sci. Rev.* **2013**, *41*, 169–173. [CrossRef] [PubMed]
66. Koopman, R.; Walrand, S.; Beelen, M.; Gijsen, A.P.; Kies, A.K.; Boirie, Y.; Saris, W.H.M.; Van Loon, L.J.C. Dietary Protein Digestion and Absorption Rates and the Subsequent Postprandial Muscle Protein Synthetic Response Do Not Differ between Young and Elderly Men. *J. Nutr.* **2009**, *139*, 1707–1713. [CrossRef] [PubMed]
67. Walrand, S.; Guillet, C.; Salles, J.; Cano, N.; Boirie, Y. Physiopathological Mechanism of Sarcopenia. *Clin. Geriatr. Med.* **2011**, *27*, 365–385. [CrossRef] [PubMed]

68. Gaffney-Stomberg, E.; Insogna, K.L.; Rodriguez, N.R.; Kerstetter, J.E. Increasing Dietary Protein Requirements in Elderly People for Optimal Muscle and Bone Health. *J. Am. Geriatr. Soc.* **2009**, *57*, 1073–1079. [CrossRef]
69. Surdykowski, A.K.; Kenny, A.M.; Insogna, K.L.; Kerstetter, E.J. Optimizing bone health in older adults: The importance of dietary protein. *Aging Health* **2010**, *6*, 345–357. [CrossRef] [PubMed]
70. Van Vliet, S.; Burd, A.N.; Van Loon, L.J. The Skeletal Muscle Anabolic Response to Plant- versus Animal-Based Protein Consumption. *J. Nutr.* **2015**, *145*, 1981–1991. [CrossRef]
71. Soop, M.; Nehra, V.; Henderson, G.C.; Boirie, Y.; Ford, G.C.; Nair, K.S. Coingestion of whey protein and casein in a mixed meal: Demonstration of a more sustained anabolic effect of casein. *Am. J. Physiol. Metab.* **2012**, *303*, E152–E162. [CrossRef]
72. Dangin, M.; Guillet, C.; Garcia-Rodenas, C.; Gachon, P.; Bouteloup-Demange, C.; Reiffers-Magnani, K.; Fauquant, J.; Ballevre, O.; Beaufrere, B. The rate of protein digestion affects protein gain differently during aging in humans. *J. Physiol.* **2003**, *549*, 635–644. [CrossRef]
73. Burd, N.A.; Yang, Y.; Moore, D.R.; Tang, J.E.; Tarnopolsky, M.A.; Phillips, S.M. Greater stimulation of myofibrillar protein synthesis with ingestion of whey protein isolate v. micellar casein at rest and after resistance exercise in elderly men. *Br. J. Nutr.* **2012**, *108*, 958–962. [CrossRef]
74. Paddon-Jones, D.; Van Loon, L.J. Nutritional Approaches to Treating Sarcopenia. In *Sarcopenia*; Wiley: Hoboken, NJ, USA, 2012; pp. 275–295.
75. Bouillanne, O.; Curis, E.; Hamon-Vilcot, B.; Nicolis, I.; Chretien, P.; Schauer, N.; Vincent, J.P.; Cynober, L.; Aussel, C. Impact of protein pulse feeding on lean mass in malnourished and at-risk hospitalized elderly patients: A randomized controlled trial. *Clin. Nutr.* **2013**, *32*, 186–192. [CrossRef] [PubMed]
76. Deutz, N.E.; Wolfe, R.R. Is there a maximal anabolic response to protein intake with a meal? *Clin. Nutr.* **2013**, *32*, 309–313. [CrossRef] [PubMed]
77. Lin, R.; Liu, W.; Piao, M.; Zhu, H. A review of the relationship between the gut microbiota and amino acid metabolism. *Amino Acids* **2017**, *49*, 2083–2090. [CrossRef] [PubMed]
78. Clark, A.; Mach, N. The Crosstalk between the Gut Microbiota and Mitochondria during Exercise. *Front. Physiol.* **2017**, *8*, 319. [CrossRef] [PubMed]
79. Ticinesi, A.; Lauretani, F.; Milani, C.; Nouvenne, A.; Tana, C.; Del Rio, D.; Maggio, M.; Ventura, M.; Meschi, T. Aging Gut Microbiota at the Cross-Road between Nutrition, Physical Frailty, and Sarcopenia: Is There a Gut–Muscle Axis? *Nutrients* **2017**, *9*, 1303. [CrossRef] [PubMed]
80. Wong, J.M.W.; De Souza, R.; Kendall, C.W.C.; Emam, A.; Jenkins, D.J.A. Colonic health: Fermentation and short chain fatty acids. *J. Clin. Gastroenterol.* **2006**, *40*, 235–243. [CrossRef] [PubMed]
81. Besten, G.D.; Lange, K.; Havinga, R.; Van Dijk, T.H.; Gerding, A.; Van Eunen, K.; Muller, M.; Groen, A.K.; Hooiveld, G.J.; Bakker, B.M.; et al. Gut-derived short-chain fatty acids are vividly assimilated into host carbohydrates and lipids. *Am. J. Physiol. Liver Physiol.* **2013**, *305*, G900–G910. [CrossRef] [PubMed]
82. Besten, G.D.; Van Eunen, K.; Groen, A.K.; Venema, K.; Reijngoud, D.J.; Bakker, B.M. The role of short-chain fatty acids in the interplay between diet, gut microbiota, and host energy metabolism. *J. Lipid Res.* **2013**, *54*, 2325–2340. [CrossRef] [PubMed]
83. Sonnenburg, J.L.; Bäckhed, F. Diet–microbiota interactions as moderators of human metabolism. *Nature* **2016**, *535*, 56–64. [CrossRef]
84. Shapiro, H.; Thaiss, A.C.; Levy, M.; Elinav, E. The cross talk between microbiota and the immune system: Metabolites take center stage. *Curr. Opin. Immunol.* **2014**, *30*, 54–62. [CrossRef]
85. Anthony, J.C.; Anthony, T.G.; Kimball, S.R.; Jefferson, L.S. Signaling pathways involved in translational control of protein synthesis in skeletal muscle by leucine. *J. Nutr.* **2011**, *131*, 856S–860S. [CrossRef] [PubMed]
86. Anthony, J.C.; Yoshizawa, F.; Anthony, T.G.; Jefferson, L.S.; Vary, T.C.; Kimball, S.R. Leucine Stimulates Translation Initiation in Skeletal Muscle of Postabsorptive Rats via a Rapamycin-Sensitive Pathway. *J. Nutr.* **2000**, *130*, 2413–2419. [CrossRef] [PubMed]
87. Nakashima, K.; Ishida, A.; Yamazaki, M.; Abé, H. Leucine suppresses myofibrillar proteolysis by down-regulating ubiquitin–proteasome pathway in chick skeletal muscles. *Biochem. Biophys. Res. Commun.* **2005**, *336*, 660–666. [CrossRef] [PubMed]
88. Katsanos, C.S.; Kobayashi, H.; Sheffield-Moore, M.; Aarsland, A.; Wolfe, R.R. Aging is associated with diminished accretion of muscle proteins after the ingestion of a small bolus of essential amino acids. *Am. J. Clin. Nutr.* **2005**, *82*, 1065–1073. [CrossRef] [PubMed]

89. Xu, Z.; Tan, Z.; Zhang, Q.; Gui, Q.; Yang, Y. The effectiveness of leucine on muscle protein synthesis, lean body mass and leg lean mass accretion in older people: A systematic review and meta-analysis. *Br. J. Nutr.* **2015**, *113*, 25–34. [CrossRef] [PubMed]
90. McDonald, C.K.; Ankarfeldt, M.Z.; Capra, S.; Bauer, J.; Raymond, K.; Heitmann, B.L. Lean body mass change over 6 years is associated with dietary leucine intake in an older Danish population. *Br. J. Nutr.* **2016**, *115*, 1556–1562. [CrossRef] [PubMed]
91. Børsheim, E.; Bui, Q.-U.T.; Tissier, S.; Kobayashi, H.; Ferrando, A.A.; Wolfe, R.R. Effect of Amino Acid Supplementation on Muscle Mass, Strength and Physical Function in Elderly. *Clin. Nutr.* **2008**, *27*, 189–195. [CrossRef]
92. Gerlinger-Romero, F.; Guimarães-Ferreira, L.; Giannocco, G.; Nunes, M. Chronic supplementation of beta-hydroxy-beta methylbutyrate (HMβ) increases the activity of the GH/IGF-I axis and induces hyperinsulinemia in rats. *Growth Horm. IGF Res.* **2011**, *21*, 57–62. [CrossRef]
93. Smith, H.J.; Mukerji, P.; Tisdale, M.J. Attenuation of proteasome-induced proteolysis in skeletal muscle by {beta}-hydroxy-{beta}-methylbutyrate in cancer-induced muscle loss. *Cancer Res.* **2005**, *65*, 277–283.
94. Smith, H.J.; Wyke, S.M.; Tisdale, M.J. Mechanism of the attenuation of proteolysis-inducing factor stimulated protein degradation in muscle by beta-hydroxy-beta-methylbutyrate. *Cancer Res.* **2004**, *64*, 8731–8735. [CrossRef]
95. HoleČek, M. Beta-hydroxy-beta-methylbutyrate supplementation and skeletal muscle in healthy and muscle-wasting conditions. *J. Cachex Sarcopenia Muscle* **2017**, *8*, 529–541. [CrossRef] [PubMed]
96. He, X.; Duan, Y.; Yao, K.; Li, F.; Hou, Y.; Wu, G.; Yin, Y. β-Hydroxy-β-methylbutyrate, mitochondrial biogenesis, and skeletal muscle health. *Amino Acids* **2016**, *48*, 653–664. [CrossRef] [PubMed]
97. Wilson, G.J.; Wilson, J.M.; Manninen, A.H. Effects of beta-hydroxy-beta-methylbutyrate (HMB) on exercise performance and body composition across varying levels of age, sex, and training experience: A review. *Nutr. Metab.* **2008**, *5*, 1. [CrossRef] [PubMed]
98. Kornasio, R.; Riederer, I.; Butler-Browne, G.; Mouly, V.; Uni, Z.; Halevy, O. β-hydroxy-β-methylbutyrate (HMB) stimulates myogenic cell proliferation, differentiation and survival via the MAPK/ERK and PI3K/Akt pathways. *Biochim. Biophys. Acta Mol. Cell Res.* **2009**, *1793*, 755–763. [CrossRef] [PubMed]
99. Van Koevering, M.; Nissen, S. Oxidation of leucine and alpha-ketoisocaproate to beta-hydroxy-beta-methylbutyrate in vivo. *Am. J. Physiol. Metab.* **1992**, *262*, 27–31. [CrossRef] [PubMed]
100. Kuriyan, R.; Lokesh, D.P.; Selvam, S.; Jayakumar, J.; Philip, M.G.; Shreeram, S.; Kurpad, A.V.; Sathyavageeswaran, S. The relationship of endogenous plasma concentrations of β-Hydroxy β-Methyl Butyrate (HMB) to age and total appendicular lean mass in humans. *Exp. Gerontol.* **2016**, *81*, 13–18. [CrossRef] [PubMed]
101. Portal, S.; Eliakim, A.; Nemet, D.; Halevy, O.; Zadik, Z. Effect of HMB supplementation on body composition, fitness, hormonal profile and muscle damage indices. *J. Pediatr. Endocrinol. Metab.* **2010**, *23*, 641–650. [CrossRef]
102. Flakoll, P.; Sharp, R.; Baier, S.; Levenhagen, D.; Carr, C.; Nissen, S. Effect of beta-hydroxy-beta-methylbutyrate, arginine, and lysine supplementation on strength, functionality, body composition, and protein metabolism in elderly women. *Nutrition* **2004**, *20*, 445–451. [CrossRef]
103. Argilés, J.M.; Campos, N.; Lopez-Pedrosa, J.M.; Rueda, R.; Rodriguez-Mañas, L. Skeletal Muscle Regulates Metabolism via Interorgan Crosstalk: Roles in Health and Disease. *J. Am. Med. Dir. Assoc.* **2016**, *17*, 789–796. [CrossRef]
104. Deutz, N.E.; Pereira, S.L.; Hays, N.P.; Oliver, J.S.; Edens, N.K.; Evans, C.M.; Wolfe, R.R. Effect of β-hydroxy-β-methylbutyrate (HMB) on lean body mass during 10 days of bed rest in older adults. *Clin. Nutr.* **2013**, *32*, 704–712. [CrossRef]
105. Fitschen, P.J.; Wilson, G.J.; Wilson, J.M.; Wilund, K.R. Efficacy of β-hydroxy-β-methylbutyrate supplementation in elderly and clinical populations. *Nutrition* **2013**, *29*, 29–36. [CrossRef] [PubMed]
106. Cynober, L. Ornithine alpha-ketoglutarate as a potent precursor of arginine and nitric oxide: A new job for an old friend. *J. Nutr.* **2004**, *134*, 2858S–2862S. [CrossRef] [PubMed]
107. Walrand, S. Ornithine alpha-ketoglutarate: Could it be a new therapeutic option for sarcopenia? *J. Nutr. Health Aging* **2010**, *14*, 570–577. [CrossRef] [PubMed]

108. Brocker, P.; Vellas, B.; Albarede, J.L.; Poynard, T. A Two-centre, Randomized, Double-blind Trial of Ornithine Oxoglutarate in 194 Elderly, Ambulatory, Convalescent Subjects. *Age Ageing* **1994**, *23*, 303–306. [CrossRef] [PubMed]
109. Segaud, F.; Combaret, L.; Neveux, N.; Attaix, D.; Cynober, L.; Moinard, C. Effects of ornithine alpha-ketoglutarate on protein metabolism in Yoshida sarcoma-bearing rats. *Clin. Nutr.* **2007**, *26*, 624–630. [CrossRef]
110. Donati, L.; Ziegler, F.; Pongelli, G.; Signorini, M.S. Nutritional and clinical efficacy of ornithine alpha-ketoglutarate in severe burn patients. *Clin. Nutr.* **1999**, *18*, 307–311. [CrossRef]
111. Wernerman, J.; Hammarqvist, F.; Von Der Decken, A.; Vinnars, E. Ornithine-alpha-ketoglutarate Improves Skeletal Muscle Protein Synthesis as Assessed by Ribosome Analysis and Nitrogen Use After Surgery. *Ann. Surg.* **1987**, *208*, 674–680. [CrossRef]
112. Visser, M.; Deeg, D.J.H.; Lips, P.; Longitudinal Aging Study Amsterdam. Low vitamin D and high parathyroid hormone levels as determinants of loss of muscle strength and muscle mass (sarcopenia): The Longitudinal Aging Study Amsterdam. *J. Clin. Endocrinol. Metab.* **2003**, *88*, 5766–5772. [CrossRef]
113. Scott, D.; Blizzard, L.; Fell, J.; Ding, C.; Winzenberg, T.; Jones, G. A prospective study of the associations between 25-hydroxy-vitamin D, sarcopenia progression and physical activity in older adults. *Clin. Endocrinol.* **2010**, *73*, 581–587. [CrossRef]
114. Johnson, M.A.; Kimlin, M.G. Vitamin D, Aging, and the 2005 Dietary Guidelines for Americans. *Nutr. Rev.* **2006**, *64*, 410–421. [CrossRef]
115. Borchers, M.; Gudat, F.; Dürmüller, U.; Stahelin, H.; Dick, W.; Bischoff-Ferrari, H.; Bischoff-Ferrari, H. Vitamin D Receptor Expression in Human Muscle Tissue Decreases With Age. *J. Bone Miner. Res.* **2004**, *19*, 265–269.
116. Ceglia, L.; Morais, M.D.S.; Park, L.K.; Morris, E.; Harris, S.S.; Bischoff-Ferrari, H.A.; Fielding, R.A.; Dawson-Hughes, B. Multi-step immunofluorescent analysis of vitamin D receptor loci and myosin heavy chain isoforms in human skeletal muscle. *J. Mol. Histol.* **2010**, *41*, 137–142. [CrossRef] [PubMed]
117. Ceglia, L. Vitamin D and skeletal muscle tissue and function. *Mol. Asp. Med.* **2008**, *29*, 407–414. [CrossRef] [PubMed]
118. Montero-Odasso, M.; Duque, G. Vitamin D in the aging musculoskeletal system: An authentic strength preserving hormone. *Mol. Asp. Med.* **2005**, *26*, 203–219. [CrossRef] [PubMed]
119. Pojednic, R.M.; Ceglia, L.; Olsson, K.; Gustafsson, T.; Lichtenstein, A.H.; Dawson-Hughes, B.; Fielding, R.A. Effects of 1, 25-dihydroxyvitamin D3 and vitamin D3 on the expression of the vitamin d receptor in human skeletal muscle cells. *Calcif. Tissue Int.* **2015**, *96*, 256–263. [CrossRef]
120. Muir, S.W.; Montero-Odasso, M.; Montero-Odasso, M.; Montero-Odasso, M. Effect of Vitamin D Supplementation on Muscle Strength, Gait and Balance in Older Adults: A Systematic Review and Meta-Analysis. *J. Am. Geriatr. Soc.* **2011**, *59*, 2291–2300. [CrossRef]
121. Beaudart, C.; Buckinx, F.; Rabenda, V.; Gillain, S.; Cavalier, E.; Slomian, J.; Petermans, J.; Reginster, J.Y.; Bruyère, O. The Effects of Vitamin D on Skeletal Muscle Strength, Muscle Mass, and Muscle Power: A Systematic Review and Meta-Analysis of Randomized Controlled Trials. *J. Clin. Endocrinol. Metab.* **2014**, *99*, 4336–4345. [CrossRef]
122. Yamada, M.; Arai, H.; Yoshimura, K.; Kajiwara, Y.; Sonoda, T.; Nishiguchi, S.; Aoyama, T. Nutritional Supplementation during Resistance Training Improved Skeletal Muscle Mass in Community-Dwelling Frail Older Adults. *J. Frailty Aging* **2012**, *1*, 64–70.
123. Kurosawa, Y.; Hamaoka, T.; Katsumura, T.; Kuwamori, M.; Kimura, N.; Sako, T.; Chance, B. Creatine supplementation enhances anaerobic ATP synthesis during a single 10 sec maximal handgrip exercise. *Guanidino Compd. Biol. Med.* **2003**, *244*, 105–112.
124. Bemben, M.G.; Lamont, H.S. Creatine supplementation and exercise performance: Recent findings. *Sports Med.* **2005**, *35*, 107–125. [CrossRef]
125. Ingwall, J.S. Creatine and the control of muscle-specific protein synthesis in cardiac and skeletal muscle. *Circ. Res.* **1976**, *38*, 115–123.
126. Lang, F.; Busch, G.L.; Ritter, M.; Völkl, H.; Waldegger, S.; Gulbins, E.; Häussinger, D. Functional Significance of Cell Volume Regulatory Mechanisms. *Physiol. Rev.* **1998**, *78*, 247–306. [CrossRef] [PubMed]
127. Burke, D.G.; Candow, D.G.; Chilibeck, P.D.; MacNeil, L.G.; Roy, B.D.; Tarnopolsky, M.A.; Ziegenfuss, T. Effect of creatine supplementation and resistance-exercise training on muscle insulin-like growth factor in young adults. *Int. J. Sport Nutr. Exerc. Metab.* **2008**, *18*, 389–398. [CrossRef] [PubMed]

128. Louis, M.; Van Beneden, R.; Dehoux, M.; Thissen, J.P.; Francaux, M. Creatine increases IGF-I and myogenic regulatory factor mRNA in C(2)C(12) cells. *FEBS Lett.* **2004**, *557*, 243–247. [CrossRef]
129. Deldicque, L.; Louis, M.; Theisen, D.; Nielens, H.; Dehoux, M.; Thissen, J.P.; Rennie, M.J.; Francaux, M. Increased IGF mRNA in Human Skeletal Muscle after Creatine Supplementation. *Med. Sci. Sports Exerc.* **2005**, *37*, 731–736. [CrossRef]
130. Deldicque, L.; Theisen, D.; Bertrand, L.; Hespel, P.; Hue, L.; Francaux, M. Creatine enhances differentiation of myogenic C(2)C(12)cells by activating both p38 and Akt/PKB pathways. *Am. J. Physiol. Physiol.* **2007**, *293*, C1263–C1271. [CrossRef] [PubMed]
131. Fujita, S.; Dreyer, H.C.; Drummond, M.J.; Glynn, E.L.; Cadenas, J.G.; Yoshizawa, F.; Volpi, E.; Rasmussen, B.B. Nutrient signalling in the regulation of human muscle protein synthesis. *J. Physiol.* **2007**, *582*, 813–823. [CrossRef]
132. Bentzinger, C.F.; Lin, S.; Romanino, K.; Castets, P.; Guridi, M.; Summermatter, S.; Handschin, C.; Tintignac, A.L.; Hall, M.N.; Ruegg, A.M. Differential response of skeletal muscles to mTORC1 signaling during atrophy and hypertrophy. *Skelet. Muscle* **2013**, *3*, 6. [CrossRef]
133. Bentzinger, C.F.; Romanino, K.; Cloëtta, D.; Lin, S.; Mascarenhas, J.B.; Oliveri, F.; Xia, J.; Casanova, E.; Costa, C.F.; Brink, M.; et al. Skeletal Muscle-Specific Ablation of raptor, but Not of rictor, Causes Metabolic Changes and Results in Muscle Dystrophy. *Cell Metab.* **2008**, *8*, 411–424. [CrossRef]
134. Zanou, N.; Gailly, P. Skeletal muscle hypertrophy and regeneration: Interplay between the myogenic regulatory factors (MRFs) and insulin-like growth factors (IGFs) pathways. *Cell. Mol. Life Sci.* **2013**, *70*, 4117–4130. [CrossRef]
135. Deldicque, L.; Theisen, D.; Francaux, M. Regulation of mTOR by amino acids and resistance exercise in skeletal muscle. *Graefe's Arch. Clin. Exp. Ophthalmol.* **2005**, *94*, 1–10. [CrossRef] [PubMed]
136. Kirwan, J.P.; Del Aguila, L.F.; Hernandez, J.M.; Williamson, D.L.; O'Gorman, D.J.; Lewis, R.; Krishnan, R.K. Regular exercise enhances insulin activation of IRS-1-associated PI3-kinase in human skeletal muscle. *J. Appl. Physiol.* **2000**, *88*, 797–803. [CrossRef] [PubMed]
137. Willoughby, D.S.; McFarlin, B.; Bois, C. Interleukin-6 Expression after Repeated Bouts of Eccentric Exercise. *Int. J. Sports Med.* **2003**, *24*, 15–21. [CrossRef] [PubMed]
138. Ferretti, R.; Moura, E.G.; Dos Santos, V.C.; Caldeira, E.J.; Conte, M.; Matsumura, C.Y.; Pertille, A.; Mosqueira, M. High-fat diet suppresses the positive effect of creatine supplementation on skeletal muscle function by reducing protein expression of IGF-PI3K-AKT-mTOR pathway. *PLoS ONE* **2018**, *13*, e0199728. [CrossRef] [PubMed]
139. Möller, P.; Bergström, J.; Fürst, P.; Hellström, K. Effect of aging on energy-rich phosphagens in human skeletal muscles. *Clin. Sci.* **1980**, *58*, 553–555. [CrossRef] [PubMed]
140. Candow, D.G. Sarcopenia: Current theories and the potential beneficial effect of creatine application strategies. *Biogerontology* **2011**, *12*, 273–281. [CrossRef]
141. Liguori, I.; Russo, G.; Curcio, F.; Bulli, G.; Aran, L.; Della-Morte, D.; Gargiulo, G.; Testa, G.; Cacciatore, F.; Bonaduce, D.; et al. Oxidative stress, aging, and diseases. *Clin. Interv. Aging* **2018**, *13*, 757–772. [CrossRef]
142. Yakes, F.M.; Van Houten, B. Mitochondrial DNA damage is more extensive and persists longer than nuclear DNA damage in human cells following oxidative stress. *Proc. Natl. Acad. Sci. USA* **1997**, *94*, 514–519. [CrossRef]
143. Marzetti, E.; Calvani, R.; Cesari, M.; Buford, T.W.; Lorenzi, M.; Behnke, B.J.; Leeuwenburgh, C. Mitochondrial dysfunction and sarcopenia of aging: From signaling pathways to clinical trials. *Int. J. Biochem. Cell Biol.* **2013**, *45*, 2288–2301. [CrossRef]
144. Howl, J.D.; Publicover, S.J. Permeabilisation of the sarcolemma in mouse diaphragm exposed to Bay K 8644 in vitro: Time course, dependence on Ca2+ and effects of enzyme inhibitors. *Acta Neuropathol.* **1990**, *79*, 438–443. [CrossRef]
145. Kim, J.S.; Wilson, J.M.; Lee, S.R. Dietary implications on mechanisms of sarcopenia: Roles of protein, amino acids and antioxidants. *J. Nutr. Biochem.* **2010**, *21*, 1–13. [CrossRef] [PubMed]
146. Lauretani, F.; Semba, R.D.; Bandinelli, S.; Dayhoff-Brannigan, M.; Lauretani, F.; Corsi, A.M.; Guralnik, J.M.; Ferrucci, L. Carotenoids as Protection Against Disability in Older Persons. *Rejuvenation Res.* **2008**, *11*, 557–563. [CrossRef] [PubMed]

147. Lauretani, F.; Semba, R.D.; Bandinelli, S.; Dayhoff-Brannigan, M.; Giacomini, V.; Corsi, A.M.; Guralnik, J.M.; Ferrucci, L. Low Plasma Carotenoids and Skeletal Muscle Strength Decline Over 6 Years. *J. Gerontol. Ser. A Biol. Sci. Med Sci.* **2008**, *63*, 376–383. [CrossRef] [PubMed]
148. Bjørnsen, T.; Salvesen, S.; Berntsen, S.; Hetlelid, K.J.; Stea, T.H.; Lohne-Seiler, H.; Rohde, G.; Haraldstad, K.; Raastad, T.; Køpp, U.; et al. Vitamin C and E supplementation blunts increases in total lean body mass in elderly men after strength training. *Scand. J. Med. Sci. Sports* **2016**, *26*, 755–763. [CrossRef] [PubMed]
149. Handy, D.E.; Loscalzo, J. Redox Regulation of Mitochondrial Function. *Antioxid. Redox Signal.* **2012**, *16*, 1323–1367. [CrossRef] [PubMed]
150. Ji, L.L. Antioxidant signaling in skeletal muscle: A brief review. *Exp. Gerontol.* **2007**, *42*, 582–593. [CrossRef]
151. Musarò, A.; Fulle, S.; Fano, G. Oxidative stress and muscle homeostasis. *Curr. Opin. Clin. Nutr. Metab. Care* **2010**, *13*, 236–242. [CrossRef] [PubMed]
152. Gutteridge, J.M.; Halliwell, B. Antioxidants: Molecules, medicines, and myths. *Biochem. Biophys. Res. Commun.* **2010**, *393*, 561–564. [CrossRef] [PubMed]
153. Ristow, M.; Zarse, K.; Oberbach, A.; Klöting, N.; Birringer, M.; Kiehntopf, M.; Stumvoll, M.; Kahn, C.R.; Blüher, M. Antioxidants prevent health-promoting effects of physical exercise in humans. *Proc. Natl. Acad. Sci. USA* **2009**, *106*, 8665–8670. [CrossRef]
154. Miller, E.; Pastor-Barriuso, R.; Dalal, D.; Riemersma, R.; Appel, L.; Guallar, E. Meta-Analysis: High-Dosage Vitamin E Supplementation May Increase All-Cause Mortality. *ACC Curr. J. Rev.* **2005**, *14*, 17. [CrossRef]
155. Bjelakovic, G.; Nikolova, D.; Gluud, L.L.; Simonetti, R.G.; Gluud, C. Mortality in Randomized Trials of Antioxidant Supplements for Primary and Secondary Prevention: Systematic Review and Meta-analysis. *JAMA* **2007**, *297*, 842. [CrossRef] [PubMed]
156. Bjelaković, G.; Nikolova, D.; Gluud, L.L.; Simonetti, R.G.; Gluud, C. Antioxidant supplements for prevention of mortality in healthy participants and patients with various diseases. *Cochrane Database Syst. Rev.* **2012**. [CrossRef] [PubMed]
157. Fusco, D.; Colloca, G.; Monaco, M.R.L.; Cesari, M. Effects of antioxidant supplementation on the aging process. *Clin. Interv. Aging* **2007**, *2*, 377–387. [PubMed]
158. Bouayed, J.; Bohn, T. Exogenous antioxidants–Double-edged swords in cellular redox state: Health beneficial effects at physiologic doses versus deleterious effects at high doses. *Oxid. Med. Cell. Longev.* **2010**, *3*, 228–237. [CrossRef] [PubMed]
159. Smith, G.I. The Effects of Dietary Omega-3s on Muscle Composition and Quality in Older Adults. *Curr. Nutr. Rep.* **2016**, *5*, 99–105. [CrossRef] [PubMed]
160. Li, K.; Huang, T.; Zheng, J.; Wu, K.; Li, D. Effect of Marine-Derived n-3 Polyunsaturated Fatty Acids on C-Reactive Protein, Interleukin 6 and Tumor Necrosis Factor α: A Meta-Analysis. *PLoS ONE* **2014**, *9*, e88103. [CrossRef] [PubMed]
161. Calder, P.C. n-3 polyunsaturated fatty acids, inflammation, and inflammatory diseases. *Am. J. Clin. Nutr.* **2006**, *83*, 1505S–1519S. [CrossRef]
162. Welch, A.A.; MacGregor, A.J.; Minihane, A.-M.; Skinner, J.; Valdes, A.A.; Spector, T.D.; Cassidy, A. Dietary Fat and Fatty Acid Profile Are Associated with Indices of Skeletal Muscle Mass in Women Aged 18–79 Years. *J. Nutr.* **2014**, *144*, 327–334. [CrossRef]
163. Robinson, S.M.; Jameson, K.A.; Batelaan, S.F.; Martin, H.J.; Syddall, H.E.; Dennison, E.M.; Cooper, C.; Sayer, A.A.; Hertfordshire Cohort Study Group. Diet and its relationship with grip strength in community-dwelling older men and women: The Hertfordshire cohort study. *J. Am. Geriatr. Soc.* **2008**, *56*, 84–90. [CrossRef]
164. Hutchins-Wiese, H.L.; Kleppinger, A.; Annis, K.; Liva, E.; Lammi-Keefe, C.J.; Durham, H.A.; Kenny, A.M. The impact of supplemental n-3 long chain polyunsaturated fatty acids and dietary antioxidants on physical performance in postmenopausal women. *J. Nutr. Health Aging* **2013**, *17*, 76–80. [CrossRef]
165. Krzymińska-Siemaszko, R.; Czepulis, N.; Lewandowicz, M.; Zasadzka, E.; Suwalska, A.; Witowski, J.; Wieczorowska-Tobis, K. The Effect of a 12-Week Omega-3 Supplementation on Body Composition, Muscle Strength and Physical Performance in Elderly Individuals with Decreased Muscle Mass. *Int. J. Environ. Res. Public Health* **2015**, *12*, 10558–10574. [CrossRef] [PubMed]
166. Jäger, S.; Trojan, H.; Kopp, T.; Laszczyk, M.N.; Scheffler, A. Pentacyclic Triterpene Distribution in Various Plants – Rich Sources for a New Group of Multi-Potent Plant Extracts. *Molecules* **2009**, *14*, 2016–2031. [CrossRef] [PubMed]

167. Kunkel, S.D.; Suneja, M.; Ebert, S.M.; Bongers, K.S.; Fox, D.K.; Malmberg, S.E.; Alipour, F.; Shields, R.K.; Adams, C.M. mRNA Expression Signatures of Human Skeletal Muscle Atrophy Identify a Natural Compound that Increases Muscle Mass. *Cell Metab.* **2011**, *13*, 627–638. [CrossRef] [PubMed]
168. Lundberg, J.O. Nitrate transport in salivary glands with implications for NO homeostasis. *Proc. Natl. Acad. Sci. USA* **2012**, *109*, 13144–13145. [CrossRef] [PubMed]
169. Buford, T.W.; Anton, S.D.; Judge, A.R.; Marzetti, E.; Wohlgemuth, S.E.; Carter, C.S.; Leeuwenburgh, C.; Pahor, M.; Manini, T.M. Models of Accelerated Sarcopenia: Critical Pieces for Solving the Puzzle of Age-Related Muscle Atrophy. *Ageing Res. Rev.* **2010**, *9*, 369–383. [CrossRef] [PubMed]
170. Larsen, F.J.; Weitzberg, E.; Lundberg, J.O.; Ekblom, B. Dietary nitrate reduces maximal oxygen consumption while maintaining work performance in maximal exercise. *Free Radic. Biol. Med.* **2010**, *48*, 342–347. [CrossRef] [PubMed]
171. Larsen, F.J.; Schiffer, T.A.; Borniquel, S.; Sahlin, K.; Ekblom, B.; Lundberg, J.O.; Weitzberg, E. Dietary Inorganic Nitrate Improves Mitochondrial Efficiency in Humans. *Cell Metab.* **2011**, *13*, 149–159. [CrossRef]
172. Siervo, M.; Oggioni, C.; Jakovljevic, D.G.; Trenell, M.; Mathers, J.C.; Houghton, D.; Celis-Morales, C.; Ashor, A.W.; Ruddock, A.; Ranchordas, M.; et al. Dietary nitrate does not affect physical activity or outcomes in healthy older adults in a randomized, cross-over trial. *Nutr. Res.* **2016**, *36*, 1361–1369. [CrossRef]
173. Jones, A.M. Dietary Nitrate Supplementation and Exercise Performance. *Sports Med.* **2014**, *44*, 35–45. [CrossRef]
174. Grosicki, G.J.; Fielding, R.A.; Lustgarten, M.S. Gut Microbiota Contribute to Age-Related Changes in Skeletal Muscle Size, Composition, and Function: Biological Basis for a Gut-Muscle Axis. *Calcif. Tissue Int.* **2018**, *102*, 433–442. [CrossRef]
175. Picca, A.; Fanelli, F.; Calvani, R.; Mulé, G.; Pesce, V.; Sisto, A.; Pantanelli, C.; Bernabei, R.; Landi, F.; Marzetti, E. Gut Dysbiosis and Muscle Aging: Searching for Novel Targets against Sarcopenia. *Mediat. Inflamm.* **2018**, *2018*, 1–15. [CrossRef] [PubMed]
176. Rampelli, S.; Candela, M.; Turroni, S.; Biagi, E.; Collino, S.; Franceschi, C.; O'Toole, P.W.; Brigidi, P. Functional metagenomic profiling of intestinal microbiome in extreme ageing. *Aging* **2013**, *5*, 902–912. [CrossRef] [PubMed]
177. Steves, C.J.; Bird, S.; Williams, F.M.K.; Spector, T.D. The Microbiome and Musculoskeletal Conditions of Aging: A Review of Evidence for Impact and Potential Therapeutics. *J. Bone Miner. Res.* **2016**, *31*, 261–269. [CrossRef] [PubMed]
178. Quigley, E.M.M. Commentary: Synbiotics and gut microbiota in older people—A microbial guide to healthy ageing. *Aliment. Pharmacol. Ther.* **2013**, *38*, 1141–1142. [CrossRef] [PubMed]
179. Caputi, V.; Marsilio, I.; Filpa, V.; Cerantola, S.; Orso, G.; Bistoletti, M.; Paccagnella, N.; De Martin, S.; Montopoli, M.; Dall'Acqua, S.; et al. Antibiotic-induced dysbiosis of the microbiota impairs gut neuromuscular function in juvenile mice. *Br. J. Pharmacol.* **2017**, *174*, 3623–3639. [CrossRef] [PubMed]
180. De Vrese, M.; Schrezenmeir, J. Probiotics, Prebiotics, and Synbiotics. *Adv. Biochem. Eng. Biotechnol.* **2008**, *111*, 1–66. [PubMed]
181. Buigues, C.; Fernández-Garrido, J.; Pruimboom, L.; Hoogland, A.J.; Navarro-Martínez, R.; Martínez-Martínez, M.; Verdejo, Y.; Mascarós, M.C.; Peris, C.; Cauli, O. Effect of a Prebiotic Formulation on Frailty Syndrome: A Randomized, Double-Blind Clinical Trial. *Int. J. Mol. Sci.* **2016**, *17*, 932. [CrossRef] [PubMed]
182. Food and Agriculture Organization of the United Nations; World Health Organization. *Probiotics in food: Health and Nutritional Properties and Guidelines for Evaluation*; Food and Agriculture Organization of the United Nations; World Health Organization: Geneva, Switzerland, 2006.
183. Rondanelli, M.; Giacosa, A.; Faliva, M.A.; Perna, S.; Allieri, F.; Castellazzi, A.M. Review on microbiota and effectiveness of probiotics use in older. *World J. Clin. Cases* **2015**, *3*, 156–162. [CrossRef]
184. Varian, B.J.; Goureshetti, S.; Poutahidis, T.; Lakritz, J.R.; Levkovich, T.; Kwok, C.; Teliousis, K.; Ibrahim, Y.M.; Mirabal, S.; Erdman, S.E. Beneficial bacteria inhibit cachexia. *Oncotarget* **2016**, *7*, 11803–11816. [CrossRef]
185. Munukka, E.; Rintala, A.; Toivonen, R.; Nylund, M.; Yang, B.; Takanen, A.; Hänninen, A.; Vuopio, J.; Huovinen, P.; Jalkanen, S.; et al. Faecalibacterium prausnitzii treatment improves hepatic health and reduces adipose tissue inflammation in high-fat fed mice. *ISME J.* **2017**, *11*, 1667–1679. [CrossRef]

186. Neyrinck, A.M.; Taminiau, B.; Walgrave, H.; Daube, G.; Cani, P.D.; Bindels, L.B.; Delzenne, N.M. Spirulina Protects against Hepatic Inflammation in Aging: An Effect Related to the Modulation of the Gut Microbiota? *Nutrients* **2017**, *9*, 633. [CrossRef] [PubMed]
187. Tiihonen, K.; Ouwehand, A.C.; Rautonen, N. Human intestinal microbiota and healthy ageing. *Ageing Res. Rev.* **2010**, *9*, 107–116. [CrossRef] [PubMed]
188. Singh, R.K.; Chang, H.W.; Yan, D.; Lee, K.M.; Ucmak, D.; Wong, K.; Abrouk, M.; Farahnik, B.; Nakamura, M.; Zhu, T.H.; et al. Influence of diet on the gut microbiome and implications for human health. *J. Transl. Med.* **2017**, *15*, 1101. [CrossRef] [PubMed]
189. Dickinson, J.M.; Volpi, E.; Rasmussen, B.B. Exercise and nutrition to target protein synthesis impairments in aging skeletal muscle. *Exerc. Sport Sci. Rev.* **2013**, *41*, 216–223. [CrossRef] [PubMed]
190. Glover, E.I.; Phillips, S.M.; Oates, B.R.; Tang, J.E.; Tarnopolsky, M.A.; Selby, A.; Smith, K.; Rennie, M.J. Immobilization induces anabolic resistance in human myofibrillar protein synthesis with low and high dose amino acid infusion. *J. Physiol.* **2008**, *586*, 6049–6061. [CrossRef] [PubMed]
191. WHO. *Global Recommendations on Physical Activity for Health*; WHO: Geneva, Switzerland, 2010.
192. Beckwée, D.; Delaere, A.; Aelbrecht, S.; Baert, V.; Beaudart, C.; Bruyere, O.; de Saint-Hubert, M.; Bautmans, I. Exercise Interventions for the Prevention and Treatment of Sarcopenia. A Systematic Umbrella Review. *J. Nutr. Health Aging* **2019**, *23*, 494–502. [CrossRef]
193. Azzolino, D.; Damanti, S.; Bertagnoli, L.; Lucchi, T.; Cesari, M. Sarcopenia and swallowing disorders in older people. *Aging Clin. Exp. Res.* **2019**, *31*, 1–7. [CrossRef]
194. Bernardelli, G.; Roncaglione, C.; Damanti, S.; Mari, D.; Cesari, M.; Marcucci, M. Adapted physical activity to promote active and healthy ageing: The PoliFIT pilot randomized waiting list-controlled trial. *Aging Clin. Exp. Res.* **2019**, *31*, 511–518. [CrossRef]
195. So, C.; Pierluissi, E. Attitudes and Expectations Regarding Exercise in the Hospital of Hospitalized Older Adults: A Qualitative Study. *J. Am. Geriatr. Soc.* **2012**, *60*, 713–718. [CrossRef]
196. West, D.W.D.; Moore, D.R.; Staples, A.W.; Prior, T.; Tang, J.E.; Rennie, M.J.; Burd, N.A.; Atherton, P.J.; Baker, S.K.; Phillips, S.M. Enhanced Amino Acid Sensitivity of Myofibrillar Protein Synthesis Persists for up to 24 h after Resistance Exercise in Young Men. *J. Nutr.* **2011**, *141*, 568–573.
197. Yang, Y.; Breen, L.; Burd, N.A.; Hector, A.J.; Churchward-Venne, T.A.; Josse, A.R.; Tarnopolsky, M.A.; Phillips, S.M. Resistance exercise enhances myofibrillar protein synthesis with graded intakes of whey protein in older men. *Br. J. Nutr.* **2012**, *108*, 1780–1788. [CrossRef] [PubMed]
198. Conn, V.S.; Minor, M.A.; Burks, K.J.; Rantz, M.J.; Pomeroy, S.H. Integrative Review of Physical Activity Intervention Research with Aging Adults. *J. Am. Geriatr. Soc.* **2003**, *51*, 1159–1168. [CrossRef] [PubMed]
199. Kruger, J.; Buchner, D.M.; Prohaska, T.R. The Prescribed Amount of Physical Activity in Randomized Clinical Trials in Older Adults. *Gerontologist* **2009**, *49*, S100–S107. [CrossRef] [PubMed]
200. Fielding, A.R. Effects of exercise training in the elderly: Impact of progressive-resistance training on skeletal muscle and whole-body protein metabolism. *Proc. Nutr. Soc.* **1995**, *54*, 665–675. [CrossRef] [PubMed]
201. Van Abbema, R.; De Greef, M.; Crajé, C.; Krijnen, W.; Hobbelen, H.; Van Der Schans, C. What type, or combination of exercise can improve preferred gait speed in older adults? A meta-analysis. *BMC Geriatr.* **2015**, *15*, 2211. [CrossRef] [PubMed]
202. Hortobagyi, T.; Lesinski, M.; Gäbler, M.; VanSwearingen, J.M.; Malatesta, D.; Granacher, U. Effects of Three Types of Exercise Interventions on Healthy Old Adults' Gait Speed: A Systematic Review and Meta-Analysis. *Sports Med.* **2015**, *45*, 1627–1643. [CrossRef] [PubMed]
203. Peterson, M.D.; Sen, A.; Gordon, P.M. Influence of Resistance Exercise on Lean Body Mass in Aging Adults: A Meta-Analysis. *Med. Sci. Sports Exerc.* **2011**, *43*, 249–258. [CrossRef]
204. Borde, R.; Hortobágyi, T.; Granacher, U. Dose–Response Relationships of Resistance Training in Healthy Old Adults: A Systematic Review and Meta-Analysis. *Sports Med.* **2015**, *45*, 1693–1720. [CrossRef]
205. Fiatarone, M.A.; Marks, E.C.; Ryan, N.D.; Meredith, C.N.; Lipsitz, L.A.; Evans, W.J. High-Intensity Strength Training in Nonagenarians. *JAMA* **1990**, *263*, 3029. [CrossRef]
206. Fiatarone, M.A.; O'Neill, E.F.; Ryan, N.D.; Clements, K.M.; Solares, G.R.; Nelson, M.E.; Kehayias, J.J.; Lipsitz, L.A.; Roberts, S.B.; Evans, W.J. Exercise Training and Nutritional Supplementation for Physical Frailty in Very Elderly People. *N. Engl. J. Med.* **1994**, *330*, 1769–1775. [CrossRef]

207. Serra-Rexach, J.A.; Bustamante-Ara, N.; Villarán, M.H.; Gil, P.G.; Ibáñez, M.J.S.; Sanz, N.B.; Santamaría, V.O.; Sanz, N.G.; Prada, A.B.M.; Gallardo, C.; et al. Short-Term, Light- to Moderate-Intensity Exercise Training Improves Leg Muscle Strength in the Oldest Old: A Randomized Controlled Trial. *J. Am. Geriatr. Soc.* **2011**, *59*, 594–602. [CrossRef] [PubMed]
208. Oettle, G.J. Effect of moderate exercise on bowel habit. *Gut* **1991**, *32*, 941–944. [CrossRef] [PubMed]
209. Vandeputte, D.; Falony, G.; Vieira-Silva, S.; Tito, R.Y.; Joossens, M.; Raes, J. Stool consistency is strongly associated with gut microbiota richness and composition, enterotypes and bacterial growth rates. *Gut* **2016**, *65*, 57–62. [CrossRef] [PubMed]
210. Zhu, L.; Liu, W.; Alkhouri, R.; Baker, R.D.; Bard, J.E.; Quigley, E.M.; Baker, S.S. Structural changes in the gut microbiome of constipated patients. *Physiol. Genom.* **2014**, *46*, 679–686. [CrossRef] [PubMed]
211. Tang, E.J.; Phillips, S.M. Maximizing muscle protein anabolism: The role of protein quality. *Curr. Opin. Clin. Nutr. Metab. Care* **2009**, *12*, 66–71. [CrossRef] [PubMed]
212. Shad, B.J.; Thompson, J.L.; Breen, L. Does the muscle protein synthetic response to exercise and amino acid-based nutrition diminish with advancing age? A systematic review. *Am. J. Physiol. Metab.* **2016**, *311*, E803–E817. [CrossRef]
213. Pennings, B.; Koopman, R.; Beelen, M.; Senden, J.M.; Saris, W.H.; van Loon, L.J. Exercising before protein intake allows for greater use of dietary protein-derived amino acids for de novo muscle protein synthesis in both young and elderly men. *Am. J. Clin. Nutr.* **2011**, *93*, 322–331. [CrossRef] [PubMed]
214. Yang, Y.; Churchward-Venne, A.T.; Burd, A.N.; Breen, L.; Tarnopolsky, A.M.; Phillips, S.M. Myofibrillar protein synthesis following ingestion of soy protein isolate at rest and after resistance exercise in elderly men. *Nutr. Metab.* **2012**, *9*, 57. [CrossRef]
215. Timmerman, K.L.; Dhanani, S.; Glynn, E.L.; Fry, C.S.; Drummond, M.J.; Jennings, K.; Rasmussen, B.B.; Volpi, E. A moderate acute increase in physical activity enhances nutritive flow and the muscle protein anabolic response to mixed nutrient intake in older adults123. *Am. J. Clin. Nutr.* **2012**, *95*, 1403–1412. [CrossRef]
216. Fujita, S.; Rasmussen, B.B.; Cadenas, J.G.; Drummond, M.J.; Glynn, E.L.; Sattler, F.R.; Volpi, E. Aerobic Exercise Overcomes the Age-Related Insulin Resistance of Muscle Protein Metabolism by Improving Endothelial Function and Akt/Mammalian Target of Rapamycin Signaling. *Diabetes* **2007**, *56*, 1615–1622. [CrossRef]
217. Cermak, N.M.; Res, P.T.; De Groot, L.C.; Saris, W.H.; Van Loon, L.J. Protein supplementation augments the adaptive response of skeletal muscle to resistance-type exercise training: A meta-analysis. *Am. J. Clin. Nutr.* **2012**, *96*, 1454–1464. [CrossRef] [PubMed]
218. Beaudart, C.; Dawson, A.; Shaw, S.C.; Harvey, N.C.; Kanis, J.A.; Binkley, N.; Reginster, J.Y.; Chapurlat, R.; Chan, D.C.; Bruyere, O.; et al. Nutrition and physical activity in the prevention and treatment of sarcopenia: Systematic review. *Osteoporos. Int.* **2017**, *28*, 1817–1833. [CrossRef] [PubMed]
219. Wilson, J.M.; Fitschen, P.J.; Campbell, B.; Wilson, G.J.; Zanchi, N.; Taylor, L.; Wilborn, C.; Kalman, D.S.; Stout, J.R.; Hoffman, J.R.; et al. International Society of Sports Nutrition Position Stand: Beta-hydroxy-beta-methylbutyrate (HMB). *J. Int. Soc. Sports Nutr.* **2013**, *10*, 6. [CrossRef] [PubMed]
220. Vukovich, M.D.; Stubbs, N.B.; Bohlken, R.M. Body composition in 70-year-old adults responds to dietary beta-hydroxy-beta-methylbutyrate similarly to that of young adults. *J. Nutr.* **2001**, *131*, 2049–2052. [CrossRef] [PubMed]
221. Silva, V.R.; Belozo, F.L.; Micheletti, T.O.; Conrado, M.; Stout, J.R.; Pimentel, G.D.; Gonzalez, A.M. β-hydroxy-β-methylbutyrate free acid supplementation may improve recovery and muscle adaptations after resistance training: A systematic review. *Nutr. Res.* **2017**, *45*, 1–9. [CrossRef] [PubMed]
222. Paddon-Jones, D.; Keech, A.; Jenkins, D. Short-term beta-hydroxy-beta-methylbutyrate supplementation does not reduce symptoms of eccentric muscle damage. *Int. J. Sport Nutr. Exerc. Metab.* **2001**, *11*, 442–450. [CrossRef] [PubMed]
223. Schiaffino, S.; Mammucari, C. Regulation of skeletal muscle growth by the IGF1-Akt/PKB pathway: Insights from genetic models. *Skelet. Muscle* **2011**, *1*, 4. [CrossRef] [PubMed]
224. Candow, D.G.; Chilibeck, P.D.; Chad, K.E.; Chrusch, M.J.; Davison, K.S.; Burke, D.G. Effect of Ceasing Creatine Supplementation while Maintaining Resistance Training in Older Men. *J. Aging Phys. Act.* **2004**, *12*, 219–231. [CrossRef] [PubMed]
225. Becque, M.D.; Lochmann, J.D.; Melrose, D.R. Effects of oral creatine supplementation on muscular strength and body composition. *Med. Sci. Sports Exerc.* **2000**, *32*, 654–658. [CrossRef] [PubMed]

226. Vandenberghe, K.; Goris, M.; Van Hecke, P.; Van Leemputte, M.; Vangerven, L.; Hespel, P. Long-term creatine intake is beneficial to muscle performance during resistance training. *J. Appl. Physiol.* **1997**, *83*, 2055–2063. [CrossRef] [PubMed]
227. Jówko, E.; Ostaszewski, P.; Jank, M.; Sacharuk, J.; Zieniewicz, A.; Wilczak, J.; Nissen, S. Creatine and beta-hydroxy-beta-methylbutyrate (HMB) additively increase lean body mass and muscle strength during a weight-training program. *Nutrition* **2001**, *17*, 558–566. [CrossRef]
228. Kreider, R.B.; Ferreira, M.; Wilson, M.; Grindstaff, P.; Plisk, S.; Reinardy, J.; Cantler, E.; Almada, A.L. Effects of creatine supplementation on body composition, strength, and sprint performance. *Med. Sci. Sports Exerc.* **1998**, *30*, 73–82. [CrossRef] [PubMed]
229. Brose, A.; Parise, G.; Tarnopolsky, M.A. Creatine Supplementation Enhances Isometric Strength and Body Composition Improvements Following Strength Exercise Training in Older Adults. *J. Gerontol. Ser. A Biol. Sci. Med. Sci.* **2003**, *58*, B11–B19. [CrossRef] [PubMed]
230. Chrusch, M.J.; Chilibeck, P.D.; Chad, K.E.; Davison, K.S.; Burke, D.G. Creatine supplementation combined with resistance training in older men. *Med. Sci. Sports Exerc.* **2001**, *33*, 2111–2117. [CrossRef] [PubMed]
231. Tarnopolsky, M.A.; Safdar, A. The potential benefits of creatine and conjugated linoleic acid as adjuncts to resistance training in older adults. *Appl. Physiol. Nutr. Metab.* **2008**, *33*, 213–227. [CrossRef] [PubMed]
232. Candow, D.G.; Little, J.P.; Chilibeck, P.D.; Abeysekara, S.; Zello, G.A.; Kazachkov, M.; Cornish, S.M.; Yu, P.H. Low-Dose Creatine Combined with Protein during Resistance Training in Older Men. *Med. Sci. Sports Exerc.* **2008**, *40*, 1645–1652. [CrossRef] [PubMed]
233. Bemben, M.; Witten, M.; Carter, J.; Eliot, K.; Knehans, A.; Bemben, D. The effects of supplementation with creatine and protein on muscle strength following a traditional resistance training program in middle-aged and older men. *J. Nutr. Health Aging* **2010**, *14*, 155–159. [CrossRef] [PubMed]
234. Eijnde, B.O.; Van Leemputte, M.; Goris, M.; Labarque, V.; Taes, Y.; Verbessem, P.; Vanhees, L.; Ramaekers, M.; Eynde, B.V.; Van Schuylenbergh, R.; et al. Effects of creatine supplementation and exercise training on fitness in men 55–75 year old. *J. Appl. Physiol.* **2003**, *95*, 818–828. [CrossRef] [PubMed]
235. Domingues-Faria, C.; Boirie, Y.; Walrand, S. Vitamin D and muscle trophicity. *Curr. Opin. Clin. Nutr. Metab. Care* **2017**, *20*, 169–174. [CrossRef]
236. Dawson-Hughes, B. Vitamin D and muscle function. *J. Steroid Biochem. Mol. Biol.* **2017**, *173*, 313–316. [CrossRef]
237. Bunout, D.; Barrera, G.; Leiva, L.; Gattás, V.; De La Maza, M.P.; Avendaño, M.; Hirsch, S. Effects of vitamin D supplementation and exercise training on physical performance in Chilean vitamin D deficient elderly subjects. *Exp. Gerontol.* **2006**, *41*, 746–752. [CrossRef] [PubMed]
238. Binder, E.F. Implementing a Structured Exercise Program for Frail Nursing Home Residents with Dementia: Issues and Challenges. *J. Aging Phys. Act.* **1995**, *3*, 383–395. [CrossRef]
239. Rodacki, C.L.; Rodacki, A.L.; Pereira, G.; Naliwaiko, K.; Coelho, I.; Pequito, D.; Fernandes, L.C. Fish-oil supplementation enhances the effects of strength training in elderly women. *Am. J. Clin. Nutr.* **2012**, *95*, 428–436. [CrossRef] [PubMed]
240. Cornish, S.M.; Chilibeck, P.D. Alpha-linolenic acid supplementation and resistance training in older adults. *Appl. Physiol. Nutr. Metab.* **2009**, *34*, 49–59. [CrossRef] [PubMed]
241. Rossato, L.T.; Schoenfeld, B.J.; De Oliveira, E.P. Is there sufficient evidence to supplement omega-3 fatty acids to increase muscle mass and strength in young and older adults? *Clin. Nutr.* **2019**. [CrossRef] [PubMed]
242. Murphy, C.H.; Roche, H.M. Nutrition and physical activity countermeasures for sarcopenia: Time to get personal? *Nutr. Bull.* **2018**, *43*, 374–387. [CrossRef]
243. Law, T.D.; Clark, L.A.; Clark, B.C. Resistance Exercise to Prevent and Manage Sarcopenia and Dynapenia. *Annu. Rev. Gerontol. Geriatr.* **2016**, *36*, 205–228. [CrossRef] [PubMed]
244. Cruz-Jentoft, A.J.; Landi, F.; Schneider, S.M.; Zúñiga, C.; Arai, H.; Boirie, Y.; Chen, L.K.; Fielding, R.A.; Martin, F.C.; Michel, J.P.; et al. Prevalence of and interventions for sarcopenia in ageing adults: A systematic review. Report of the International Sarcopenia Initiative (EWGSOP and IWGS). *Age Ageing* **2014**, *43*, 748–759. [CrossRef]
245. Zão, A. Exercise for Sarcopenia in the Elderly: What Kind, Which Role? *Res. Investig. Sports Med.* **2018**, 2. [CrossRef]
246. Helms, E.R.; Cronin, J.; Storey, A.; Zourdos, M.C. Application of the Repetitions in Reserve-Based Rating of Perceived Exertion Scale for Resistance Training. *Strength Cond. J.* **2016**, *38*, 42–49. [CrossRef]

247. Molina, R.G.; Ruíz-Grao, M.C.; García, A.N.; Reig, M.M.; Víctor, M.E.; Izquierdo, M.; Abizanda, P.; Grao, M.C.R.; Redín, M.I.; Soler, P.A. Benefits of a multicomponent Falls Unit-based exercise program in older adults with falls in real life. *Exp. Gerontol.* **2018**, *110*, 79–85. [CrossRef] [PubMed]
248. Chalé, A.; Cloutier, G.J.; Hau, C.; Phillips, E.M.; Dallal, G.E.; Fielding, R.A. Efficacy of whey protein supplementation on resistance exercise-induced changes in lean mass, muscle strength, and physical function in mobility-limited older adults. *J. Gerontol. A Biol. Sci. Med. Sci.* **2013**, *68*, 682–690. [CrossRef] [PubMed]
249. Reeves, N.D.; Maganaris, C.N.; Narici, M.V. Effect of strength training on human patella tendon mechanical properties of older individuals. *J. Physiol.* **2003**, *548*, 971–981. [CrossRef] [PubMed]
250. Singh, N.A.; Quine, S.; Clemson, L.M.; Williams, E.J.; Williamson, D.A.; Stavrinos, T.M.; Grady, J.N.; Perry, T.J.; Lloyd, B.D.; Smith, E.U.; et al. Effects of High-Intensity Progressive Resistance Training and Targeted Multidisciplinary Treatment of Frailty on Mortality and Nursing Home Admissions after Hip Fracture: A Randomized Controlled Trial. *J. Am. Med Dir. Assoc.* **2012**, *13*, 24–30. [CrossRef] [PubMed]
251. Liao, C.D.; Chen, H.C.; Huang, S.W.; Liou, T.H. The Role of Muscle Mass Gain Following Protein Supplementation Plus Exercise Therapy in Older Adults with Sarcopenia and Frailty Risks: A Systematic Review and Meta-Regression Analysis of Randomized Trials. *Nutrients* **2019**, *11*, 1713. [CrossRef] [PubMed]
252. Volkert, D.; Beck, A.M.; Cederholm, T.; Cruz-Jentoft, A.; Goisser, S.; Hooper, L.; Kiesswetter, E.; Maggio, M.; Raynaud-Simon, A.; Sieber, C.C.; et al. ESPEN guideline on clinical nutrition and hydration in geriatrics. *Clin. Nutr.* **2019**, *38*, 10–47. [CrossRef] [PubMed]

3

Prevention and Treatment of Sarcopenic Obesity in Women

Maria L. Petroni [1,*], Maria T. Caletti [1], Riccardo Dalle Grave [2], Alberto Bazzocchi [3], Maria P. Aparisi Gómez [4] and Giulio Marchesini [1]

1 Unit of Metabolic Diseases and Clinical Dietetics, Sant'Orsola-Malpighi Hospital, "Alma Mater" University, via G. Massarenti 9, 40138 Bologna, Italy; maria.caletti@studio.unibo.it (M.T.C.); giulio.marchesini@unibo.it (G.M.)

2 Department of Eating and Weight Disorders, Villa Garda Hospital, via Monte Baldo 89, 37016 Garda (VR), Italy; rdalleg@tin.it

3 Diagnostic and Interventional Radiology, IRCCS Istituto Ortopedico Rizzoli, via G.C. Pupilli 1, 40136 Bologna, Italy; abazzo@inwind.it

4 Department of Radiology, Auckland City Hospital, Park Road, Grafton, 1023 Auckland, New Zealand; pilucaparisi193@gmail.com

* Correspondence: marialetizia.petroni@unibo.it.

Abstract: Sarcopenic obesity (SO) is referred to as the combination of obesity with low skeletal muscle mass and function. However, its definition and diagnosis is debated. SO represents a sizable risk factor for the development of disability, possibly with a worse prognosis in women. The present narrative review summarizes the current evidence on pharmacological, nutrition and exercise strategies on the prevention and/or treatment of SO in middle-aged and older-aged women. A literature search was carried out in Medline and Google Scholar between 29th January and 14th March 2019. Only controlled intervention studies on mid-age and older women whose focus was on the prevention and/or treatment of sarcopenia associated with obesity were included. Resistance training (RT) appears effective in the prevention of all components of SO in women, resulting in significant improvements in muscular mass, strength, and functional capacity plus loss of fat mass, especially when coupled with hypocaloric diets containing at least 0.8 g/kg body weight protein. Correction of vitamin D deficit has a favorable effect on muscle mass. Treatment of SO already established is yet unsatisfactory, although intense and prolonged RT, diets with higher (1.2 g/kg body weight) protein content, and soy isoflavones all look promising. However, further confirmatory research and trials combining different approaches are required.

Keywords: sarcopenic obesity; aging; hormone replacement treatment; phytoestrogens; nutrition; exercise; physical therapy; body composition

---

1. Introduction

In Europe, the prevalence of obesity in older adults has already reached epidemic proportions. In 2013, 19.9% of European women ≥ 50 years were affected by obesity, with a peak prevalence (21.6%) between 70 and 79 years [1]. In other non-European countries, obesity prevalence rates >20% in middle-age and elderly women have been reported [2]. Obesity in the elderly is associated with more advanced clinical disease stages and may in fact result in a significant number of years spent in chronic poor health.

The term 'sarcopenic obesity' (SO) has been proposed to identify obesity with low skeletal muscle function and mass [3]. The concept stems from the study of sarcopenia in the geriatric population, since aging is accompanied by alterations in body composition. SO may lead to frailty, disability, and increased morbidity and mortality, which represent a significant burden on the health and social insurance systems.

Many uncertainties still surround the condition of SO in terms of its definition, adverse short- and long-term health effect and clinical management [4]. As a matter of fact, studies on SO prevention and treatment are widely heterogeneous in terms of the definition of SO and methodologies employed for diagnosis, study design and outcome measures. A recently published systematic review on the effect of exercise alone or combined with dietary supplements included eight randomized controlled trials studies for a total of 604 patients [5]. As a consequence of the diversity of the methodologies employed and of the results observed, no clear conclusion or recommendation could be inferred. Alternatively, narrative reviews address a specific topic; the recent narrative review by Trouwborst and coll. [6] focused on nutrition and physical activity interventions in the prevention and/or treatment of SO, and the authors concluded that a combination of a moderate weight loss diet with concurrent exercise and a relatively high protein intake was able to ameliorate some parameters of SO. This review did not specifically report results about the impact of gender and did not include pharmacological treatment.

The purpose of the present narrative review was to identify and summarize all that has been published so far about the prevention and/or treatment of SO limited to middle-aged and more mature women and to highlight new research areas not addressed so far.

1.1. *Age-Related and Obesity-Related Changes in Muscle Composition, Structure and Function in Women*

There is some controversy about the time of onset of age-related changes in fat-free mass—composed mostly of skeletal muscle—in women. Some authors [7] showed that body fat-free mass, measured by bioelectric impedance analysis (BIA), starts to decrease from 45 years onwards; for others [8], the decline in lean mass measured by dual-energy x-ray absorptiometry (DEXA) starts from age 58. Data from the NHANES cohort showed that women of European American and African American descent lose less than 1% total fat-free mass—measured by DEXA—during menopause but this figure decreases to −12 and −9% respectively between the age group of 40–49 and >75 years [9].

While in men hormonal changes have a pivotal role in the reduction of muscle mass, cross-sectional studies do not fully support the hypothesis that sarcopenia is mainly linked to estrogen deficiency in women, as is osteoporosis [10]. Parallel to changes in fat-free mass with aging, there is also a redistribution of fat mass mainly in the visceral component, but fat deposits are also observed in skeletal muscles and in the liver. Primary metabolic abnormalities have been described such as systemic and muscle oxidative stress, inflammation and insulin resistance, and adipose tissue derangement due to increased lipid storage. These alterations—which are interrelated—promote catabolic processes as well as a state of "anabolic resistance" to nutrients in the skeletal muscle [11]. Metabolic lipotoxicity secondary to ectopic fat accumulation in muscle tissue, mitochondrial dysfunction and muscle stem cell dysfunction with trans-differentiation into adipose cells have also been described [12]. Decreased resting metabolic rate as a consequence of loss of metabolically active fat-free mass, reduced physical activity and increased sedentary time all contribute to the development of obesity in women from mid- to old-age.

Ageing in general is associated with lower muscle volume, decreased muscle fascicle pennation angle, decreased isometric and concentric contractile function but maintenance of eccentric function [13]. Middle-aged women with obesity (41–65 years) were noted to have a significantly lower peak knee extensor isokinetic torque than their younger counterparts (18–40 years) [14]. Elderly women with obesity have been found to have a larger lower limb muscle size and increased pennation angle [15,16]. Also, they have greater absolute maximum muscle strength compared to non-obese persons of same age [16]. However, they develop a lower force per unit of skeletal muscle than their normal-weight counterparts [13,16,17] and have a greater fat content in muscle. The likely explanation is that increased adiposity and body mass on one side load the antigravity muscles limbs—increasing muscle size and strength similarly to resistance training—but at the same time result in unfavorable muscle composition and architecture.

Indeed, most changes in muscle function associated with ageing and obesity are similar, since obesity can result in a phenotype typical of ageing even in relatively young individuals. Obesity and ageing have common mechanistic determinants such as chronic inflammation, decreased muscle protein synthesis and innervation, and impaired intramyocellular calcium metabolism. This explains why obesity-related changes may exacerbate the physiological muscle ageing process [13]. Further research is needed in order to understand the effects of obesity on skeletal muscle ageing.

1.2. Risk Factors for Sarcopenic Obesity and Related Disability

Excess weight burden leads to a vicious circle causing the reduction of physical activity, osteoarthritis and accretion of adipose tissue as well as the deterioration of muscle mass and function. SO has been shown to precede the onset of instrumental activities of daily living (IADL) disability in the community-dwelling elderly with a risk approximately 2.5 times higher than in individuals with non-SO [10]. The impact of SO on disability in different sexes has not been fully elucidated; some studies showed no difference in incidence [10], others showed a worse prognosis in women [18].

A number of risk factors for the development of SO have been highlighted. A putative role for the polymorphisms of TP53 Arg/Arg and for 308 G/A TNF-α in sarcopenia and in SO has been proposed [19,20]. Also, low vitamin D status exerts a detrimental effect on muscle function, while there is evidence for a beneficial effect of vitamin D supplementation on muscle strength, physical performance and the prevention of falls in the elderly female population [21]. Obese individuals are often deficient in vitamin D, especially women due to their relative larger adipose tissue mass than their male counterparts. Epidemiological data suggest a role for vitamin D deficit in SO development [22]. Weight loss (intentional and non-intentional) and weight cycling represent other potential risk factors. With weight change in old age, significantly more lean mass is lost with weight loss than is built up with weight gain [23]. This suggests that weight loss and weight cycling could accelerate sarcopenia in older women with overweight/obesity as well as in men [24]. As a consequence, strategies to counteract loss of muscle mass during weight loss have been advocated.

2. Methods of Narrative Review

A literature search was carried out in Medline and Google Scholar in order to identify relevant articles. The search was carried out between 29th January and 14th March 2019. English language papers were included if they were published in a peer-reviewed journal.

To start with, the following search strategy was used: ("sarcopenic obesity") OR ("sarcopenia" AND "obesity") AND (drug* OR pharmacological OR hormone replacement therapy OR supplement* OR amino acid* OR diet OR nutrition OR nutraceutical* OR protein OR vitamin OR mineral OR exercise OR physical activity OR gait speed OR walking speed OR handgrip strength OR strength). Additionally, the following keywords were used: "energy restriction OR weight loss" AND "skeletal muscle OR body composition". The limitations "human", "female" and "middle-aged AND aged (>45 year)" were applied to the search parameters. Further publications of potential interest were identified as citations in the articles retrieved during the first search. Only controlled intervention studies were included. Those involving procedural therapies (endoscopic treatments or bariatric surgery) or carried out in subjects who had been treated for oncological conditions over the previous 12 months were excluded because of potential confounders. Acute and short-term (i.e., $\leq$1 week) treatments were also excluded.

The search strategy was further refined by including only intervention studies in which the focus was on the prevention and/or treatment of sarcopenia (or the prevention of fat-free mass loss during intentional weight reduction) associated with obesity and/or with SO. All selected studies could be retrieved as full papers. Since the search targeted mid-age and older women, investigations involving subjects younger than 45 without a separate analysis for age groups were excluded, as were those that enrolled men only. Studies incorporating both male and female populations were included only if there was a predominant (subjectively defined as $\geq$ 80% enrolled subjects) presence of women—alternatively, if a separated analysis for differences between sexes had at least partly been carried out. Studies that enrolled overweight subjects (defined as BMI between 25 and 30 kg/m^2) together with obese subjects were also included. The publication date of the retrieved studies ranges between 2001 and 2019. The review comprises 24 papers including 1820 women (90%) out of a total number of 2014 enrolled subjects.

3. Definition of Sarcopenic Obesity

The identification of SO is a currently debated issue, since BMI and waist circumference are inadequate to evaluate muscle mass loss in the elderly population. SO is currently defined as the combination of sarcopenia (see below) and obesity, the latter defined as a body mass index (BMI) ≥ 30 kg/m^2 (in certain ethnic groups ≥ 27.5 kg/m^2). BMI is not useful for identifying the status of obesity or as an outcome measure and should be abandoned as it inaccurate [25]. Alternatively, obesity could be diagnosed by cutoffs of percent body fat or other adiposity indices. Regrettably, once more, there is heterogeneity about the level of fat mass to be used as a cut-off [26], since most published values range between 30 and 40% or even higher. In 2015, fat mass ≥ 32% in women (measured by DEXA) has been proposed as a consensus cut-off [27]. A combination of body mass index and adiposity measures, i.e., fat mass index (FMI) and fat-free mass index (FFMI), has also been reported in epidemiological studies [25].

A number of methods for evaluating body composition, based on the assessment of both adiposity and muscle mass, are currently being used. Computed tomography (CT) and magnetic resonance imaging (MRI) represent the gold standard for estimating total and segmental fat mass (especially visceral fat), as well as muscle mass (cross-sectional area and volume) in the research setting [28]. They additionally allow the evaluation of muscle density (which relates to intramyocellular lipid deposits) as well as intramuscular and subcutaneous adipose tissue accumulation. Air displacement plethysmography measures body volume and body density, providing a non-invasive estimation of total lean mass and fat mass and can equally be applied to patients with morbid obesity [29]. DEXA provide estimates of the lean and fat mass of the entire body or in specific body regions, e.g., the appendicular region. It is relatively inexpensive, and it also provides the advantage of estimating bone mass and density, thus allowing the diagnosis of the triad of bone, muscle, and adipose tissue impairment, i.e., osteosarcopenic obesity [30].

However, in individuals with overweight/obesity, the appendicular skeletal muscle mass (ASM) either expressed as centile or normalized by the square of the height (h^2) can underestimate sarcopenia [25,30], and other criteria, e.g., ASM adjusted for total fat mass or adjusted for height and body fat mass (residuals method), have been proposed [31,32]. Bioelectrical impedance analysis (BIA) is a simple and low-cost technique, but its estimation of body composition is indirect, through measurement of whole body and segmental reactance and resistance affected by fluid retention and disease-related conditions. For these reasons, despite its widespread use also in clinical trials, the use of BIA as an assessment tool of muscle mass for diagnosing sarcopenia has been unrecommended in a consensus statement [33]. A further level of complexity is represented by infiltrated fat in muscle and bone, which contributes to limb adiposity, but it can be concealed and therefore hard to detect [25].

While the assessment of body composition is adequate for the diagnosis of obesity, this does not suffice for the diagnosis of sarcopenia according to a forthcoming evidence-based definition of sarcopenia [34]. Unlike diagnosis based on DEXA alone, the diagnosis of sarcopenia based on grip strength is associated with mortality, hip fracture, falls, mobility disability and IADL disability. Cut-off points in grip strength or grip strength/BMI are the best tools to identify women (and men) at risk for mobility disability.

A clinical diagnosis of "sarcopenia" might also include functional limitations such as slow walking, difficulty in rising from a chair without hands or walking up stairs. This is especially relevant for decision-making about interventions other than physical activity or other lifestyle changes [34].

As a consequence, the definition of sarcopenia in women according to the European Working Group on Sarcopenia in Older People (EWGSOP1) [35] has recently been updated (EWGSOP2) and it is based on three criteria: 1) low muscle strength; 2) low muscle quantity or quality; 3) low physical performance [36]. Low muscle strength is defined as grip strength below 16 kg (27 kg in males) and/or chair stand >15 s for five rises. Low muscle quantity or quality is defined as appendicular skeletal muscle mass (ASM) < 15 kg (20 kg in males) or ASM/height^2 less than 6.0 kg/m^2 (7.0 kg/m^2 in males). The cutoffs for low physical performance are:

- Gait speed ≤ 0.8 m/s
- Short Physical Performance Battery (SPPB) ≤ 8-point score
- Timed-Up and Go test (TUG) ≥ 20 s
- Non-completion or ≥ 6 min for completion of the 400-m walk test.

Criterion 1 identifies probable sarcopenia. Diagnosis is confirmed by additional documentation of Criterion 2. If all three criteria are met, sarcopenia is considered severe. Note that these criteria are different from those identified in 2010 (EWGSOP1), i.e., skeletal muscle index less than 6.76 kg/m^2; gait speed less than 1 m/s; grip strength below 20 kg [35], and those which have been used in some intervention studies reported in the present review.

The EWGSOP2 document, however, remarks that sarcopenic obesity represents a distinct condition [36] and the lack of consensus on its definition and diagnosis represents a recognized limitation requiring widespread coordinated action among researchers and clinicians [12]. In a recent paper from El Ghoch and coll., the six-minute walking test was the only independent test associated with low lean body mass, but the 4-m gait-speed test was shown to represent an accurate functional test for SO screening in female patients [37].

4. Prevention of Sarcopenic Obesity

Prevention of SO can be defined in terms of interventions aimed at preserving skeletal muscle function and mass in obesity [12]. It is, however, difficult to entirely differentiate between those interventions aimed at prevention and those aimed at the treatment of SO in mid-age and old-age women. This is because in most research articles, a clear-cut differentiation of sarcopenic from non-SO is missing and often only indirect markers (e.g., physical independency) are provided to exclude overt severe sarcopenia. Other studies have explicitly enrolled women with a condition of pre-sarcopenia or with some functional impairment. In a few cases, non-sarcopenic and sarcopenic women with obesity have been enrolled in intervention protocols and pooled results have been reported. When SO is present, it is questionable whether intervention aimed at preserving muscle mass while inducing loss of fat mass represent secondary prevention (i.e., aimed at reducing the impact of the already present disease) or treatment itself.

Intervention strategies have either been nutritional or pharmacological or exercise-based or a combination of the above. For the purpose of clarity, interventions based on a single strategy are separated from those combining two or more intervention regimens.

4.1. Single Interventions

4.1.1. Nutrition

Two studies—from the same research group—have investigated the effect of nutritional strategies alone for the prevention of weight loss-related sarcopenia in women with obesity (Table 1.) Porter Starr et al. [38] studied the effect of a 6-month moderately hypocaloric diet (~500 kcal energy deficit) with either normal protein (0.8 g/kg) or high protein (1.2 g/kg) content in the frail elderly—mean age 68 years, mainly women—with obesity and functional impairment. Both interventions reduced body weight by approximately 8% on average and improved handgrip strength and short physical performance battery (SPPB) score as compared to baseline; notably, the amelioration of SPPB in the high protein group was greater than in the normal protein group. However, in a subsequent trial carried out in a younger (mean age 60 years) all-female population, both weight reduction diets (average weight loss, 6%) proved to be safe and effective in improving physical function with no added benefit from a higher protein content in the diet [39]. Moreover, in these studies, a modest but significant loss of lean mass (between –10% and –24% of total mass loss) was observed with both diets, with a non-significant trend for a lower reduction in the high protein group. A noteworthy observation is that in the latter study, black elderly females lost less body weight and experienced lower improvement in the 6-min walking test (6MWT) than white participants [39], confirming previous reports in the literature suggesting a reduced effectiveness of weight loss interventions in black women [40,41].

4.1.2. Pharmacotherapy

Two studies in which pharmacological intervention was carried out as the sole treatment for the prevention of SO have been identified (Table 2). The effect of hormone replacement therapy (HRT) on body composition in post-menopausal women has been compared versus placebo in a small cross-over study on 16 subjects [42]. Despite the short-term intervention (12 weeks), HRT—aside from the favorable well-known effect on bone density—was apparently not only able to prevent the loss of lean body mass occurring during placebo intake, but also to increase it in absolute terms. At the same time, HRT decreased abdominal fat mass, while total body weight was unchanged.

In the second study, the effect of the supplementation of vitamin D (cholecalciferol 10.000 UI or placebo three times a week) was tested in a gender-mixed population of pre-sarcopenic subjects (obese and non-obese) with vitamin D deficit. Cholecalciferol administration had no effect on handgrip strength. However, it was associated with increased appendicular skeletal muscle mass (ASMM). When data were analyzed to account for subgroups and the interaction between vitamin D and obesity on ASMM, the effect size of vitamin D on muscle mass was much higher in subjects without vs. subjects with obesity. Unlike non-obese subjects in whom a higher percent change in ASMM was observed in males compared to females, no sex-related effect was observed in the group with pre-sarcopenic obesity [43].

4.1.3. Exercise

Two studies from Brazil met the inclusion criteria on the effect of exercise alone for the prevention of SO (Table 3). Cunha et al. studied the effect of resistance training (RT) three times/week at two different levels (1 or 3 sets of 10–15 repetitions maximum for each exercise, i.e., 30- and 50-min duration, respectively) vs. controls (no exercise) on components of SO and on bone density in a sample of non-disabled women aged 60 and over. Both RT strategies similarly increased skeletal muscle mass vs. controls, but the 50-min sessions resulted in a significantly higher increase in strength and a modestly greater reduction in fat mass than the 30-min sessions [44]. Beneficial effects of RT were found in the study by de Oliveira Silva et al. comparing non-sarcopenic with sarcopenic women with obesity; in the non-sarcopenic subgroup RT resulted in the amelioration of functional tests and strength as well as a reduction in fat mass compared to pre-training values [45]. Two additional studies evaluating aerobic exercise (AE) as the sole intervention fulfilled the inclusion criteria for the present review. In the study by Davidson et al. AE was compared with RT alone and with the combination of both [46]. This study included both men and women, who were analyzed separately, but unfortunately only pooled results were presented, since no sex-related differences were found. The authors conclude that AE improved tests of functional limitation in similar fashion to RT alone but combined AE + RT was superior to both. Increased skeletal muscle mass was only observed following both RT and RT+AE and an improvement of cardiorespiratory fitness only occurred following AE. The other study investigated AE and hypocaloric diet in the framework of a weight loss intervention. However, one of the trial arms consisted of an AE intervention without diet and will be reported in paragraph 4.2.1 [47].

4.2. *Combined Interventions*

Five studies of combined interventions for the prevention of SO were identified. Of these, four included a weight loss intervention, while one did not (Table 4).

4.2.1. Exercise Plus Nutritional Therapy

The largest prevention study on weight loss so far carried out enrolled overweight or obese postmenopausal, mainly (83%) non-sarcopenic, sedentary women. They were randomized to dietary modification (goals of 1200–2000 kcal/day and 10% loss of baseline weight within six months followed by weight maintenance), to moderate-to-intense AE (AE-5 sessions/week for a total of 225 min/week), to diet + exercise or to no intervention (control group) for a 12-month period [47]. At 12 months, the weight changes averaged −2.4% ($p = 0.03$) in the exercise group, −8.5% ($p = 0.001$) in the diet group, and −10.8% ($p = 0.001$) in diet + exercise group, compared with −0.8% among controls. Hypocaloric diet alone resulted in a significant loss of both total (−1.1 kg, $p < 0.001$) and appendicular (−0.5 kg, $p = 0.02$) fat-free mass. Both measures of fat-free mass remained unchanged over the limited weight loss in the AE alone group. Despite the largest weight loss occurring in the AE + diet group, there were only modest losses in total (−0.4 kg) and appendicular fat-free mass (−0.2 kg), and significantly lower losses ($p < 0.01$) than in the diet-only group. However, in women who were not sarcopenic at baseline, no between-group differences in the incidence of sarcopenia were found at 12 months (between 7% and 10%).

Table 1. Prevention of Sarcopenic Obesity—Nutritional Intervention.

Ref.	No. Subjects Age (years)	Inclusion Criteria	Design	Type of Intervention	Intervention Effect	Notes
[38]	67 (80% women) Mean age, 68	BMI ≥ 30 kg/m^2, functionally impaired (SPPB score of 4–10 out of 12)	Parallel group (n = 2) RCT Duration 6 months	Normal protein (NP, 0.8 g/kg) or high protein (HP, 1.2 g/kg), moderately hypocaloric diet No exercise	WL (kg): −7.5 ± 6.2 (NP); −8.7 ± 7.4 (HP), both $p <$ 0.001 vs. BL Lean mass (kg): −1.8 (NP) −1.1 (HP), both $p < 0.01$ vs. BL Total SPPB score: +0.9 (NP), $p < 0.01$ vs. BL; +2.4 (HP), $p = 0.02$ vs. NP, $p < 0.001$ vs. BL HGS (kg): +1.3 (NP) +1.1 (HP), both $p < 0.01$ vs. BL	Mean BMI = 37.1 kg/m^2 Body composition measured by air displacement plethysmography
[39]	80 women ≥ 45 years (48.8% white) Mean age, 60	BMI ≥ 30 kg/m^2	Parallel group (n = 2) RCT Duration 6 months	Normal protein (NP, 0.8 g/kg) or high protein (HP, 1.2 g/kg) moderately hypocaloric diet No exercise	WL (kg): −6.2 (NP), −6.4 (HP), both $p < 0.001$ vs. BL. WL greater in white (−7.2) than in black women (−4.0), $p < 0.04$ Lean mass (kg): −1.0 (NP) −0.6 (HP), both $p < 0.01$ vs. BL Total SPPB score: +1.2 (NP); +1.0 (HP), $p < 0.001$ vs. BL 6MWT (m): +46.8 (NP) +46.9 (HP), both $p < 0.001$ vs. BL	Mean BMI = 37.8 kg/m^2 Body composition measured by air displacement plethysmography

AE—aerobic exercise; BL—baseline; BMI—body mass index; HGS—handgrip strength; 6MWT—6-min walking test; PL—placebo; RCT—randomized controlled trial; SPPB—short physical performance battery; WL—weight loss.

Table 2. Prevention of Sarcopenic Obesity—pharmacological interventions.

Ref.	No. Subjects Age (years)	Inclusion Criteria	Design	Type of Intervention	Intervention Effect	Notes
[42]	16 post-menopausal women Mean age, 55	BMI ≥ 25kg/m^2	Cross-over PL-controlled RCT 3-month washout in-between	HRT (12 weeks) Placebo (PL) (12 weeks) No diet or exercise advice	FFM (kg): HRT + 0.35, $p < 0.05$ vs. PL; PL: −1.0, $p < 0.05$ vs. pre-treatment Total bone mineral density (g/cm^2): HRT +8.6, $p < 0.05$ vs. PL; PL−3.9 $p < 0.05$ vs. BL Abdominal fat mass (kg): HRT −0.19, $p < 0.05$ vs. BL; PL +0.25 $p < 0.05$ vs. BL	Mean BMI = 27 kg/m^2 Mean BF = 43% Body composition measured by DEXA
[43]	Subjects (62 men, 66 women) pre-sarcopenic and deficient in vitamin D w/wo associated obesity Mean age, 73	Presarcopenia as skeletal muscle mass/height^2 <5.45 kg/m^2 for women Serum level of 25(OH)D < 20 ng/mL Obesity defined as BMI ≥ 30 kg/m^2	Parallel group (n = 2) controlled RCT Duration, 6 months	10,000 IU cholecalciferol 3/week (vitamin D) Placebo (PL)	HS: no difference in vitamin D vs. PL Appendicular skeletal muscle mass (ASMM): increased in vitamin D group ($p < 0.001$ vs. PL); (two-way ANOVA) effect of vitamin D on ASMM much higher in non-obese vs. obese subjects. (1.57 vs. 1.32, $p < 0.001$). No sex-related effect was observed in the presarcopenic obese group	Obesity in 49% of study population Body composition measured by DEXA

AE—aerobic exercise; BF-body fat; BL—baseline; BMI—body mass index; BF—body fat; DEXA—dual-energy x-ray absorptiometry; FFM—fat-free mass; HGS—handgrip strength; HRT—hormone replacement therapy; RCT—randomized controlled trial.

Table 3. Prevention of Sarcopenic Obesity—exercise and physical therapy.

Ref.	No. Subjects	Inclusion Criteria	Design	Type of Intervention	Intervention Effect	Notes
[44]	62 sedentary women aged ≥60 Mean age, 67	Physical independency Obesity not mentioned	Parallel groups ($n = 3$) RCT Duration,12 weeks	RT 1 set (30 min) 3/week (GS1) RT 3 sets (50 min) 3/week (GS3) Control (no exercise – C)	Strength (%): GS1 + 18.5, GS3 + 25, both $p < 0.05$ vs. C (−7.2); GS3 $p < 0.05$ vs. GS1 SMM (kg): GS1 +0.9, GS3 +1.1, both $p < 0.05$ vs. C (+0.2) Body fat (%): GS1: −0.4, GS3 −2.5, both $p < 0.05$ vs. C (+0.6); GS3 $p < 0.05$ vs. GS1	Mean BMI = 27 kg/m^2 Body composition measured by DEXA
[45]	41 sedentary obese non- sarcopenic women aged ≥ 60 years Mean age, 66	Body fat > 32% AFFM above a population specific cut-off	Parallel groups ($n = 2$) RCT comparing non-sarcopenic with SO Duration 16 weeks	RT (2 sessions of 40–50 min/week) All subjects advised not to change usual diet	In the subgroup of non-sarcopenic obese: BF: −0,6 kg, $p = 0{,}03$ vs. BL. No changes in AFFM vs. BL 30 s chair stand-up and timed-up-and-go: improved vs. BL ($p = 0.000$) Strength parameters: improved (moderate effect size) vs. BL ($p \leq 0.01$)	Mean BMI 28 kg/m^2 Body composition measured by DEXA
[46]	74 women out of 136 abdominally obese adults aged 60–80 Mean age, 67	WC ≥ 88 cm in women No conditions incompatible with exercise engagement	Parallel groups ($n = 2$) RCT Duration 6 months	Control, no exercise AE (150 min/week) RT (60 min/week) AE + RT (150 min/week) All on isocaloric diet	Combined z-score of tests for functional limitation improved AE, RT, RT + AE $p < 0.05$ vs. control; RT + AE $p < 0.05$ vs. AE and RT Oxygen consumption (peak VO2) increased in AE and RT + AE vs. RT ($p < 0.05$) and vs. control ($p < 0.05$) Skeletal muscle increased in RT and RT + AE vs. AE ($p < 0.05$) and vs. control ($p < 0.05$)	Mean BMI = 30 kg/m^2 Women-specific data not provided (responses not different between sexes within treatment groups) Body composition measured by MRI

AE—aerobic exercise; AFFM—appendicular fat-free mass; BL—baseline; BMI—body mass index; BF—body fat; DEXA—dual-energy x-ray absorptiometry; MRI—magnetic resonance imaging; RCT—randomized controlled trial; SMM—skeletal muscle mass; WC—waist circumference.

Table 4. Prevention of Sarcopenic Obesity—combined interventions.

Ref.	No. Subjects Age (years)	Inclusion Criteria	Design	Type of Intervention	Intervention Effect	Notes
[47]	439 overweight or obese post-menopausal sedentary women Mean age, 58	BMI ≥ 25.0 kg/m^2 (≥23.0 if Asian American) Sarcopenia as SMI ≤ 5.67 kg/m^2	Parallel groups (n = 4) RCT Duration 12 months	Moderately hypocaloric diet (D) Exercise (AE – 225 min/week) Combined (D + AE) Control (C-no intervention)	Total FFM (kg): D: −1.1 vs. −0.1 C, $p < 0.01$; AE: no significant changes; D + AE: −0.6 kg, $p > 0.01$ vs. AE Appendicular FFM (kg): D −0.5, $p = 0.02$ vs. control; AE 0.0 kg (not significant vs. C), D + AE – 0.2, ($p < 0.01$ vs. D) No differences in sarcopenia incidence among non-sarcopenic women	17% at BL (mean BMI 31 kg/m^2) had sarcopenia Body composition measured by DEXA
[48]	31 overweight or obese, postmenopausal women Mean age, 65	BMI ≥ 28 kg/m^2	parallel group (n = 2) RCT Duration 6 months	Hypocaloric diet + whey protein (2 × 25 g/day) (PRO) Hypocaloric diet supplemented with maltodextrine (CARB) Mild exercise (flexibility + aerobic 40′–50′ sessions 2–3/week) in both groups	Whole body mass (kg): CARB −3.6, PRO −7.7; ($p = 0.051$ vs. CARB) Thigh muscle mass (%): CHO +4.5, PRO +10.3 ($p = 0.049$ vs. CARB) Intermuscular adipose tissue (cm^2): CARB −1.0, PRO −9.2; ($p = 0.03$ vs. CARB) No differences in changes in strength, balance, or physical performance measures between PRO and CARB	Mean BMI = 33.4 kg/m^2 Body composition measured by DEXA and MRI
[49]	54 overweight and obese sedentary women aged 60–75 Mean age, 66	BMI ≥ 27 kg/m^2 and/or body fat percentage above 35%	Parallel groups (n = 3) RCT Duration 14 weeks	Exercise (RT, 3/week), no diet (Ex) Ex + low-calorie high-CHO diet (ExHC) Ex + low-calorie high-protein diet (ExHP)	No reduction in FFM in all groups Percent BF: Ex −2.0%; ExHC −4.3; ExHP −6.3%; $p = 0.002$ vs. Ex and HP Strength increased in all groups with no group interaction	Mean BMI 30 kg/m^2 Target HC diet: 55% HC, 15% P, 30% fat Target HP diet: P 1.2 g/kg, 30% fat Body composition by DEXA
[50]	94 post-menopausal sedentary women Age range 40–65	Being either on HRT (n = 39) or not HRT (n = 55)	Parallel groups (n = 4) RCT (2 × 2 factorial design) Duration, 12 months	Exercise (RT + weight bearing training) 3/week + HRT Exercise, no HRT No exercise, HRT No exercise, no HRT	Exercise groups: FFM total (+12%), arm (+15%), leg (+11%; strength (+9–20%); % BF (−1.9%) vs. BL ($p < 0.001$); No significant differences in no-exercise groups No interaction effects of HRT	Mean BF = 38% at BL Body composition measured by DEXA
[51]	40 women and 48 men nondiabetic overweight/obese aged 65–79 Mean age, 70	SPPB 3–10 (values < 10 predictive of mobility and disability risk)	Parallel groups RCT (n = 4) with 2 × 2 factorial design Duration 16 weeks	Hypocaloric diet (D) + Resistance Training (RT) D + RT + pioglitazone 30 mg (PIO) D + PIO D only	Women overall: WL −6.5%; FM −9.7%; LM -4.1% (all $p < 0.05$ vs. BL) Thigh muscle volume (cm^3): RT −34 vs. no–RT 59, $p = 0.040$ Thigh subcutaneous fat (cm^3): PIO −104 vs. no-PIO−298; mean difference 194, $p = 0.002$	Women BMI = 33 kg/m^2 Unlike women, PIO significantly reduced abdominal fat in men Body composition by DEXA and CT

AE—aerobic exercise; BL—baseline; BMI—body mass index; BF—body fat; DEXA—dual-energy x-ray absorptiometry; FFM—fat-free mass; HRT—hormone replacement therapy; RCT—randomized controlled trial; RT—resistance training.

Another study evaluated the effects of whey protein (25 g t.i.d.) or isoenergetic carbohydrate supplements to hypocaloric diets coupled with mild exercise (flexibility and aerobic 40′–50′ sessions 2–3/week) [48]. Whey protein supplementation resulted in a borderline significant ($p = 0.051$) greater weight loss but also in a significantly greater absolute fat-free mass loss. However, after correction for weight loss, the relative muscle volume showed a greater net gain of muscle in the protein-supplemented diet as compared to the carbohydrate-supplement group ($p = 0.049$). A greater loss of intramuscular adipose tissue ($p = 0.03$) was also observed. However, no differences in changes in strength, balance, or physical performance measures were found between diets, possibly because of the limited sample size.

Galbreath et al. studied the effect of a 6-month RT (3 times/week) intervention coupled with a moderately hypocaloric diet (1st week 1200 kcal, 2nd to 12th week 1600 kcal/day) either normal protein (0.8 g/kg) or high protein (1.2 g/kg). A third group had RT only. All three groups underwent significant improvements in muscular strength, muscular endurance, aerobic performance, balance and functional capacity [49].

4.2.2. Exercise Plus Pharmacotherapy

The prevention of changes in body composition following menopause was the scope of a trial aimed to study the interaction between hormone replacement therapy (HRT) and exercise training. Post-menopausal women aged 40–65 were randomized to exercise (resistance + weight bearing training) or to no-exercise according to their HRT status [50]. Exercise was reported to provide a significant improvement in body composition (increase of total and appendicular fat-free mass, decrease of body fat) and strength, as compared to no-exercise; however, in the exercise groups, women who were already on HRT did not gain further benefit as compared to women who were not on HRT.

Resistance training coupled with the PPARγ-agonist pioglitazione—an antidiabetic medication shown to reduce abdominal visceral adipose tissue—was tested on body composition changes in non-diabetic elderly overweight/obese of both sexes at risk of mobility disability [51]. During a weight reduction diet (15% protein, ~500 kcal energy deficit), women who received RT (with or without pioglitazione) lost less thigh muscle volume than those who did not received RT. To be noted, in women—unlike in men—pioglitazone not only did not contribute to visceral fat loss but also contrasted with the loss of subcutaneous fat.

5. Treatment of Sarcopenic Obesity

The definition of the treatment targets in SO is yet unclear. The joint statement of the European Society for Clinical Nutrition and Metabolism (ESPEN) and European Association for the Study of Obesity (EASO) focuses on improvement of skeletal muscle function and mass [12]. Both reduced burden of disabilities and comorbidities, as well as improved quality of life represent treatment targets far more important from patients' perspectives. Unfortunately, very few data in this area have been published so far. This issue is particularly critical in elderly women, at high risk of SO per se, where any effort aimed at weight loss may produce untoward, negative effects [52]. Strategies aiming at preserving (rather than increasing) muscle mass during weight loss in clearly defined SO have also been reported in the present section. Most intervention studies in women include exercise training or physical therapy. However, nutritional and pharmacological strategies have also been studied, as single treatment modality or in various combinations.

5.1. *Single Treatment*

5.1.1. Nutrition

Applicable studies are summarized in Table 5. Adding a high-quality protein food (210 g of ricotta cheese daily for 3 months) to habitual diet did not improve appendicular skeletal mass or strength in both women and men with sarcopenia, most of whom with concurrent obesity; interestingly, more favorable trends were observed for men [53]. The impact of proteins on the preservation of skeletal mass and function during weight loss in women has been studied in two separate trials. Muscariello et al. [54] reported that a high protein (1.2 g/kg) hypocaloric diet over three months resulted in the preservation of arm muscle mass, while a normal protein diet produced a modest but significant loss (-5.7 cm^2, $p < 0.001$ vs. baseline). Muscle mass index—as measured by BIA—significantly increased ($p < 0.01$ vs. baseline) following the high protein but decreased following the normal protein diet ($p < 0.01$ vs. baseline). Handgrip strength was maintained with both diets. Sammarco et al. confirmed the favorable effect of high-protein hypocaloric diet by the use of BIA [55]. In this pilot trial, women with SO on a hypocaloric diet were randomized either to protein supplementation (to reach 1.2–1.4 g/kg) or to placebo. Women in the placebo group showed higher loss of lean body mass compared to those in the protein-enriched diet group (−1.3 kg vs. −0.5 kg; $p < 0.05$). Handgrip strength improved in the high protein diet group (+1.6 kg; $p = 0.01$ vs. baseline), while it was unchanged in the placebo group. The general health domain of quality of life (Short Form-36 Questionnaire) also improved significantly in the high protein group, while no change was observed for other categories or for the score of SPPB.

5.1.2. Pharmacotherapy

The effect of a 6-month administration of soy isoflavones as compared to placebo on changes in body composition was assessed in a sample of 18 post-menopausal women with SO [56]. Isoflavones proved significantly superior to placebo in increasing leg ($p = 0.016$) and appendicular ($p = 0.034$) lean mass, as well as muscle mass index ($p = 0.037$) (Table 6).

5.1.3. Exercise and Physical Therapy

Seven studies that used exercise (RT alone or associated with aerobic training) as the sole treatment modality in women with SO were identified (Table 7). Among studies with a no-exercise arm for comparison, Gadelha et al. showed that RT (3/week over 24 weeks) improved strength-related variables ($p < 0.001$ vs. baseline and vs. controls), appendicular FFM (+0.29 kg; $p < 0.001$ vs. control), and total FFM mass (+0.6 kg; $p < 0.01$ vs. baseline and vs. controls) [57].

The differential and additive effect of RT and AE (2/week over 8 weeks) was studied in a population with a large majority of women (83%) [58]. All exercise groups (RT alone, AE alone, RT + AE) improved back extensor strength vs. controls. Only RT as the sole treatment modality increased handgrip strength (+3.5 kg; $p < 0.05$ vs. all other groups). Similarly, improvement in strength, not in functional performance, was found in the small subgroup of women with SO in the RT treatment arm, in the study by de Olivera Silva et al., who also had a low frequency of exercise (2 session/week) [45]. On the contrary, Park et al. [59] found that combined RT and AE training (5/week for 24 weeks) resulted in increased handgrip strength (+2.5 kg; $p < 0.001$ vs. baseline and vs. control) and walking speed (+0.15 m/s; $p < 0.01$ vs. baseline and vs. control). A reduction in fat mass (−2.0 kg; $p < 0.01$ vs. control) was also observed, with no effect on appendicular lean mass.

Two studies evaluated elastic band RT, an exercise modality that is simple, inexpensive and can be carried out at home without the need of attending a gym. Liao et al. carried out a 12-week intervention.

study followed by a further follow up at 6 months after the end of rehabilitation intervention [60 Elastic band RT proved effective on all sarcopenia components (muscle mass measured by BIA, strength, mobility) and also in improving quality of life. Moreover, the effects of RT were clinically significant and sustained over time at 9-month follow-up: in RT vs. controls, there was an increase in absolute muscle mass (+0.72 kg; $p < 0.01$), in global physical capacity score (+4.22; $p < 0.001$), in the physical component score of the short-form 36 questionnaire (SF-36) (+15.06; $p < 0.001$). These results were not confirmed in a study on the effects of elastic band exercise training (3/week) as compared to standard home exercise on body composition measured by DEXA [61]. No effects of RT were demonstrated on appendicular lean mass, while fat mass was reduced, and bone density increased vs. controls. The reasons for non-univocal outcomes between the two studies—which were comparable in terms of mean age and BMI—could be ascribed to differences in control interventions (non-active vs. active control group), treatment protocols, and body composition assessment modalities (BIA vs. DEXA).

One study compared two modalities of RT for 15 weeks: standard strength hypertrophy training with high-speed power training circuit [62]. Only power training improved the physical function (SPPB) of 20% ($p = 0.02$ vs. baseline). However, exercise did not improve body composition, 6MWT and handgrip strength vs. baseline, and produced only negligible-to-small improvement in IADL tasks. The small sample size (eight subjects for each group) limits the significance of these negative results.

5.2. *Combined Treatments*

Three controlled studies have examined the combination of nutritional intervention and exercise and/or physical therapy in sarcopenic women (Table 8). In two of them, a hypocaloric diet was part of the treatment.

Kemmler et al. tested the effect of weekly sessions of whole-body electromyostimulation (WB-EMS) over 26 weeks with/without protein and vitamin D supplementation vs. with a non-training control group while on an isocaloric diet [63]. In both WB-EMS groups, an increase of skeletal muscle mass index was found: WB-EMS +0.14 kg/m^2, WB-EMS plus protein +0.11 (both <0.001 vs. control). A marginal, although statistically significant, increase in gait speed was observed only in the WB-EMS group (+0.08 m/s; $p = 0.026$ vs. control). No significant changes in body fat or handgrip strength were demonstrated in all treatment groups. In a 4-arm RCT of 12-week duration, Kim et al. investigated the effect of twice weekly RT plus AE alone vs. nutritional intervention (3 g of essential amino acids plus catechins plus vitamin D supplementation) alone vs. combination of exercise and nutrition vs. control. Reduction in body fat mass was significant vs. control only in the combined treatment, −1.0 kg ($p = 0.036$). Both exercise groups increased step length vs. control. No significant changes in SMI and grip strength were found among groups [64].

Finally, in a subgroup of women with SO, in the study by Mason and coll. [47], the 12-month effect of intense (225 min/week) AE alone or combined with/without a moderately hypocaloric diet was compared with a control group of no intervention. At the end of the study, 14% of cases in the control group, 8% in the diet group, 50% in the exercise group, 35% in the diet + exercise group no longer met the criteria for sarcopenia by 12 months (no subgroup-specific statistical analysis was provided).

No studies combining RT with nutrition intervention have been reported at the time of the present review.

Table 5. Treatment of Sarcopenic Obesity—Nutritional (diet and/or supplements).

Ref.	No. Subjects Age (years)	SO Definition	Design	Type of Intervention	Intervention Effect	Notes
[53]	Analysis by sex of 23 women and 17 men Mean age, 76	Sarcopenia diagnosed by the residual method Overweight or obesity were not inclusion criteria High prevalence with cases with elevated %BF	Parallel group (n = 2) RCT Duration 12 weeks	Intervention: Protein supplements (210 g/day of ricotta cheese) plus the habitual diet Control: habitual diet	No significant effect of protein supplementation on ASMM or strength in both sexes	Mean BF in women 41% Body composition measured by DEXA
[54]	104 women aged > 65 years with SO Mean age, 66	BMI ≥ 30.0 kg/m^2, or WC > 88.0 cm or FM% ≥ 35.0%, or FM index ≥ 9.5 kg/m^2 Sarcopenia defined by MM index, MM/height^2 (kg/m^2), as <2SD the obesity-derived cut-off score (7.3 kg/m^2-class 2)	Parallel group (n = 2) RCT Duration 12 weeks	High protein (1.2 g/kg) low-calorie diet (HP) Normal protein (0.8 g/kg bw reference) low-calorie diet (NP)	BMI (kg/m^2): NP −1.3; HP −0.8, both $p < 0.001$ vs. BL MM index (kg/m^2): NP −0.2, $p < 0.01$ vs. BL; HP +0.2, $p < 0.01$ vs. BL Arm-muscle area (cm^2): NP −5.7, $p < 0.001$ vs. BL; HP −0.5, n.s. No significant difference in HGS vs. BL	Mean BMI = 31.5 kg/m^2 Body composition measured by BIA and anthropometry
[55]	18 women aged 41–74 years with SO Mean age, 55	Obesity defined FM >34.8%; Sarcopenia defined by lean body mass <90% of the subject's ideal FFM	Parallel group (n = 2) RCT (pilot)	Low-calorie high-protein diet (1.2–1.4 g/ kg bw reference/day) (HP) Low-calorie diet plus placebo (control)	WL: HP −3.9 kg (p = 0.01 vs. BL); control −3.8 kg (p = 0.05 vs. BL) FFM: HP +2.3 kg (p = 0.05 vs. control); control +0.6 kg (n.s) FM: HP −9.7 kg (p = 0.01 vs. BL); control −7.3 kg (p = 0.03 vs. BL) HGS: HP +1.6 kg (p = 0.01 vs. BL); control: n.s. No significant change in SPPB for both groups	Body composition measured by BIA

ASMM—appendicular skeletal muscle mass; BIA—bioelectrical impedance analysis; BL—baseline; BF—body fat; BMI—body mass index; DEXA—dual-energy x-ray absorptiometry; FFM—fat-free mass; FM—fat mass; HGS—handgrip strength; MM—muscle mass; PL—placebo; RCT—randomized controlled trial; SPPB—short physical performance battery; WC—waist circumference; WL—weight loss.

Table 6. Treatment of sarcopenic obesity—Pharmacological interventions.

Ref.	No. Subjects Age (years)	SO Definition	Design	Type of Intervention	Main Intervention Effect	Notes
[56]	18 post- menopausal women with SO aged 50–70 Mean age, 58	Muscle mass (MM) index <6.87 kg Appendicular FFM/m^2 FM > 40%	Parallel group (n = 2) PL-controlled RCT Duration 6 months	Isoflavones 70 mg (ISO) (n = 12) Placebo (PL) (n = 6)	Leg FFM (kg): ISO +0.29 vs. PL −0.62, p = 0.034 Appendicular FFM (kg): ISO +0.53, PL −0.78, p = 0.016 MM index: ISO +0.26, PL−0.27, p = 0.037	BMI = 29 kg/m^2 Body composition by DEXA

BMI—body mass index; DEXA—dual-energy x-ray absorptiometry; FFM—fat-free mass; FM—fat mass; MM—muscle mass; PL—placebo; RCT—randomized controlled trial.

Table 7. Treatment of sarcopenic obesity—Exercise and physical therapy.

Ref.	No. Subjects Age (years)	SO Definition	Design	Type of Intervention	Intervention Effect (Main Findings)	Notes
[57]	113 overweight and obese elderly women Mean age, 67	BMI ≥ 25 kg/m^2 appendicular FFM by residual values method including height and FM	Parallel groups (n = 2) RCT	Resistance exercise (RE) 3/week Control (C − no exercise) Duration 24 weeks	Total FFM (kg): RE: +0.6; p < 0.01 vs. BL and vs. C Appendicular FFM (kg): RE: +0.29; p < 0.01 vs. BL and vs. control Strength (Isokinetic relative peak torque 60°) (Nm/kg × 100) RE: + 20.6; p < 0.01 vs. BL and vs. C	BMI (27.1–29.1 kg/m^2) Body composition measured by DEXA
[58]	60 sarcopenic overweight and obese elderly (83% women) Mean age, 69	BMI ≥ 25 kg/m^2 and visceral fat area ≥ 100 cm plus skeletal MM ≤ 25.7% b.w.	Parallel groups (n = 4) RCT	Resistance/Aerobic Exercise (RT or AE) Combination (AE + RT) Control (C − no exercise) All sessions 2/week Duration 8 weeks	HGS (kg): RT: +3.5, p < 0.05 vs. all other groups, no changes in AE and RT + AE Skeletal MM (kg): RT: +0.1, AE: +0.1, RT+AE: +0.2 (in all p < 0.05 vs. C) FM (kg): RT: −1., AE: −0.7, RT + AE: −1.1 (in all p < 0.05 vs. C) Back extensor (kg): RT: +9.0, AE: +7.9, RT + AE: + 10.0 (in all p < 0.05 vs. C)	BMI (26.8–29.0kg/m^2) Body composition measured by BIA Effect persisted 4 weeks after end of intervention
[45]	8 sedentary women with obesity aged ≥ 60 years Mean age, 66	body fat % > 32 Appendicular fat-free mass less than population- specific cut-off	Parallel group (n = 2) RCT of women w/wo SO Duration 16 weeks	RT (2 sessions of 40–50 min/week)	In the subgroup of women with SO: no difference in %BF, 30 s chair stand-up, timed-up-and-go vs. BL Improved strength vs. BL (p ≤ 0.01) with trivial effect sizes	Mean BMI = 28 kg/m^2 Body composition measured by DEXA
[59]	50 women aged ≥ 65 years with SO Mean age, 74	BMI ≥ 25.0 kg/m^2 + ASMM/weight < 25.1 %	Parallel groups (n = 2) RCT Duration 24 weeks	Combined RT and AE 5/week (Ex) Control (C − no exercise)	BF (%): Ex −2.0, p < 0.01 vs. BL; C: n.s. No effect on appendicular lean mass. HGS (kg): Ex +2.5, p < 0.001 vs. BL and vs. C; C −0.5, p < 0.05 vs. BL Maximum walking speed (m/s): Ex +0.15, p < 0.01 vs. BL and vs. C; C −0.04, p < 0.01 vs. BL	Body composition by BIA Improvement in carotid artery IMT and flow velocity
[60]	35 women aged 60–80 years with SO Mean age, 67	BF > 30% SMI <7.15 kg/m^2	Parallel groups (n = 2) RCT Duration 12 weeks (intervention) + follow- up at 9 months	Elastic band resistance training (RT) 3 times/week Control (C-no exercise)	Results are reported at 9-mo follow-up. Absolute muscle mass: RT +0.72 kg, p < 0.01 vs. C); similar results for appendicular lean mass and SMI Global physical capacity score: RT + 4.22, p < 0.001 vs. C). Clinically significant improvement in all functional tests. Physical component score (SF-36): RT +15.06, p < 0.001 vs. C)	Mean BMI = 28 kg/m^2 Body composition measured by BIA
[61]	35 women aged ≥ 60 years with SO Mean age, 69	BF > 30% SMI <27.6%	Parallel groups (n = 2) RCT Duration 12 weeks	Elastic band resistance training (RT) 3 times/week Control (home exercise)	Total BF: RT −0.58 kg, p = 0.03; control: n.s. Total bone density: RT +0.06 g/cm^2, p = 0.026; control: n.s. No effect on lean appendicular mass	Mean BMI = 28 kg/m^2 Body composition measured by BIA (screening) and DEXA (treatment)
[62]	17 SO subjects (95% women) aged ≥ 60 years Mean age, 71	BMI > 30 kg/m^2 plus EWGSOP1 criteria	Parallel groups (n = 2) RCT	High-speed power training circuit (HSC) Standard strength hypertrophy training (ST) 2-week adaptation before treatment Duration 15 weeks	HSC improved physical function (SPPB) by 20% ($_{adj}$mean difference 1.1; p = 0.02, effect size g = 0.6 with no changes in ST group No change for SMI, BF %, 6MWT, HGS vs. BL in both groups. Few IADL tasks with negligible to small changes for either HSC or ST	Adherence rates > 80% Lower ratings of perceived exertion in HSC vs. ST Subjects in ST with mild to moderate acute joint pain.

AE—aerobic exercise; ASMM—appendicular skeletal muscle mass; BF—body fat; BIA—bioelectrical impedance analysis; BL—baseline; BMI—body mass index; DEXA—dual-energy x-ray absorptiometry; EWGSOP1—European Working Group on Sarcopenia in Older People 1 (2010 criteria); FFM—fat free mass; FM—fat mass; HGS—handgrip strength; IADL—Instrumental Activities of Daily Living; IMT—intima-media thickness; MM—muscle mass; 6MWT—6-min walking test; RT—resistance training; RCT—randomized controlled trial; SF-36—Short-Form 36 Questionnaire; SMI—skeletal muscle index.

Table 8. Treatment of sarcopenic obesity—Combined interventions.

Ref.	No. Subjects Age (years)	SO Definition	Design	Type of Intervention	Intervention Effect	Notes
[47] *see also Table 4*	Subgroup of 76 post menopausal sedentary women with SO Mean age, 58	BMI ≥ 25.0 (or ≥23.0 kg/m^2 if Asian American) Sarcopenia defined as SMI ≤ 5.67 kg/m^2	Parallel groups (n = 4) RCT Duration 12 months	Moderately hypocaloric diet (D) Aerobic exercise (AE) Combined D +AE Control (C-no intervention)	14% in C, 8% in D, 50% in AE, 35% in the D + AE no longer met the sarcopenia criteria by 12 months. No subgroup-specific statistical analysis was provided.	17% with sarcopenia (mean BMI = 31 kg/m^2) Body composition measured by DEXA
[63]	75 women aged ≥ 60 years with SO Mean age, 77	Obesity as > 35% BF Sarcopenia as SMI < 5.75 kg/m^2	Parallel groups (n = 3) RCT Duration 26 weeks	Whole-body electro-myostimulation (WB-EMS, 1/week) WB-EMS + protein + vitamin D supplements (WB-EMS&P) Non-training controls (C)	SMI (kg/m^2): WB-EMS +0.14, WB-EMS&P + 0.11; both p < 0.001 vs. C. Gait speed: WB-EMS 0.08 m/s, p = 0.026 vs. C; WB-EMS&P n.s. No significant changes in BF or HGS in all treatment groups	Mean body fat = 37% All groups were supplemented with vitamin D Body composition by DEXA
[64]	139 women aged ≥ 70 years with SO Mean age, 81	BF ≥32% and SMI < 5.67 kg/m^2 or HGS < 17.0 kg or walking speed < 1.0 m/s.	Parallel groups (n = 4) RCT Duration 12 weeks	Exercise (RT + AE – 2/week) + EAA (3 g) + catechins + vitamin D) (ExNu) Exercise only (Ex) Nutritional intervention only (N) Control (health education)	Body FM decreased significantly in all groups vs. BL; ExNU −1.0 kg (p = 0.036 vs. N) Step length: ExNu +3.2 cm; Ex +3.5 cm (p = 0.007 vs. N); both significantly increased vs. BL No significant changes in SMI and HGS among groups	Body composition measured by DEXA (screening) and BIA (treatment)

AE—aerobic exercise; BIA—bioelectrical impedance analysis; BL—baseline; BF—body fat; BMI—body mass index; DEXA—dual-energy x-ray absorptiometry; EAA, essential amino acids; FM—fat mass; HGS—handgrip strength; RT—resistance training; RCT—randomized controlled trial; SMI—skeletal muscle index; WB-EMS—whole-body electromyostimulation.

6. Discussion

Women with obesity and low muscle mass/function are at increased risk of frailty and disability. Metabolic and lifestyle abnormalities [65] compromise the ability to preserve muscle function and mass, especially when chronic diseases co-exist with obesity. Insulin resistance has been shown to contribute to muscle weakness and to the "dynapenic obesity" phenotype of middle-aged women with the metabolic syndrome [66]. Muscle fat accumulation linked to insulin resistance reduces muscle density and quality with lower contractile protein content per mass unit [66].

Weight loss regimens represent a further leading risk factor for the development or worsening of SO [67]. In a retrospective analysis of a caloric restriction and exercise weight loss intervention in postmenopausal women, Bopp et al. found that the average loss of lean mass was clinically significant, representing approximately one-third of the total mass lost at a protein intake of 15–20% of energy (approximately 0.62 g/kg body weight/day). Additionally, they found that participants lost 0.62 kg less lean mass for every 0.1 g/kg body weight/day increase in dietary protein beyond the standard [68].

Effective strategies are urgently required to reduce the burden of morbidity and mortality in a rapidly increasing obese population [12]. Nutritional, pharmacological and exercise/physical activity treatment are available to prevent SO as well as to reduce the burden of SO in post-menopausal and elderly women, and are summarized in Figure 1.

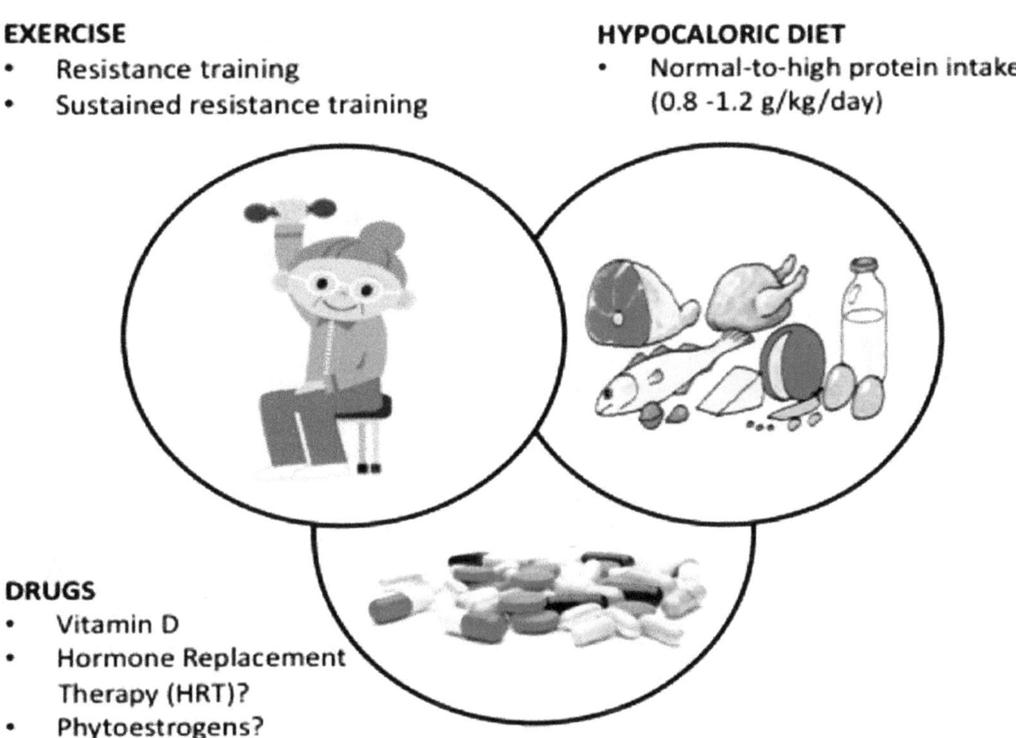
EXERCISE
• Resistance training
• Sustained resistance training
HYPOCALORIC DIET
• Normal-to-high protein intake
(0.8 -1.2 g/kg/day)
DRUGS
• Vitamin D
• Hormone Replacement
Therapy (HRT)?
• Phytoestrogens?

Figure 1. Overview of interventions for the prevention and/or treatment of sarcopenic obesity in women based on a non-systematic review of 24 papers including 1820 women. The three layers of intervention are superimposed to show that they are not mutually exclusive. Resistance training is the most effective strategy with effects directly related to its frequency and duration; when coupled with hypocaloric diets with normal-to-high protein content the effects on both prevention and treatment are amplified. Vitamin D deficit should be corrected whenever present. Evidence on HRT and phytoestrogens needs confirmation by future research.

6.1. Prevention of Sarcopenic Obesity

Most RCTs in non-sarcopenic women with obesity have focused on the prevention of sarcopenia during hypocaloric diets for weight loss. Altogether, they suggest that hypocaloric diets (500 kcal deficit) with a protein content of at least 0.8 g/kg provide significant weight and fat loss at the same time as improving physical function. A higher (1.2 g/kg) protein diet is expected to generate possible added benefits in contrasting lean mass reduction. Adding AE to a normal-protein hypocaloric diet reduces lean mass wasting but does not totally prevent the development of sarcopenia. Whey protein supplements do not seem to provide benefit when coupled with mild exercise only. These findings might not be generalizable to mixed (female and male) populations. Backx et al. failed to demonstrate a significant effect of a very high protein diet (1.7 g/kg) on the prevention of lean mass loss in a mixed-gender elderly population [69]. On the contrary, Beavers et coll. found a sparing effect of high-protein diet on lean mass over 6 months in the elderly (74% women) with obesity, with no detrimental effect on gait speed [70].

The only intervention that was definitely effective in the prevention of all components of sarcopenia was the combination of RT (thrice weekly) with either a normal (0.8 g/kg) or high protein (1.2 g/kg) hypocaloric diet, leading to significant improvements in muscular strength, endurance, aerobic capacity, balance and functional capacity [49]. Also, in the absence of dietary intervention, RT reduces fat mass, increases muscle strength and improves functional capacity in women at risk of SO. On the contrary, AE alone ameliorates functional capacity, not strength or lean mass. Physical therapies (muscle electrostimulation and vibrations) are either ineffective or add little to exercise.

The results are confirmed in mixed-gender trials. Elderly subjects of both sexes with obesity and mild-to-moderate frailty lose less lean mass and gain more strength when RT alone [71] or RT + AE is added to a hypocaloric diet [60,62,72]. Nicklas et al. also found that RT coupled with a hypocaloric diet improved mobility and strength, despite the calorie restriction-related loss of lean mass [65]. Houston et al. recalled a random sample of 60 older adults (mean age at randomization, 67.3 years; 69% women) who had been randomized to caloric restriction plus exercise or exercise only in five RCTs on average 3.5 years before. They found that physical performance was similarly maintained in both exercise groups, whereas the favorable changes in weight and body composition were not [73].

In a small-scale study, hormone replacement therapy (HRT) showed some advantage in preventing the negative body composition changes of post-menopausal age, increasing lean body mass and decreasing abdominal fat mass, without changes in total body weight [42]. In another study using exercise as strategy, HRT did not gain further benefit as compared to women who were not on HRT [50]. Regrettably, no additional studies are available, possibly because of the concern about an increased risk of cancer linked to estrogens in obesity. Correction of vitamin D deficiency—which is often present in obesity—can produce beneficial effects on lean mass [43] and should routinely be carried out.

6.2. Treatment of Sarcopenic Obesity

In women with sarcopenic obesity, there is concordance among RCTs that a higher protein content in the diet may effectively contrast lean mass loss and may yield some benefit on strength during hypocaloric diets but cannot ameliorate SO during isocaloric diets.

On the whole, RT—delivered with different regimens and possibly combined with aerobic training—improves strength and physical function, especially if intense (≥ 3 sessions/week) and prolonged (≥ 3 months). A beneficial effect on muscle mass was not consistent across the studies. The scarcity and heterogeneity of RCTs prevent any firm conclusion about the efficacy of the combination of nutritional intervention (with either hypocaloric and isocaloric diet) and exercise on SO.

Only one RCT on pharmacological treatment used soy isoflavones in post-menopausal obese sarcopenic women [56] and showed a beneficial effect on muscle mass, but data require confirmative trials due to the limited number of patients.

6.3. Sex-Related Aspects

Sex hormones have pivotal roles in maintaining skeletal muscle homeostasis. Under normal conditions, the different roles of estrogens and androgens contribute to sex differences in skeletal muscle morphology and function. Testosterone is a powerful anabolic factor promoting protein synthesis and muscular regeneration, mainly via increased muscular expression of insulin-growth factor-1 (IGF-I). Estradiol reduces the progressive muscle atrophy in postmenopausal women, suggesting an anti-inflammatory and anti-catabolic influence of estrogens on skeletal muscle in women, especially after exercise. However, further research is awaited to support a significant effect of estrogens on muscle mass [74].

Oikawa and colleagues have recently highlighted sex-based differences in the ability to recover muscle strength in the elderly. Two weeks of combined calorie restriction (with maintenance of normal protein intake) plus reduced physical activity resulted in decreased muscle isometric strength in older men and women. However, upon resumption of physical activity and caloric intake, women did not recover strength as measured by maximum voluntary contraction, while men did [75]. In the male sex, single muscle fiber power and isometric tension were unchanged or paradoxically increased (muscle biopsies were not carried out in women). This finding suggests impaired resiliency, which could result in greater functional impairment over time. Whether estrogens as HRT or soy phytoestrogens may overcome this defect warrants assessment by future studies.

The present review does not provide a definite answer about which sex responds best to exercise and nutritional strategies targeting sarcopenic obesity. Only two studies were identified including a comparison between sexes. In the study by Davidson and coll. [46], skeletal muscle mass—measured by MRI—muscle strength measures and changes in functional limitations did not reveal any differences among gender following the exercise interventions. The sole exception was a greater reduction of total and visceral fat in men than women in the aerobic exercise group only. Similarly, a trend towards increased appendicular muscle mass measured by DEXA in men but not in women was found in the cheese protein supplementation study by Aleman-Mateo and coll. [53] which did not attain statistical significance possibly due to the small number of study subjects.

Pharmacological agents other than estrogen have demonstrated sex-specific effects on body and muscle composition. For example, pioglitazone resulted in significant sex-based differences in abdominal fat, where abdominal fat loss was significantly greater in men, with no change in women [51]. Vitamin D supplementation showed a gender effect by increasing ASMM only in presarcopenic non-obese male subjects, while no sex-related difference was found in obese subjects [43].

7. Conclusions

SO in women represents a condition under research scrutiny with regard to definition, diagnostic criteria and optimal treatment. At present, intense and prolonged RT has definite efficacy in the prevention and/or treatment of SO. Adequate protein content in the diet and correction of vitamin D deficiency are also required. This conclusion supports the ESPEN/EASO recommendation of coordinating action aimed at reaching consensus on optimal treatment with particular regard to nutritional therapy [12]. However, more research on optimal nutritional strategies in weight loss protocols and combined approaches is required.

Author Contributions: Conceptualization, M.L.P, A.B., G.M.; methodology, M.L.P, M.P.A.G; literature search, M.L.P., M.T.C; data analysis, M.L.P, G.M.; writing—original draft preparation, M.L.P, G.M; writing—review and editing, A.B.; R.D.G, M.P.A.G, M.T.C; supervision, G.M.

Abbreviations

6MWT	6-min walking test
AE	Aerobic exercise
ASMM	Appendicular skeletal muscle mass
BIA	Bioelectrical impedance analysis
CT	Computerized tomography
DEXA	Dual-energy x-ray absorptiometry
EAA	Essential amino acids
EWGSOP1	European Working Group on Sarcopenia in Older People 1 (2010 criteria)
EWGSOP2	European Working Group on Sarcopenia in Older People 2 (2019 criteria)
FFM	Fat-free mass
HGS	Handgrip strength
HRT	Hormone replacement treatment
IADL	Instrumental activities of daily living
MRI	Magnetic resonance imaging
RCT	Randomized controlled trial
RT	Resistance training
SBBP	Short physical performance battery
SF-36	Short form-36 questionnaire
SMI	Skeletal muscle index
SO	Sarcopenic obesity
WB-EMS	Whole-body electromyostimulation

References

1. Peralta, M.; Ramos, M.; Lipert, A.; Martins, J.; Marques, A. Prevalence and trends of overweight and obesity in older adults from 10 European countries from 2005 to 2013. *Scand. J. Public Health* **2018**, *46*, 522–529. [CrossRef] [PubMed]
2. Samper-Ternent, R.; Al Snih, S. Obesity in Older Adults: Epidemiology and implications for Disability and Disease. *Rev. Clin. Gerontol.* **2012**, *22*, 10–34. [CrossRef] [PubMed]
3. Zamboni, M.; Mazzali, G.; Fantin, F.; Rossi, A.; Di Francesco, V. Sarcopenic obesity: A new category of obesity in the elderly. *Nutr. Metab. Cardiovasc. Dis.* **2008**, *18*, 388–395. [CrossRef] [PubMed]
4. El Ghoch, M.; Calugi, S.; Dalle Grave, R. Sarcopenic obesity: Definition, health consequences and clinical management. *Open Nutr. J.* **2018**, *12*, 70–73. [CrossRef]
5. Martínez-Amat, A.; Aibar-Almazán, A.; Fábrega-Cuadros, R.; Cruz-Díaz, D.; Jiménez-García, J.D.; Pérez-López, F.R.; Achalandabaso, A.; Barranco-Zafra, R.; Hita-Contreras, F. Exercise alone or combined with dietary supplements for sarcopenic obesity in community-dwelling older people: A systematic review of randomized controlled trials. *Maturitas* **2018**, *110*, 92–103. [CrossRef] [PubMed]
6. Trouwborst, I.; Verreijen, A.; Memelink, R.; Massanet, P.; Boirie, Y.; Weijs, P.; Tieland, M. Exercise and Nutrition Strategies to Counteract Sarcopenic Obesity. *Nutrients* **2018**, *10*, 605. [CrossRef] [PubMed]
7. Chumlea, W.C.; Guo, S.S.; Kuczmarski, R.J.; Flegal, K.M.; Johnson, C.L.; Heymsfield, S.B.; Lukaski, H.C.; Friedl, K.; Hubbard, V.S. Body composition estimates from NHANES III bioelectrical impedance data. *Int. J. Obes. Relat. Metab. Disord.* **2002**, *26*, 1596–1609. [CrossRef] [PubMed]
8. Welch, G.W.; Sowers, M.R. The interrelationship between body topology and body composition varies with age among women. *J. Nutr.* **2000**, *130*, 2371–2377. [CrossRef]
9. Tian, S.; Morio, B.; Denis, J.-B.; Mioche, L. Age-related changes in segmental body composition by ethnicity and history of weight change across the adult lifespan. *Int. J. Environ. Res. Public Health* **2016**, *13*, 821. [CrossRef]
10. Baumgartner, R.N.; Wayne, S.J.; Waters, D.L.; Janssen, I.; Gallagher, D.; Morley, J.E. Sarcopenic obesity predicts instrumental activities of daily living disability in the elderly. *Obes. Res.* **2004**, *12*, 1995–2004. [CrossRef]

11. Burd, N.A.; Gorissen, S.H.; van Loon, L.J.C. Anabolic resistance of muscle protein synthesis with aging. *Exerc. Sport Sci. Rev.* **2013**, *41*, 169–173. [CrossRef] [PubMed]
12. Barazzoni, R.; Bischoff, S.; Boirie, Y.; Busetto, L.; Cederholm, T.; Dicker, D.; Toplak, H.; Van Gossum, A.; Yumuk, V.; Vettor, R. Sarcopenic obesity: Time to meet the challenge. *Obes. Facts* **2018**, *11*, 294–305. [CrossRef] [PubMed]
13. Tallis, J.; James, R.S.; Seebacher, F. The effects of obesity on skeletal muscle contractile function. *J. Exp. Biol.* **2018**, *221 Pt 13*. [CrossRef] [PubMed]
14. Hulens, M.; Vansant, G.; Lysens, R.; Claessens, A.L.; Muls, E. Assessment of isokinetic muscle strength in women who are obese. *J. Orthop. Sports Phys. Ther.* **2002**, *32*, 347–356. [CrossRef] [PubMed]
15. Tomlinson, D.J.; Erskine, R.M.; Winwood, K.; Morse, C.I.; Onambélé, G.L. The impact of obesity on skeletal muscle architecture in untrained young vs. old women. *J. Anat.* **2014**, *225*, 675–684. [CrossRef] [PubMed]
16. Rastelli, F.; Capodaglio, P.; Orgiu, S.; Santovito, C.; Caramenti, M.; Cadioli, M.; Falini, A.; Rizzo, G.; Lafortuna, C.L. Effects of muscle composition and architecture on specific strength in obese older women. *Exp. Physiol.* **2015**, *100*, 1159–1167. [CrossRef] [PubMed]
17. Tomlinson, D.J.; Erskine, R.M.; Morse, C.I.; Winwood, K.; Onambélé-Pearson, G. The impact of obesity on skeletal muscle strength and structure through adolescence to old age. *Biogerontology* **2016**, *17*, 467–483. [CrossRef]
18. Gretebeck, K.A.; Sabatini, L.M.; Black, D.R.; Gretebeck, R.J. Physical activity, functional ability, and obesity in older adults: A gender difference. *J. Gerontol. Nurs.* **2017**, *43*, 38–46. [CrossRef]
19. Di Renzo, L.; Gratteri, S.; Sarlo, F.; Cabibbo, A.; Colica, C.; De Lorenzo, A. Individually tailored screening of susceptibility to sarcopenia using p53 codon 72 polymorphism, phenotypes, and conventional risk factors. *Dis. Markers* **2014**, 743634. [CrossRef]
20. Di Renzo, L.; Sarlo, F.; Petramala, L.; Iacopino, L.; Monteleone, G.; Colica, C.; De Lorenzo, A. Association between −308 G/A TNF-alpha polymorphism and appendicular skeletal muscle mass index as a marker of sarcopenia in normal weight obese syndrome. *Dis. Markers* **2013**, *35*, 615–623. [CrossRef]
21. Anagnostis, P.; Dimopoulou, C.; Karras, S.; Lambrinoudaki, I.; Goulis, D.G. Sarcopenia in post-menopausal women: Is there any role for vitamin D? *Maturitas* **2015**, *82*, 56–64. [CrossRef] [PubMed]
22. Oh, C.; Jho, S.; No, J.-K.; Kim, H.-S. Body composition changes were related to nutrient intakes in elderly men but elderly women had a higher prevalence of sarcopenic obesity in a population of Korean adults. *Nutr. Res.* **2015**, *35*, 1–6. [CrossRef] [PubMed]
23. Newman, A.B.; Lee, J.S.; Visser, M.; Goodpaster, B.H.; Kritchevsky, S.B.; Tylavsky, F.A.; Nevitt, M.; Harris, T.B. Weight change and the conservation of lean mass in old age: The Health, Aging and Body Composition Study. *Am. J. Clin. Nutr.* **2005**, *82*, 872–878. [CrossRef] [PubMed]
24. Rossi, A.P.; Rubele, S.; Caliari, C.; Pedelini, F.; Calugi, S.; Soave, F.; Chignola, E.; Bazzani, P.V.; Dalle Grave, R.; Zamboni, M. Weight cycling as a risk factor for low muscle mass and strength in a population of males and females with obesity. *Obesity* **2019**. [CrossRef]
25. Kelly, O.J.; Gilman, J.C.; Boschiero, D.; Ilich, J.Z. Osteosarcopenic Obesity: Current Knowledge, Revised Identification Criteria and Treatment Principles. *Nutrients* **2019**, *11*, 747. [CrossRef] [PubMed]
26. Prado, C.M.; Wells, J.C.; Smith, S.R.; Stephan, B.C.; Siervo, M. Sarcopenic obesity: A critical appraisal of the current evidence. *Clin. Nutr.* **2012**, *31*, 583–601. [CrossRef] [PubMed]
27. American Society of Bariatric Physicians (ASBP) Obesity Algorithm. 2015. Available online: http://www.asbp.org/obesityalgorithm.html (accessed on 26 May 2019).
28. Cesari, M.; Fielding, R.A.; Pahor, M.; Goodpaster, B.; Hellerstein, M.; Van Kan, G.A.; Anker, S.D.; Rutkove, S.; Vrijbloed, J.W.; Isaac, M.; et al. Biomarkers of sarcopenia in clinical trials-recommendations from the International Working Group on Sarcopenia. *J. Cachexia Sarcopenia Muscle* **2012**, *3*, 181–190. [CrossRef]
29. Petroni, M.L.; Bertoli, S.; Maggioni, M.; Morini, P.; Battezzati, A.; Tagliaferri, M.A. Feasibility of air plethysmography (BOD POD) in morbid obesity: A pilot study. *Acta Diabetol.* **2003**, *40*, S59–S62. [CrossRef]
30. Ilich, J.Z.; Kelly, O.J.; Inglis, J.E. Osteosarcopenic Obesity Syndrome: What Is It and How Can It Be Identified and Diagnosed? *Curr. Gerontol. Geriatr. Res.* **2016**, *2016*, 7325973. [CrossRef]
31. Newman, A.B.; Kupelian, V.; Visser, M.; Simonsick, E.; Goodpaster, B.; Nevitt, M.; Kritchevsky, S.B.; Tylavsky, F.A.; Rubin, S.M.; Harris, T.B.; et al. Sarcopenia: Alternative definitions and associations with lower extremity function. *J. Am. Geriatr. Soc.* **2003**, *51*, 1602–1609. [CrossRef]

32. Domiciano, D.S.; Figueiredo, C.P.; Lopes, J.B.; Caparbo, V.F.; Takayama, L.; Menezes, P.R.; Bonfa, E.; Pereira, R.M. Discriminating sarcopenia in community-dwelling older women with high frequency of overweight/obesity: The São Paulo Ageing & Health Study (SPAH). *Osteoporos. Int.* **2013**, *24*, 595–603. [CrossRef] [PubMed]
33. Morley, J.E.; Abbatecola, A.M.; Argiles, J.M.; Baracos, V.; Bauer, J.; Bhasin, S.; Cederholm, T.; Coats, A.J.S.; Cummings, S.R.; Evans, W.J.; et al. Sarcopenia with limited mobility: An international consensus. *J. Am. Med. Dir. Assoc.* **2011**, *12*, 403–409. [CrossRef] [PubMed]
34. Cawthon, P.M.; Travison, T.G.; Manini, T.M.; Patel, S.; Pencina, K.M.; Fielding, R.A.; Magaziner, J.M.; Newman, A.B.; Brown, T.; Kiel, D.P.; et al. Establishing the link between lean mass and grip strength cut-points with mobility disability and other health outcomes: Proceedings of the Sarcopenia Definition and Outcomes Consortium Conference. *J. Gerontol. A Biol. Sci. Med. Sci.* **2019**. [CrossRef]
35. Cruz-Jentoft, A.J.; Baeyens, J.P.; Bauer, J.M.; Boirie, Y.; Cederholm, T.; Landi, F.; Martin, F.C.; Michel, J.P.; Rolland, Y.; Schneider, S.M.; et al. Sarcopenia: European consensus on definition and diagnosis: Report of the European Working Group on Sarcopenia in Older People. *Age Ageing* **2010**, *39*, 412–423. [CrossRef] [PubMed]
36. Cruz-Jentoft, A.J.; Bahat, G.; Bauer, J.; Boirie, Y.; Bruyère, O.; Cederholm, T.; Cooper, C.; Landi, F.; Rolland, Y.; Sayer, A.A.; et al. Writing Group for the European Working Group on Sarcopenia in Older People 2 (EWGSOP2), and the Extended Group for EWGSOP2. Sarcopenia: Revised European consensus on definition and diagnosis. *Age Ageing* **2019**, *48*, 16–31. [CrossRef] [PubMed]
37. El Ghoch, M.; Rossi, A.P.; Calugi, S.; Rubele, S.; Soave, F.; Zamboni, M.; Chignola, E.; Mazzali, G.; Bazzani, P.V.; Dalle Grave, R. Physical performance measures in screening for reduced lean body mass in adult females with obesity. *Nutr. Metab. Cardiovasc. Dis.* **2018**, *28*, 917–921. [CrossRef] [PubMed]
38. Porter Starr, K.N.; Pieper, C.F.; Orenduff, M.C.; McDonald, S.R.; McClure, L.B.; Zhou, R.; Payne, M.E.; Bales, C.W. Improved function with enhanced protein intake per meal: A pilot study of weight reduction in frail, obese older adults. *J. Gerontol. A Biol. Sci. Med. Sci.* **2016**, *71*, 1369–1375. [CrossRef]
39. Bales, C.W.; Porter Starr, K.N.; Orenduff, M.C.; McDonald, S.R.; Molnar, K.; Jarman, A.K.; Onyenwoke, A.; Mulder, H.; Payne, M.E.; Pieper, C.F. Influence of protein intake, race, and age on responses to a weight-reduction intervention in obese women. *Curr. Dev. Nutr.* **2017**, *1*, e000703. [CrossRef] [PubMed]
40. DeLany, J.P.; Jakicic, J.M.; Lowery, J.B.; Hames, K.C.; Kelley, D.E.; Goodpaster, B.H. African American women exhibit similar adherence to intervention but lose less weight due to lower energy requirements. *Int. J. Obes.* **2014**, *38*, 1147–1152. [CrossRef] [PubMed]
41. Wingo, B.C.; Carson, T.L.; Ard, J. Differences in weight loss and health outcomes among African Americans and whites in multicentre trials. *Obes. Rev.* **2014**, *15* (Suppl. 4), 46–61. [CrossRef]
42. Sorensen, M.B.; Rosenfalck, A.M.; Hojgaard, L.; Ottesen, B. Obesity and sarcopenia after menopause are reversed by sex hormone replacement therapy. *Obes. Res.* **2001**, *9*, 622–626. [CrossRef] [PubMed]
43. El Hajj, C.; Fares, S.; Chardigny, J.M.; Boirie, Y.; Walrand, S. Vitamin D supplementation and muscle strength in pre-sarcopenic elderly Lebanese people: A randomized controlled trial. *Arch. Osteoporos.* **2019**, *14*, 4. [CrossRef] [PubMed]
44. Cunha, P.M.; Ribeiro, A.S.; Tomeleri, C.M.; Schoenfeld, B.J.; Silva, A.M.; Souza, M.F.; Nascimento, M.A.; Sardinha, L.B.; Cyrino, E.S. The effects of resistance training volume on osteosarcopenic obesity in older women. *J. Sports Sci.* **2018**, *36*, 1564–1571. [CrossRef] [PubMed]
45. De Oliveira Silva, A.; Dutra, M.; de Moraes, W.M.; Funghetto, S.; Lopes de Farias, D.; dos Santos, P.H.F.; Vieira, D.C.L.; da Cunha Nascimento, D.; Orsano, V.S.M.; Schoenfeld, B.J.; et al. Resistance training-induced gains in muscle strength, body composition, and functional capacity are attenuated in elderly women with sarcopenic obesity. *Clin. Interv. Aging* **2018**, *13*, 411–417. [CrossRef] [PubMed]
46. Davidson, L.E.; Hudson, R.; Kilpatrick, K.; Kuk, J.L.; McMillan, K.; Janiszewski, P.M.; Lee, S.; Lam, M.; Ross, R. Effects of exercise modality on insulin resistance and functional limitation in older adults: A randomized controlled trial. *Arch. Intern. Med.* **2009**, *169*, 122–131. [CrossRef] [PubMed]
47. Mason, C.; Xiao, L.; Imayama, I.; Duggan, C.R.; Foster-Schubert, K.E.; Kong, A.; Neuhouser, M.L.; Alfano, C.M. Influence of diet, exercise, and serum vitamin d on sarcopenia in postmenopausal women. *Med. Sci. Sports Exerc.* **2013**, *45*, 607–614. [CrossRef] [PubMed]

48. Mojtahedi, M.C.; Thorpe, M.P.; Karampinos, D.C.; Johnson, C.L.; Layman, D.K.; Georgiadis, J.G.; Evans, E.M. The effects of a higher protein intake during energy restriction on changes in body composition and physical function in older women. *J. Gerontol. A Biol. Sci. Med. Sci.* **2011**, *66A*, 1218–1225. [CrossRef]
49. Galbreath, M.; Campbell, B.; LaBounty, P.; Bunn, J.; Dove, J.; Harvey, T.; Hudson, G.; Gutierrez, J.; Levers, K.; Galvan, E.; et al. Effects of adherence to a higher protein diet on weight loss, markers of health, and functional capacity in older women participating in a resistance-based exercise program. *Nutrients* **2018**, *10*, 1070. [CrossRef]
50. Figueroa, A.; Going, S.B.; Milliken, L.A.; Blew, R.M.; Sharp, S.; Teixeira, P.J.; Lohman, T.G. Effects of exercise training and hormone replacement therapy on lean and fat mass in postmenopausal women. *J. Gerontol. A Biol. Sci. Med. Sci.* **2003**, *58*, 266–270. [CrossRef]
51. Shea, M.K.; Nicklas, B.J.; Marsh, A.P.; Houston, D.K.; Miller, G.D.; Isom, S.; Miller, M.E.; Carr, J.J.; Lyles, M.F.; Harris, T.B.; et al. The effect of pioglitazone and resistance training on body composition in older men and women undergoing hypocaloric weight loss. *Obesity* **2011**, *19*, 1636–1646. [CrossRef]
52. Corica, F.; Bianchi, G.; Corsonello, A.; Mazzella, N.; Lattanzio, F.; Marchesini, G. Obesity in the context of aging: Quality of lfe considerations. *Pharmacoeconomics* **2015**, *33*, 655–672. [CrossRef] [PubMed]
53. Aleman-Mateo, H.; Macias, L.; Esparza-Romero, J.; Astiazaran-Garcia, H.; Blancas, A.L. Physiological effects beyond the significant gain in muscle mass in sarcopenic elderly men: Evidence from a randomized clinical trial using a protein-rich food. *Clin. Interv. Aging* **2012**, *7*, 225–234. [CrossRef] [PubMed]
54. Muscariello, E.; Nasti, G.; Siervo, M.; Di Maro, M.; Lapi, D.; D'Addio, G.; Colantuoni, A. Dietary protein intake in sarcopenic obese older women. *Clin. Interv. Aging* **2016**, *11*, 133–140. [CrossRef] [PubMed]
55. Sammarco, R.; Marra, M.; Di Guglielmo, M.L.; Naccarato, M.; Contaldo, F.; Poggiogalle, E.; Donini, L.M.; Pasanisi, F. Evaluation of hypocaloric diet with protein supplementation in middle-aged sarcopenic obese women: A pilot study. *Obes. Facts* **2017**, *10*, 160–167. [CrossRef] [PubMed]
56. Aubertin-Leheudre, M.; Lord, C.; Khalil, A.; Dionne, I.J. Six months of isoflavone supplement increases fat-free mass in obese–sarcopenic postmenopausal women: A randomized double-blind controlled trial. *Eur. J. Clin. Nutr.* **2007**, *61*, 1442–1444. [CrossRef] [PubMed]
57. Gadelha, A.B.; Paiva, F.M.; Gauche, R.; de Oliveira, R.J.; Lima, R.M. Effects of resistance training on sarcopenic obesity index in older women: A randomized controlled trial. *Arch. Gerontol. Geriatr.* **2016**, *65*, 168–173. [CrossRef] [PubMed]
58. Chen, H.-T.; Chung, Y.-C.; Chen, Y.-J.; Ho, S.-Y.; Wu, H.-J. Effects of different types of exercise on body composition, muscle strength, and IGF-1 in the elderly with sarcopenic obesity. *J. Am. Geriatr. Soc.* **2017**, *65*, 827–832. [CrossRef]
59. Park, J.; Kwon, Y.; Park, H. Effects of 24-week aerobic and resistance training on carotid artery intima-media thickness and flow velocity in elderly women with sarcopenic obesity. *J. Atheroscler. Thromb.* **2017**, *24*, 1117–1124. [CrossRef]
60. Liao, C.-D.; Tsauo, J.-Y.; Huang, S.-W.; Ku, J.-W.; Hsiao, D.-J.; Liou, T.-H. Effects of elastic band exercise on lean mass and physical capacity in older women with sarcopenic obesity: A randomized controlled trial. *Sci. Rep.* **2018**, *8*, 2317. [CrossRef]
61. Huang, S.-W.; Ku, J.-W.; Lin, L.-F.; Liao, C.-D.; Chou, L.-C.; Liou, T.-H. Body composition influenced by progressive elastic band resistance exercise of sarcopenic obesity elderly women: A pilot randomized controlled trial. *Eur. J. Phys. Rehabil. Med.* **2017**, *53*, 556–563. [CrossRef]
62. Balachandran, A.; Krawczyk, S.N.; Potiaumpai, M.; Signorile, J.F. High-speed circuit training vs. hypertrophy training to improve physical function in sarcopenic obese adults: A randomized controlled trial. *Exp. Gerontol.* **2014**, *60*, 64–71. [CrossRef] [PubMed]
63. Kemmler, W.; Teschler, M.; Weissenfels, A.; Bebenek, M.; von Stengel, S.; Kohl, M.; Freiberger, E.; Goisser, S.; Jakob, F.; Sieber, C.; et al. Whole-body electromyostimulation to fight sarcopenic obesity in community-dwelling older women at risk. Results of the randomized controlled FORMOsA-sarcopenic obesity study. *Osteoporos. Int.* **2016**, *27*, 3261–3270. [CrossRef] [PubMed]
64. Kim, H.; Kim, M.; Kojima, N.; Fujino, K.; Hosoi, E.; Kobayashi, H.; Somekawa, S.; Niki, Y.; Yamashiro, Y.; Yoshida, H. Exercise and nutritional supplementation on community-dwelling elderly Japanese women with sarcopenic obesity: A randomized controlled trial. *J. Am. Med. Dir. Assoc.* **2016**, *17*, 1011–1019. [CrossRef] [PubMed]

65. Nicklas, B.J.; Chmelo, E.; Delbono, O.; Carr, J.J.; Lyles, M.F.; Marsh, A.P. Effects of resistance training with and without caloric restriction on physical function and mobility in overweight and obese older adults: A randomized controlled trial. *Am. J. Clin. Nutr.* **20151**, *101*, 991–999. [CrossRef] [PubMed]
66. Poggiogalle, E.; Migliaccio, S.; Lenzi, A.; Donini, L.M. Treatment of body composition changes in obese and overweight older adults: Insight into the phenotype of sarcopenic obesity. *Endocrine* **2014**, *47*, 699–716. [CrossRef] [PubMed]
67. Cava, E.; Yeat, N.C.; Mittendorfer, B. Preserving muscle mass during weight loss. *Adv. Nutr.* **2017**, *8*, 511–519. [CrossRef]
68. Bopp, M.J.; Houston, D.K.; Lenchik, L.; Easter, L.; Kritchevsky, S.B.; Nicklas, B.J. Lean mass loss is associated with low protein intake during dietary-induced weight loss in postmenopausal women. *J. Am. Diet. Assoc.* **2008**, *108*, 1216–1220. [CrossRef]
69. Backx, E.M.; Tieland, M.; Borgonjen-van den Berg, K.J.; Claessen, P.R.; van Loon, L.J.; de Groot, L.C. Protein intake and lean body mass preservation during energy intake restriction in overweight older adults. *Int. J. Obes.* **2016**, *40*, 299–304. [CrossRef]
70. Beavers, K.M.; Nesbit, B.A.; Kiel, J.R.; Sheedy, J.L.; Arterburn, L.M.; Collins, A.E.; Ford, S.A.; Henderson, R.M.; Coleman, C.D.; Beavers, D.P. Effect of an energy-restricted, nutritionally complete, higher protein meal plan on body composition and mobility in older adults with obesity: A randomized controlled trial. *J. Gerontol. A Biol. Sci. Med. Sci.* **2018**. [CrossRef]
71. Villareal, D.T.; Aguirre, L.; Gurney, A.B.; Waters, D.L.; Sinacore, D.R.; Colombo, E.; Armamento-Villareal, R.; Qualls, C. Aerobic or resistance exercise, or both, in dieting obese older adults. *N. Engl. J. Med.* **2017**, *376*, 1943–1955. [CrossRef]
72. Frimel, T.N.; Sinacore, D.R.; Villareal, D.T. Exercise attenuates the weight-loss-induced reduction in muscle mass in frail obese older adults. *Med. Sci. Sports Exerc.* **2008**, *40*, 1213–1219. [CrossRef] [PubMed]
73. Houston, D.K.; Miller, M.E.; Kitzman, D.W.; Rejeski, W.J.; Messier, S.P.; Lyles, M.F.; Kritchevsky, S.B.; Nicklas, B.J. Long-term effects of randomization to a weight loss intervention in older adults: A pilot study. *J. Nutr. Gerontol. Geriatr.* **2019**, *38*, 83–99. [CrossRef] [PubMed]
74. Anderson, L.J.; Liu, H.; Garcia, J.M. Sex Differences in Muscle Wasting. In *Sex and Gender Factors Affecting Metabolic Homeostasis, Diabetes and Obesity*; Mauvais-Jarvis, F., Ed.; Springer International Publishing: Cham, Switzerland, 2017; pp. 153–197. [CrossRef]
75. Oikawa, S.Y.; Callahan, D.M.; McGlory, C.; Toth, M.J.; Phillips, S.M. Maintenance of skeletal muscle function following reduced daily physical activity in healthy older adults: A pilot trial. *Appl. Physiol. Nutr. Metab.* **2019**. [CrossRef] [PubMed]

4

An Update on Protein, Leucine, Omega-3 Fatty Acids and Vitamin D in the Prevention and Treatment of Sarcopenia and Functional Decline

Anne-Julie Tessier [1,2] **and Stéphanie Chevalier** [1,2,3,*]

1 School of Human Nutrition, McGill University, 21111 Lakeshore Rd, Ste-Anne-de-Bellevue, QC H9X 3V9, Canada; anne-julie.tessier@mail.mcgill.ca

2 Research Institute of the McGill University Health Centre, 1001 Décarie Blvd, Montreal, QC H4A 3J1, Canada

3 Department of Medicine, McGill University, 845 Sherbrooke St. W, Montreal, QC H3A 0G4, Canada

* Correspondence: stephanie.chevalier@mcgill.ca.

Abstract: Aging is associated with sarcopenia and functional decline, leading to frailty and disability. As a modifiable risk factor, nutrition may represent a target for preventing or postponing the onset of these geriatric conditions. Among nutrients, high-quality protein, leucine, vitamin D, and omega-3 polyunsaturated fatty acids (*n*-3 PUFA) are of particular interest for their demonstrated effects on skeletal muscle health. This narrative review aims to examine the recent observational and interventional evidence on the associations and the role of these nutrients in the muscle mass, strength, mobility, and physical function of free-living older adults, who are either healthy or at risk of frailty. Recent evidence supports a higher protein intake recommendation of 1.0–1.2 g/kg/day in healthy older adults; an evenly distributed mealtime protein intake or minimal protein per meal may be beneficial. In addition, vitamin D supplementation of 800–1000 IU, particularly when vitamin D status is low, and doses of ~3 g/day of *n*-3 PUFA may be favorable for physical function, muscle mass, and strength. Reviewed studies are highly heterogenous, yet the quantity, quality, and timing of intakes should be considered when designing intervention studies. Combined protein, leucine, vitamin D, and *n*-3 PUFA supplements may convey added benefits and may represent an intervention strategy in the prevention of sarcopenia and functional decline.

Keywords: protein; leucine; vitamin D; omega-3 fatty acids; sarcopenia; muscle strength; physical performance; older adults; frailty

---

1. Introduction

Sarcopenia is defined as the generalized and progressive loss of muscle mass and strength [1,2], leading to declines in physical function and mobility. These are integral components of frailty defined by a decrease in the function of several physiological and psychological systems, which increases vulnerability to stressors [2]. In addition to reducing the quality of life [3], these age-related conditions increase risks of morbidity [4,5], hospitalization [6] and its associated costs [7], and mortality [8]. Sarcopenia has a multifactorial etiology, namely neuromotor dysfunction, chronic low-grade inflammation, physical inactivity, decreased endocrine function, and poor nutritional status [1]. The latter, resulting from a reduction in dietary intake among other causes, was previously associated with lower physical function and frailty among older adults from various settings (hospitals, community, rehabilitation) [9–11]. Approximately two-third of older adults are estimated as malnourished or at risk of becoming malnourished [12]. Adding to a poor nutritional status in a context of advanced age is the presence of anabolic resistance, which is characterized by a reduced response to anabolic stimuli including dietary protein, leading to higher protein needs compared to those of younger adults [13].

As a modifiable risk factor, nutrition is a potential target to improve or prevent the loss of physical function in older adults (Figure 1). Specific nutrients are of particular interest for their demonstrated role on the muscular system, and have been the object of earlier and more recent studies, either as single supplements or in combination with other supplements. These include proteins, especially those rich in leucine, which is the most potent branched-chain amino acid at stimulating muscle protein synthesis (MPS) [14], vitamin D, and *n*-3 polyunsaturated fatty acids (*n*-3 PUFAs). This narrative review aims to examine the latest observational and interventional (supplementation alone, without physical exercise) evidence on the associations and the role of these nutrients in the muscle mass, strength, mobility, and physical function of free-living older adults, who are either healthy, frail, or at risk of functional decline.

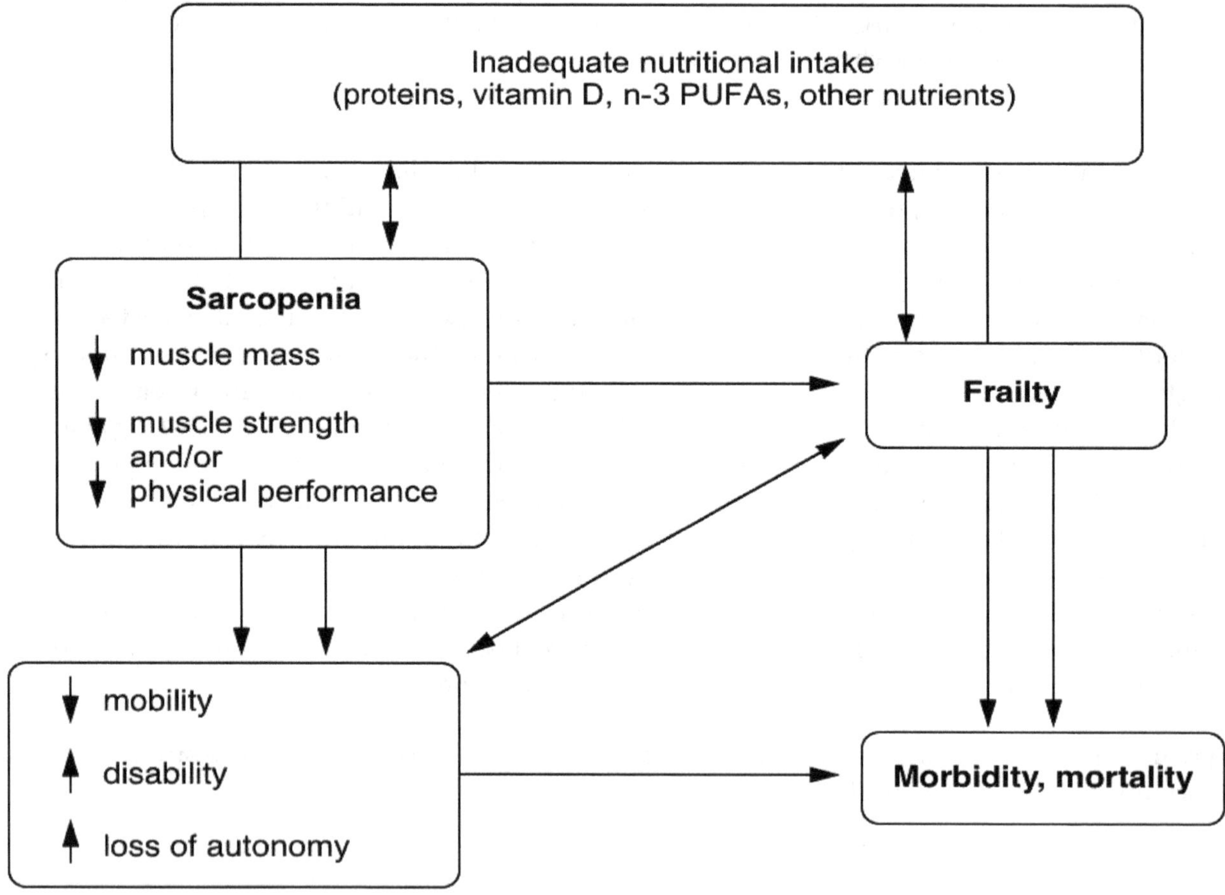

Figure 1. Potential role of nutrition on the physical health of older adults. Short arrows within boxes: increase or decrease. Long arrows between boxes: may lead to. Double-sided arrows: the relationship may be bidirectional. Arrows passing through boxes: factors in box could be mediators.

2. Proteins and Amino Acids

2.1. Total Dietary Protein Intake

Inadequate dietary protein intake is generally recognized as an etiologic factor contributing to sarcopenia [1]. In an effort to prevent sarcopenia and maintain physical function and long-term optimal health, in 2013 and 2014, large international groups of experts issued a consensus to increase protein recommendations to 1.0–1.2 g/kg/day for healthy individuals, 1.2 g/kg/day for active individuals, and 1.2–1.5 g/kg/day for those with chronic or acute diseases (except renal) [15,16] from the current recommended daily allowance (RDA) of 0.83 g/kg/day [17]. This consensus was based on substantial evidence emanating from metabolic, interventional, and observational studies that were then available, and continues to be supported by more recent evidence, comprehensively reviewed elsewhere [18]. In brief, metabolic studies concur to show greater requirements than previously estimated by nitrogen balance, and the majority of observation studies concur to show higher lean or muscle mass and strength and lesser risk of losses and functional decline in subgroups of the older population consuming more dietary protein.

Interventional studies. On the other hand, randomized clinical trials of protein or amino acid supplements have reported opposing results on muscle mass or strength. From nine trials included in a recent meta-analysis, no significant effect of supplements was found on lean body mass, leg strength, or handgrip strength [19]. Heterogeneity was evident for trials that differed in the studied population (healthy, frail, diabetic, or sarcopenic individuals), duration, and supplement forms and doses. Importantly, usual dietary protein intake was not measured in all of the studies, therefore limiting data interpretation as to additional protein effect. The issue of compliance, which is difficult to measure with precision, is also to be considered, since these supplements are not always palatable and become monotonous over long periods of time. In that respect, Mitchell et al. (2017) conducted a well-controlled feeding study of 35 healthy older men (>70 years old), providing all prepared foods to test a diet at the current protein RDA against twice the RDA, i.e., 0.8 g/kg/day or 1.6 g/kg/day, for 10 weeks [20]. While the appendicular lean mass (ALM) remained unchanged in individuals following the 1.6 g/kg/day diet, it decreased in the RDA group. This strengthens the higher protein needs for the maintenance of muscle mass with aging. With regards to functional outcomes, benefits in favor of supplements versus placebo were reported as increased grip strength [21], improvement in functional limitations [22], the absence of deterioration [23], or an improvement [24] in physical performance (Short Physical Performance Battery score, SPPB) whereas no improvement was observed in others [20,25].

Again, this general lack of effect of protein supplements as opposed to positive associations between protein intake and muscle mass and function observed in cohort studies could be due to the type, dose, and timing of supplements, as well as compliance, and the population studied. Indeed, from the above studies, beneficial effects of protein supplements on physical function appear to be seen especially in frail, malnourished individuals or those at risk of malnutrition.

2.2. Meal Distribution of Dietary Protein

Beyond total daily protein intake, the effect of its mealtime distribution is a topic of emerging interest in the field of sarcopenia research. To equally distribute protein intake across the three daily meals is based on the concept of reaching a per-meal anabolic threshold [26,27]. A combination of factors such as insulin resistance [28–30], sedentary lifestyle or short-term immobilization [31,32], inflammation, lipotoxicity, and oxidative stress [33] are thought to cause anabolic resistance [27,33]. An elevated anabolic threshold translates into greater needs to achieve maximal stimulation of MPS in older compared to younger individuals [34–36]. Earlier studies agreed upon a desirable dose of 25–30 g of high-quality protein per meal, providing $\geq$15 g of essential amino acids, which are recognized as the main amino acids responsible for stimulating MPS [37].

Interventional studies. The even distribution hypothesis was first confirmed in a crossover study in young adults (n = 8) comparing a seven-day diet of evenly (30/30/30 g) versus unevenly (11/16/63 g) distributed protein intake. MPS measured by incorporation of $^{13}C_6$-phenylalanine over 24 h was significantly higher following the diet with an even distribution [38]. In contrast, a randomized trial testing the distribution at two levels of intake (0.8 g/kg/day and 1.5 g/kg/day) over four days in older adults (52–75 years old) concluded that quantity of dietary protein intake, but not distribution, resulted in an increased MPS and net protein balance [39]. These studies were of too short duration to demonstrate effects on muscle mass or strength. To date, only the longer-term intervention study (42 days) testing distribution has been conducted in malnourished hospitalized elderly patients. They consumed on average 1.3 g/kg/day from a diet that provided either >70% of proteins at lunch (bolus) or an amount that was divided into four meals (spread; $n = 30–36$/group). Lean body mass significantly increased in the group that was fed the protein bolus diet. No change in grip strength was reported in neither of the groups [40]. It is possible that none of the four meals in the spread diet provided enough protein to reach the anabolic threshold, which would theoretically be higher in these malnourished and inactive patients. Clearly, the response to protein intake may differ according to health status, which justifies further research in vulnerable persons at risk of malnutrition.

Observational studies. We examined the loss of lean mass related to protein intake distribution using data from 351 and 361 free-living men and women aged 67–84 years of the Quebec Longitudinal Study on Nutrition and Successful Aging (NuAge) [41]. We found that a more evenly distributed protein intake, regardless of quantity, was associated with higher lean mass at baseline and two-year follow-up after adjustment for relevant covariates [42]. However, neither total intake nor protein distribution were related to the rate of loss over the two-year follow-up, which is a period that was perhaps not long enough to detect association with a marginal decline (2% across two years). Muscle strength and mobility were also studied in this cohort ($n = 1741$; three-year follow-up). A composite score was created for each of these parameters, embedding handgrip, arm strength, and leg strength, and timed-up-and-go (TUG), chair-stand, and walking speed, respectively. In both sexes, a more evenly distributed protein intake was positively associated with muscle strength throughout the study, but not with mobility, and did not predict strength or mobility rate of decline [43]. A recent and smaller cross-sectional study ($n = 140$) reported a positive association between a more even protein distribution and gait speed, but not with total SPPB and its other single components. Muscle mass and strength were not measured [44]. Finally, no such associations were found in a small cross-sectional study ($n = 99$) of successful agers. However, these results did not represent a broad range of functional capacity, thus pointing to dietary protein intake and distribution perhaps having more impact on those with impaired muscle health [45]. Since both total and mealtime distribution of protein may influence muscle mass and function, a per-meal minimal intake has been advocated [46]. Testing this rationale in 4123 adults >50 years old in the 2011–2014 National Health and Nutrition Examination Survey (NHANES), grip strength was positively associated with consumption of ≥25 g protein/meal on two or more eating occasions compared to only one eating occasion of the same amount. This relationship disappeared when adjusted for multiple covariates, including total daily protein intake, which was related with grip strength [47]. In contrast, in 1081 older adults (50–85 years) of the 1999–2002 NHANES, Loenneke et al. (2016) found that participants consuming at least two meals containing 30–45 g protein/meal had the greatest leg lean mass and strength, and those consuming at least one meal/day of ≥30 g protein/meal had greater responses than those with no meal reaching the 30 g threshold [48]. Adjusted models included age, sex, ethnicity, smoking, physical activity, total carbohydrate intake, total fat intake, and relative protein intake (g/kg). It appears that a threshold of 30 g versus 25 g may explain discrepancies between studies, but it was more likely that lower limb muscles respond more to protein intake due to solicitation for mobility than handgrip strength.

In summary, in healthy older adults, mealtime protein distribution may have more of an impact when other anabolic stimuli are minimal, i.e., at low total protein intakes and physical activity levels, which remains to be investigated in longer-term intervention studies. To date, per-meal protein doses sufficient to generate anabolism in persons at risk of malnutrition and sarcopenia are still unknown.

3. Leucine

Leucine is the most potent amino acid to stimulate MPS from activation of the nutrient and growth factor-sensing mammalian target of rapamycin complex 1 (mTORC1) and in turn, its downstream targets ribosomal protein S6 kinase 1, translation initiation factor 4EBP-1, and elongation factor 2 [49,50]. Though not fully elucidated, mTORC1 activation by leucine is thought to occur at the lysosome through a cascade involving Ragulator Rag GTPases and vacuolar H+-ATPase [51,52]. Three to fourfold increments in plasma leucine appear to be required to elevate intracellular concentrations and augment MPS [53] provided that other essential amino acids are also available to sustain greater protein synthesis [54].

Interventional studies. Very few cohort studies have associated dietary leucine intake to muscle mass. Since leucine is ubiquitously found in all proteins, though in animal more than plant proteins, its intake is practically impossible to dissociate from total protein intake from foods. Thus, most of the evidence on leucine's effect has been accrued from supplement studies, most of which were of short-term duration. Two meta-analyses published in 2015 concluded differently [55,56]. The one from Xu et al. (2015) included nine randomized controlled trials (RCTs), four testing acute post-challenge responses (three in healthy, one in cancer participants), and five longer-term, ranging from 10 days to six months (in participants who were either healthy, had type 2 diabetes, or had polymyalgia, and were on bed rest, or exercising) [56]. A pooled effect of 1.08 (95% CI: 0.50–1.67) was found on acutely increasing MPS, but no effect was observed on lean body mass or leg lean mass from longer-term interventions. The meta-analysis by Komar et al. (2015) included 16 studies testing leucine-rich supplements in a wider variety of participants, who were also frail, sarcopenic, and institutionalized [55]. Subgroup analysis revealed a mean effect of 1.14 kg (95% CI: 0.55–1.74) increase in lean body mass in favor of leucine-rich supplements in sarcopenic, but not in healthy participants. In both meta-analyses, leucine was either given as pure crystalline powder, or as part of essential amino acid drinks, complete medical formula, or whey protein, at doses ranging from 2 g/day to 17.6 g/day. This considerable heterogeneity in population, study design, and the type of supplements studied precludes firm conclusions, but points to plausible effects in persons having or at risk of sarcopenia. The question as to why the acute stimulation of MPS by leucine supplements does not seem to translate into measurable changes in lean body mass in healthy older adults remains open. Insufficient usual dietary protein intake, poor long-term compliance, and perhaps habituation to a sustained stimulus may explain negative findings.

More recent studies from Phillips et al. have revived a promising anabolic role for leucine [57–59]. Using an integrative measure of myofibrillar protein synthesis (MyoPS) over three days in well-controlled crossover feeding studies, providing all foods to older men, 5 g of leucine that was added to each of the three daily meals resulted in augmented MyoPS in both the rested leg and the one submitted to unilateral resistance exercise [59]. Interestingly, this effect was seen at both low (0.8 g/kg/day) and higher (1.2 g/kg/day) daily protein intakes. In healthy older women, 10 g of whey protein added with 3 g of leucine were compared to 25 g of whey protein intrinsically containing 3 g of leucine, taken twice daily for six days. Results showed that the lower protein, leucine-matched supplement was as effective as the 25-g protein dose at increasing acute and integrated MyoPS, which could represent a practical alternative for older women with typical low appetite [57]. Lastly, Devries et al. (2018) tested the twice daily consumption of 15 g of a milk protein drink containing 4.2 g of leucine against 15 g of mixed protein drink containing 1.3 g of leucine, as part of a diet providing 1 g protein/kg/day, under the same protocol in older women [58]. Greater acute postprandial and integrated MyoPS responses over six days were found with the higher leucine-containing drink. Altogether, these positive results obtained in rigorous conditions are promising and warrant corroboration in longer-term interventions to demonstrate potential benefits of leucine for preserving muscle mass and function.

4. Vitamin D

4.1. Vitamin D, Physical Function, and Muscle Mass and Strength

Vitamin D is a key nutrient in musculoskeletal health. In adults, vitamin D deficiency is associated with bone diseases including osteomalacia, osteopenia, and osteoporosis, and increases the risk of fractures [60]. However, bone health is not the only physiological dimension to be impacted by vitamin D, since its involvement has been evidenced in cardiovascular disease, autoimmune diseases, and cancer prevention [61], among others. There has been growing interest in the implications of vitamin D status in the physical function of older adults given the high prevalence of vitamin D deficiency in this population [62]. The ubiquity of vitamin D receptors (VDR) in various tissues, including muscles, is well recognized [63]. From its binding to VDRs, vitamin D mediates genomic and non-genomic effects in muscle cells; it namely promotes muscle contractility through calcium influx, myoblast differentiation, and the insulin sensitivity of muscles [64]. The current RDA for vitamin D intake is 600 IU/day for persons aged 1–70 years, and 800 IU/day for older adults (≥71 years), which translates into serum 25-hydroxyvitamin D (25(OH)D) level ≥50 nmol/L for skeletal health [65].

Observational studies. While large cross-sectional studies corroborate a relationship between insufficient level of serum 25(OH)D (<50 nmol/L) and low physical performance [66–71], mobility [66,68–70], muscle strength [66,67,69,70,72,73], and greater disability [66,73] in free-living older adults, the association with muscle strength was not found in a cohort of older women (>90% with vitamin D insufficiency) [74]. In 2017, a meta-analysis of 17 cross-sectional and five longitudinal studies (n = 54–4100) provided fair evidence that seniors with low vitamin D status, regardless of the cut-point used for its definition, had a slower usual gait speed compared to those with normal status (−0.18 m/s in vitamin D deficient; ≤25 nmol/L) [75]. Physical performance (by TUG) was also associated with vitamin D deficiency. More recently, Vaes et al. (2018) confirmed cross-sectional associations between vitamin D insufficiency, gait speed (n = 745), and TUG (n = 488) in older men and women aged ≥65 years; interestingly, frail individuals were at higher risk of being vitamin D insufficient compared to non-frail individuals [76], which is an association that has also been ascertained in a meta-analysis [77]. No link with muscle strength was found in this cohort.

Vitamin D insufficiency has also been longitudinally associated with greater risks of disability [69,78,79], decline in physical performance [71,80], and handgrip strength [81] in healthy older adults. However, few groups did not find such associations (n = 988–2099; 2.5 to six years follow-up) [69,82]. Since then, Granic et al. (2017) studied very old adults (n = 845, age ≥85 years old) and found a greater handgrip strength decline in men of the lowest 25(OH)D season-specific quartile over five years, but this was not seen in women [83]. Although causal effect cannot be concluded from these observational studies, altogether the evidence suggests that interventions should aim at targeting at risk populations, namely individuals with vitamin D insufficiency or deficiency, and frail seniors to favor better mobility or delay the onset of disabilities.

Interventional studies. Systematic reviews and meta-analyses examined the benefits of vitamin D supplementation on physical performance, muscle mass, and strength in community and/or institution-dwelling seniors [84–87]. The importance of considering baseline serum 25(OH)D concentrations has been emphasized, since individuals with vitamin D deficiency appear to be more responsive to supplementation [84]. Modest mean differences in TUG (3 studies; n = 551) and postural sway (three studies; n = 413) independent of doses were reported following vitamin D supplementation in a first meta-analysis; yet authors observed that all of the studies providing high daily vitamin D doses (i.e., 800 IU to 1000 IU) supported beneficial effects on balance and lower extremity muscle strength [85]. A second meta-analysis's age subgroup analysis showed a favorable effect of vitamin D supplementation, with or without calcium, on muscle strength in older adults ≥65 years old and especially, greater improvement in institutionalized compared to free-living individuals [87]. In line with these previous studies, the most recent meta-analysis of RCTs (2017) conducted in community-dwelling older adults confirmed a slight improvement of −0.3 s (95% CI: −0.1 to −0.5; 5 studies; n = 1260) in the TUG test following supplementation, but no overall increase in handgrip strength was detected (seven studies; n = 1452) [86]. The included RCTs assessing TUG performance provided doses ranging from 800 IU to 2000 IU/day between 10 weeks and 20 months, and one study provided 150,000 IU every three months for a nine-month period. The latter revealed an effect in favor of the placebo [88], and no effect was found from 2000 IU/day for 10 weeks [89]. Further, one additional study by Bischoff-Ferrari et al. (2016) that was not included in the abovementioned meta-analysis established a null effect of monthly doses of 24,000 IU + calcifediol and 60,000 IU on lower extremity function (by SPPB) after one year, and led to higher fall incidence compared to

24,000 IU/month [90]. This finding strengthens that benefits are observed with vitamin D doses within the range of 800–1000 IU/day, but not necessarily at higher doses.

Heterogeneity between RCTs (doses and type of supplement, duration of the intervention, participants' baseline vitamin D status) and few discrepancies among meta-analyses with regard to selection criteria makes comparison between studies difficult. Nonetheless, in light of the pooled evidence, vitamin D supplementation should be considered to improve physical performance in older adults and perhaps for muscle strength in most likely frail seniors.

4.2. Vitamin D and Fall Prevention

Unintentional falls are the leading cause of injury death in seniors aged ≥65 years in the United States (US) [91]. Beyond musculoskeletal-related functions, risk factors for falls belong to multiple intrinsic (biological) and extrinsic (socio-economic, environmental, and behavioral) dimensions; these include balance, gait abnormalities, chronic conditions such as neurological disorders, cognitive impairment, vision, fear of falling, use of medications, and environmental hazards, all of which contribute to the occurrence of falls [92].

Interventional studies. Vitamin D and falls is an area that has been extensively studied; trials have tested the impact of vitamin D supplementation on the prevention of falls and numerous meta-analyses have examined the overall reported effects. However, due to substantial differences in selection criteria between meta-analyses [93], conflicting results remain. In their high-quality meta-analysis of 14 trials and 27,522 participants, Bolland et al. reported a non-meaningful effect of vitamin D, with or without calcium, on the relative risk (0.96; 95% CI: 0.91–1.01), and highlighted that it would unlikely change with additional future studies [94,95].

In 2018, an updated evidence report and systematic review of fall prevention interventions in community-dwelling older adults was published for the US Preventive Service Task Force. From the seven studies of vitamin D supplementation included in the review, the authors found inconsistent results, which was possibly due to high heterogeneity [96]. Also, one trial in older women showed the deleterious effects of an annual 500,000 IU vitamin D3 dose on falls and fractures [97]. Following this report, the new recommendation advises against vitamin D supplementation for fall prevention in community-dwelling non-osteoporotic and non-vitamin D deficient older adults ≥65 years old [98].

5. N-3 Polyunsaturated Fatty Acids

N-3 PUFAs are consumed as eicosapentaenoic acid (EPA; 20:5 *n*-3) and docosahexaenoic acid (DHA; 22:6 *n*-3) or as alpha-linolenic acid (ALA; 18:3 *n*-3), of which a very limited fraction is converted to EPA (8 and 21% conversion rates) and DHA (~0 and 9%) in men and women, respectively [99,100]. N-3 PUFAs are well-known for their anti-inflammatory properties and their role in the development and maintenance of neurocerebral functions [101–103]. In a large prospective cohort study of older adults, plasma *n*-3 PUFA levels were associated with a 27% reduction in total mortality risk across quintiles, increasing the life expectancy of individuals in the highest quintile by ~2 years [104]. This association with mortality was essentially ascribed to docosapentaenoic acid (DPA; 22:5 *n*-3), DHA, and EPA status, and was more pronounced for cardiovascular disease mortality, including coronary heart disease and ischemic stroke. No RDA recommendations exist for *n*-3 PUFA, only adequate intake (AI) was established for ALA (1.6 g/day for men and 1.1 g/day for women, aged ≥14 years) [17]; however, the majority of expert groups endorse intakes of 250–500 mg/day EPA and DHA for cardiovascular health, which translates into ~2 servings (140 g, 5 oz) of fatty fish per week [105]. Although older adults tend to consume more fish that are high in n-3 PUFA compared to younger adults, their intake remains suboptimal, with a mean of 0.19 ± 0.02 oz/day [106]. Although still elusive, the anabolic role of n-3 PUFAs on skeletal muscle is thought to be owed to a reduction in pro-inflammatory cytokines, myosteatosis, an improvement of insulin sensitivity [107], the stimulation of muscle protein synthesis via the mTOR-p70S6k signaling pathway [108], and a diminution of mitochondrial reactive oxygen species emission [109].

Observational studies. Inconsistent associations were found between n-3 PUFA dietary intakes and muscle function from scarce cross-sectional evidence [110,111], and to our knowledge, no study has examined this relationship since then. Previous evidence showed higher plasma n-3 PUFA levels, which is an objective biomarker of dietary intake [112], to be associated with better physical performance and gait speed in healthy older adults at baseline and with a lower risk of poor physical performance (odds ratio, OR = 0.21, 95% CI: 0.08–0.53; n = 884) over three years (relationship owing to EPA and DHA) [113]. This cross-sectional association with gait speed was also confirmed recently [114]; however, one study did not find red blood cell membrane EPA and DHA levels to be associated with physical performance in participants at risk of cognitive decline after controlling for covariates [115]. As for muscle strength, the relationship is unclear, as evidenced by one study reporting no association with plasma n-3 PUFA once adjusted for covariates [116].

Longitudinal analyses with follow-up periods ranging from three to five years were performed on the cohorts cited above. One study found baseline total plasma n-3 PUFAs and DHA to be associated with incidences of self-reported mobility disability after five years in healthy older women only (OR = 0.48, 95% CI: 0.25–0.93), suggesting that there may be a sex-specific biological role for DHA in mobility [117]. However, other studies found no relationship with the relative change in muscular parameters [116], decline in gait speed [117,118], or decline in physical performance [118] after three and five years. As frequently encountered with longitudinal studies, the decline in the main outcome or the incidence of the condition being looked at may not have been sufficient to detect significant associations. Also, considering the limited evidence available, it can only be concluded that cross-sectional and longitudinal associations of plasma or erythrocyte n-3 PUFA concentrations and muscle mass or function remain uncertain. In future studies, analysis with EPA and DHA levels should consistently be reported, as detected relationships with total n-3 PUFA were driven by these specific fatty acids.

Interventional studies. One study previously reported a modest effect of a six-month, 1.2 g/day n-3 PUFA (720 mg EPA and 480 mg DHA) supplementation on gait speed in 126 seniors aged ≥65 years, but not on body composition and strength [119]. Three additional recent studies have tested daily 1.1–3.36 g EPA and DHA supplementation over three to six months. Following a six-month, 4 g/d n-3 PUFA supplementation (1.86 g EPA, 1.5 g DHA) compared to corn oil placebo, Smith et al. (2015) detected gains of 2.3 kg in handgrip strength (95% CI: 0.8, 3.7 kg) and of 3.6% (95% CI: 0.2, 7.0%) in thigh muscle volume in community-dwelling older adults (n = 60; aged 60 to 85 years) [120]. The authors estimated that these beneficial changes would result in a two to three-year prevention of muscle mass and function decline normally associated with aging. Similarly, Logan et al. (2015) reported a 4% increase (1.6 kg ± 0.7 kg, p = 0.01) in muscle mass as measured by bioelectrical impedance analysis BIA and a 7% improvement in the TUG in the intervention group (5 g/day fish oil; 2 g of EPA, 1 g of DHA) compared to an olive oil placebo after three months (n = 24 healthy women aged 60–76 years; those who consumed >1 meal of fish per week or took n-3 supplements were excluded) [121]. Yet, another three-month trial showed no effect of a 1.3 g/day n-3 PUFA supplementation (660 mg of EPA, 440 mg of DHA) on body composition (by BIA), TUG, handgrip strength, and gait speed in 53 older adults (age ≥65 years) at risk (1 SD below the mean ALM index of a reference population) or having low lean mass at baseline [122]. This absence of effect is possibly due to the low EPA and DHA doses provided and the relatively short duration of the intervention [119,122]. Although a biomarker measure of n-3 PUFA was not reported in the latter study, those that provided doses of 3.0 g and 3.36 g of EPA and DHA effectively increased serum and red blood cells' n-3 PUFA concentrations after three [121] and six [120] months, respectively, versus no change in the control groups. The effect of doses between 1.1–3.0 g was not tested in untrained older adults.

It is of note that the methodologies of these trials used different approaches to body composition assessment, the duration of interventions, measures of n-3 PUFA status, and doses of supplements, which prevents direct comparison of studies. Future trials should report at least one measure of n-3 PUFA circulating levels as well as its changes to allow proper interpretation of the efficacy of the supplement [112]. Yet, a three-month intervention appears long enough to see improvements, but only doses ≥3.0 g/day showed a compelling increment in functional measures and muscle mass and volume [120,121]. While *n*-3 PUFA may prevent sarcopenia in healthy older adults, its effect in sarcopenic seniors and those losing autonomy remains to be investigated.

6. Combined Supplements of Protein, Leucine, Vitamin D, and *n*-3 PUFA

While increased protein intakes and supplements in leucine, vitamin D, and *n*-3 PUFA support potential gains in muscle mass and function when consumed individually, the combination of these nutrients may provide further benefits. Four recent, randomized, double-blind placebo-controlled studies tested a combined supplement of high-quality protein and vitamin D, without exercise intervention, on lean mass, strength, and physical performance [123–126]; two of them included added leucine to the mix [124,126], and one included *n*-3 PUFA, and creatine [125]. A 13-week multicenter study conducted in 380 sarcopenic older individuals aged ≥65 years with high disability risk found a beneficial effect of a 800 IU vitamin D, 3 g of leucine, and 20 g of whey protein supplement, given twice daily, on the chair-stand time (−1.01 s, 95% CI: −1.77, −0.19), but not on physical performance, mobility, and strength compared to the control group receiving an isocaloric placebo [126]. A very slight increase in ALM (0.17 kg, 95% CI: 0.004, 0.338) was reported, although it was within the 1.2% lean body mass measurement error by dual-energy X-ray absorptiometry DXA [127]. The same supplement was provided before breakfast only to 24 healthy older men, and similarly showed a modest gain in ALM (estimate difference of 0.37 kg) and leg lean mass after six weeks [124]. Interestingly, dietary protein intake was displaced by the supplement in the intervention group, as shown by the same total protein intake between groups when accounting for the supplement. The modest improvement in outcomes may be attributable to the change in meal protein intake distribution, as breakfast protein consumption was higher in the intervention group at the end of the trial, with an average of >25 g at each meal compared to ~10 g at breakfast, at baseline, and in the control group. Again, the supplement did not show any improvement on handgrip strength and physical performance. Bell et al. examined the effect of a similar multinutrient supplement that had 30 g of whey protein, 2.5 g of creatine, 500 IU of vitamin D, 400 mg of calcium, and 1.5 g of *n*-3 PUFA, 700 mg of EPA, 445 mg of DHA, and was consumed twice per day (1 h after breakfast and 1 h before going to bed) against a placebo of 22 g of maltodextrin, on strength and lean mass in 49 healthy older men (aged 73 ± 1 years) during six weeks alone and in combination with high-intensity interval trainings during the 12 following weeks [125]. After six weeks of supplementation alone, both lean mass and strength increased in the intervention group; the authors reported gains of 0.4 kg for ALM and 3% for the sum of isotonic strength, but the intervention was only superior to the control for the latter. Similarly, Bo et al. found an improvement in handgrip strength (1.91 ± 4.24 kg, $p = 0.020$) from a long, six-month intervention of 22 g of whey protein, 702 IU of vitamin D, and 109 mg of vitamin E consumed before breakfast and dinner, in 60 sarcopenic men and women aged 65–80 years (versus an isocaloric placebo). Although participants receiving the treatment did not gain muscle mass, a declining trend was seen in the control group, suggesting that the supplementation was protective of muscle mass loss over six months. The authors did not find any effect from the intervention on mobility and physical performance.

Importantly, none of these studies reported serious adverse effects from supplements. Combined supplements showed favorable effects on muscle mass, but may be more effective at stimulating MPS in healthy older adults, and promoting muscle mass maintenance in sarcopenic older adults. Their impact on muscle strength is inconsistent, and no improvement in physical performance was observed. Although isolating the effect of each nutrient from a combined supplement is impossible, providing high-quality proteins, leucine, vitamin D, and *n*-3 PUFA all together appears to be promising in the prevention of sarcopenia, while also being safe. Indeed, more longer-term (i.e., >six weeks) research of multinutrient supplementation involving populations at risk of greater muscle mass decline, such as frail individuals and those losing autonomy, is needed.

7. Conclusions

Proteins, leucine, vitamin D, and *n*-3 PUFAs may individually play a protective role in skeletal muscle health. Therefore, inadequate intakes of these nutrients could lead to several prejudicial conditions such as sarcopenia, frailty, loss of mobility and physical function, morbidity, and mortality. Groups of authors recommend protein intakes of 1.0–1.2 g/kg/day for older adults, which is higher than the currently established RDA, but may not always be achievable through dietary sources for some individuals with reduced appetite. The manifestation of anabolic resistance associated with aging explains, among other factors, the increase in protein requirements. In addition, an even distribution of proteins throughout the day may favor the reach of the anabolic threshold to maximally stimulate MPS. However, this effect remains to be confirmed by long-term intervention studies, and may differ between healthy and malnourished individuals. The effect of vitamin D on physical function seems to be essentially beneficial in individuals with prior vitamin D deficiency. Also, doses of 800–1000 IU/day appear to be more effective compared to lower doses. With respect to *n*-3 PUFAs, recent evidence suggests that EPA + DHA doses of ~3 g/day may have a positive impact on physical performance, muscle strength, and muscle mass in older adults, and this minimal amount may be required for beneficial effects when provided alone, i.e., not combined to other nutrients. Heterogeneity makes comparison of studies difficult, such that future studies should have standardized methods.

Key nutrient supplementation in older adults is of interest in the prevention of sarcopenia and frailty, since it is a simple, low-cost treatment approach without major side effects. Intervention studies testing a combined nutritional supplement are to be explored given the potentially additive effects of proteins, vitamin D, and *n*-3 PUFAs in the prevention of muscle mass and function loss.

Author Contributions: Both authors contributed to the literature review, drafting and editing of manuscript.

Abbreviations

MPS	Muscle protein synthesis
n-3 PUFA	*n*-3 polyunsaturated fatty acids
RDA	Recommended Dietary Allowance
ALM	Appendicular lean mass
MyoPS	Myobfibrillar protein synthesis
RCT	Randomized controlled trials
SPPB	Short Physical Performance Battery
VDR	Vitamin D receptor
EPA	Eicosapentaenoic acid
DHA	Docosahexaenoic acid
TUG	Timed-Up-and-Go
DXA	Dual-energy X-ray absorptiometry
BIA	Bioelectrical impedance

References

1. Cruz-Jentoft, A.J.; Baeyens, J.P.; Bauer, J.M.; Boirie, Y.; Cederholm, T.; Landi, F.; Martin, F.C.; Michel, J.P.; Rolland, Y.; Schneider, S.M.; et al. Sarcopenia: European consensus on definition and diagnosis: Report of the european working group on sarcopenia in older people. *Age Ageing* **2010**, *39*, 412–423. [CrossRef] [PubMed]
2. Morley, J.E.; Baumgartner, R.N.; Roubenoff, R.; Mayer, J.; Nair, K.S. Sarcopenia. *J. Lab. Clin. Med.* **2001**, *137*, 231–243. [CrossRef] [PubMed]
3. Woo, T.; Yu, S.; Visvanathan, R. Systematic literature review on the relationship between biomarkers of sarcopenia and quality of life in older people. *J. Frailty Aging* **2016**, *5*, 88–99. [CrossRef] [PubMed]

4. Delmonico, M.J.; Harris, T.B.; Lee, J.S.; Visser, M.; Nevitt, M.; Kritchevsky, S.B.; Tylavsky, F.A.; Newman, A.B. Health, Aging and Body Composition Study. Alternative definitions of sarcopenia, lower extremity performance, and functional impairment with aging in older men and women. *J. Am. Geriatr. Soc.* **2007**, *55*, 769–774. [CrossRef] [PubMed]
5. Morley, J.E. Diabetes, sarcopenia, and frailty. *Clin. Geriatr. Med.* **2008**, *24*, 455–469. [CrossRef] [PubMed]
6. Cawthon, P.M.; Fox, K.M.; Gandra, S.R.; Delmonico, M.J.; Chiou, C.F.; Anthony, M.S.; Sewall, A.; Goodpaster, B.; Satterfield, S.; Cummings, S.R.; et al. Do muscle mass, muscle density, strength, and physical function similarly influence risk of hospitalization in older adults? *J. Am. Geriatr. Soc.* **2009**, *57*, 1411–1419. [CrossRef] [PubMed]
7. Janssen, I.; Shepard, D.S.; Katzmarzyk, P.T.; Roubenoff, R. The healthcare costs of sarcopenia in the united states. *J. Am. Geriatr. Soc.* **2004**, *52*, 80–85. [CrossRef] [PubMed]
8. Landi, F.; Cruz-Jentoft, A.J.; Liperoti, R.; Russo, A.; Giovannini, S.; Tosato, M.; Capoluongo, E.; Bernabei, R.; Onder, G. Sarcopenia and mortality risk in frail older persons aged 80 years and older: Results from ilsirente study. *Age Ageing* **2013**, *42*, 203–209. [CrossRef] [PubMed]
9. Bollwein, J.; Volkert, D.; Diekmann, R.; Kaiser, M.J.; Uter, W.; Vidal, K.; Sieber, C.C.; Bauer, J.M. Nutritional status according to the mini nutritional assessment (mna(r)) and frailty in community dwelling older persons: A close relationship. *J. Nutr. Health Aging* **2013**, *17*, 351–356. [CrossRef] [PubMed]
10. Dorner, T.E.; Luger, E.; Tschinderle, J.; Stein, K.V.; Haider, S.; Kapan, A.; Lackinger, C.; Schindler, K.E. Association between nutritional status (mna(r)-sf) and frailty (share-fi) in acute hospitalised elderly patients. *J. Nutr. Health Aging* **2014**, *18*, 264–269. [CrossRef] [PubMed]
11. Chevalier, S.; Saoud, F.; Gray-Donald, K.; Morais, J.A. The physical functional capacity of frail elderly persons undergoing ambulatory rehabilitation is related to their nutritional status. *J. Nutr. Health Aging* **2008**, *12*, 721–726. [CrossRef] [PubMed]
12. Kaiser, M.J.; Bauer, J.M.; Ramsch, C.; Uter, W.; Guigoz, Y.; Cederholm, T.; Thomas, D.R.; Anthony, P.S.; Charlton, K.E.; Maggio, M.; et al. Frequency of malnutrition in older adults: A multinational perspective using the mini nutritional assessment. *J. Am. Geriatr. Soc.* **2010**, *58*, 1734–1738. [CrossRef] [PubMed]
13. Wall, B.T.; Gorissen, S.H.; Pennings, B.; Koopman, R.; Groen, B.B.; Verdijk, L.B.; van Loon, L.J. Aging is accompanied by a blunted muscle protein synthetic response to protein ingestion. *PLoS ONE* **2015**, *10*, e0140903. [CrossRef] [PubMed]
14. Dodd, K.M.; Tee, A.R. Leucine and mTORC1: A complex relationship. *Am. J. Physiol. Endocrinol. Metab.* **2012**, *302*, E1329–E1342. [CrossRef] [PubMed]
15. Bauer, J.; Biolo, G.; Cederholm, T.; Cesari, M.; Cruz-Jentoft, A.J.; Morley, J.E.; Phillips, S.; Sieber, C.; Stehle, P.; Teta, D.; et al. Evidence-based recommendations for optimal dietary protein intake in older people: A position paper from the prot-age study group. *J. Am. Med. Dir. Assoc.* **2013**, *14*, 542–559. [CrossRef] [PubMed]
16. Deutz, N.E.; Bauer, J.M.; Barazzoni, R.; Biolo, G.; Boirie, Y.; Bosy-Westphal, A.; Cederholm, T.; Cruz-Jentoft, A.; Krznaric, Z.; Nair, K.S.; et al. Protein intake and exercise for optimal muscle function with aging: Recommendations from the espen expert group. *Clin. Nutr.* **2014**, *33*, 929–936. [CrossRef] [PubMed]
17. Institute of Medicine. *Dietary Reference Intakes for Energy, Carbohydrate, Fiber, Fat, Fatty Acids, Cholesterol, Protein, and Amino Acids*; The National Academies Press: Washington, DC, USA, 2005; p. 1358.
18. Traylor, D.A.; Gorissen, S.H.M.; Phillips, S.M. Perspective: Protein requirements and optimal intakes in aging: Are we ready to recommend more than the recommended daily allowance? *Adv. Nutr.* **2018**, *9*, 171–182. [CrossRef] [PubMed]
19. Tieland, M.; Franssen, R.; Dullemeijer, C.; van Dronkelaar, C.; Kyung Kim, H.; Ispoglou, T.; Zhu, K.; Prince, R.L.; van Loon, L.J.C.; de Groot, L. The impact of dietary protein or amino acid supplementation on muscle mass and strength in elderly people: Individual participant data and meta-analysis of rct's. *J. Nutr. Health Aging* **2017**, *21*, 994–1001. [CrossRef] [PubMed]
20. Mitchell, C.J.; Milan, A.M.; Mitchell, S.M.; Zeng, N.; Ramzan, F.; Sharma, P.; Knowles, S.O.; Roy, N.C.; Sjodin, A.; Wagner, K.H.; et al. The effects of dietary protein intake on appendicular lean mass and muscle function in elderly men: A 10-wk randomized controlled trial. *Am. J. Clin. Nutr.* **2017**, *106*, 1375–1383. [CrossRef] [PubMed]
21. Cawood, A.L.; Elia, M.; Stratton, R.J. Systematic review and meta-analysis of the effects of high protein oral nutritional supplements. *Ageing Res. Rev.* **2012**, *11*, 278–296. [CrossRef] [PubMed]

22. Neelemaat, F.; Bosmans, J.E.; Thijs, A.; Seidell, J.C.; van Bokhorst-de van der Schueren, M.A. Oral nutritional support in malnourished elderly decreases functional limitations with no extra costs. *Clin. Nutr.* **2012**, *31*, 183–190. [CrossRef] [PubMed]
23. Kim, C.O.; Lee, K.R. Preventive effect of protein-energy supplementation on the functional decline of frail older adults with low socioeconomic status: A community-based randomized controlled study. *J. Gerontol. A Biol. Sci. Med. Sci.* **2013**, *68*, 309–316. [CrossRef] [PubMed]
24. Tieland, M.; van de Rest, O.; Dirks, M.L.; van der Zwaluw, N.; Mensink, M.; van Loon, L.J.; de Groot, L.C. Protein supplementation improves physical performance in frail elderly people: A randomized, double-blind, placebo-controlled trial. *J. Am. Med. Dir. Assoc.* **2012**, *13*, 720–726. [CrossRef] [PubMed]
25. Zhu, K.; Kerr, D.A.; Meng, X.; Devine, A.; Solah, V.; Binns, C.W.; Prince, R.L. Two-year whey protein supplementation did not enhance muscle mass and physical function in well-nourished healthy older postmenopausal women. *J. Nutr.* **2015**, *145*, 2520–2526. [CrossRef] [PubMed]
26. Paddon-Jones, D.; Rasmussen, B.B. Dietary protein recommendations and the prevention of sarcopenia. *Curr. Opin. Clin. Nutr. Metab. Care* **2009**, *12*, 86–90. [CrossRef] [PubMed]
27. Dardevet, D.; Remond, D.; Peyron, M.A.; Papet, I.; Savary-Auzeloux, I.; Mosoni, L. Muscle wasting and resistance of muscle anabolism: The "anabolic threshold concept" for adapted nutritional strategies during sarcopenia. *Sci. World J.* **2012**, *2012*, 269531. [CrossRef] [PubMed]
28. Chevalier, S.; Gougeon, R.; Choong, N.; Lamarche, M.; Morais, J.A. Influence of adiposity in the blunted whole-body protein anabolic response to insulin with aging. *J. Gerontol. A Biol. Sci. Med. Sci.* **2006**, *61*, 156–164. [CrossRef] [PubMed]
29. Fujita, S.; Glynn, E.L.; Timmerman, K.L.; Rasmussen, B.B.; Volpi, E. Supraphysiological hyperinsulinaemia is necessary to stimulate skeletal muscle protein anabolism in older adults: Evidence of a true age-related insulin resistance of muscle protein metabolism. *Diabetologia* **2009**, *52*, 1889–1898. [CrossRef] [PubMed]
30. Chevalier, S.; Goulet, E.D.B.; Burgos, S.A.; Wykes, L.J.; Morais, J.A. Protein anabolic responses to a fed steady state in healthy aging. *J. Gerontol. Ser. A* **2011**, *66A*, 681–688. [CrossRef] [PubMed]
31. Glover, E.I.; Phillips, S.M.; Oates, B.R.; Tang, J.E.; Tarnopolsky, M.A.; Selby, A.; Smith, K.; Rennie, M.J. Immobilization induces anabolic resistance in human myofibrillar protein synthesis with low and high dose amino acid infusion. *J. Physiol.* **2008**, *586*, 6049–6061. [CrossRef] [PubMed]
32. Breen, L.; Stokes, K.A.; Churchward-Venne, T.A.; Moore, D.R.; Baker, S.K.; Smith, K.; Atherton, P.J.; Phillips, S.M. Two weeks of reduced activity decreases leglean mass and induces "anabolic resistance" of myofibrillar protein synthesis n healthy elderly. *J. Clin. Endocrinol. Metab.* **2013**, *98*, 2604–2612. [CrossRef] [PubMed]
33. Boirie, Y. Fighting sarcopenia in older frail subjects: Protein fuel for strength, exercise for mass. *J. Am. Med. Dir. Assoc.* **2013**, *14*, 140–143. [CrossRef] [PubMed]
34. Katsanos, C.S.; Kobayashi, H.; Sheffield-Moore, M.; Aarsland, A.; Wolfe, R.R. Aging is associated with diminished accretion of muscle proteins after the ingestion of a small bolus of essential amino acids. *Am. J. Clin. Nutr.* **2005**, *82*, 1065–1073. [CrossRef] [PubMed]
35. Paddon-Jones, D.; Sheffield-Moore, M.; Zhang, X.J.; Volpi, E.; Wolf, S.E.; Aarsland, A.; Ferrando, A.A.; Wolfe, R.R. Amino acid ingestion improves muscle protein synthesis in the young and elderly. *Am. J. Physiol. Endocrinol. Metab.* **2004**, *286*, E321–E328. [CrossRef] [PubMed]
36. Moore, D.R.; Churchward-Venne, T.A.; Witard, O.; Breen, L.; Burd, N.A.; Tipton, K.D.; Phillips, S.M. Protein ingestion to stimulate myofibrillar protein synthesis requires greater relative protein intakes in healthy older versus younger men. *J. Gerontol. A Biol. Sci. Med. Sci.* **2015**, *70*, 57–62. [CrossRef] [PubMed]
37. Volpi, E.; Kobayashi, H.; Sheffield-Moore, M.; Mittendorfer, B.; Wolfe, R.R. Essential amino acids are primarily responsible for the amino acid stimulation of muscle protein anabolism in healthy elderly adults. *Am. J. Clin. Nutr.* **2003**, *78*, 250–258. [CrossRef] [PubMed]
38. Mamerow, M.M.; Mettler, J.A.; English, K.L.; Casperson, S.L.; Arentson-Lantz, E.; Sheffield-Moore, M.; Layman, D.K.; Paddon-Jones, D. Dietary protein distribution positively influences 24-h muscle protein synthesis in healthy adults. *J. Nutr.* **2014**. [CrossRef] [PubMed]
39. Kim, I.Y.; Schutzler, S.; Schrader, A.; Spencer, H.; Kortebein, P.; Deutz, N.E.; Wolfe, R.R.; Ferrando, A.A. Quantity of dietary protein intake, but not pattern of intake, affects net protein balance primarily through differences in protein synthesis in older adults. *Am. J. Physiol. Endocrinol. Metab.* **2015**, *308*, E21–E28. [CrossRef] [PubMed]

40. Bouillanne, O.; Curis, E.; Hamon-Vilcot, B.; Nicolis, I.; Chretien, P.; Schauer, N.; Vincent, J.P.; Cynober, L.; Aussel, C. Impact of protein pulse feeding on lean mass in malnourished and at-risk hospitalized elderly patients: A randomized controlled trial. *Clin. Nutr.* **2013**, *32*, 186–192. [CrossRef] [PubMed]
41. Gaudreau, P.; Morais, J.A.; Shatenstein, B.; Gray-Donald, K.; Khalil, A.; Dionne, I.; Ferland, G.; Fulop, T.; Jacques, D.; Kergoat, M.J.; et al. Nutrition as a determinant of successful aging: Description of the Quebec longitudinal study nuage and results from cross-sectional pilot studies. *Rejuvenation Res.* **2007**, *10*, 377–386. [CrossRef] [PubMed]
42. Farsijani, S.; Morais, J.A.; Payette, H.; Gaudreau, P.; Shatenstein, B.; Gray-Donald, K.; Chevalier, S. Relation between mealtime distribution of protein intake and lean mass loss in free-living older adults of the nuage study. *Am. J. Clin. Nutr.* **2016**, *104*, 694–703. [CrossRef] [PubMed]
43. Farsijani, S.; Payette, H.; Morais, J.A.; Shatenstein, B.; Gaudreau, P.; Chevalier, S. Even mealtime distribution of protein intake is associated with greater muscle strength, but not with 3-y physical function decline, in free-living older adults: The Quebec longitudinal study on nutrition as a determinant of successful aging (nuage study). *Am. J. Clin. Nutr.* **2017**, *106*, 113–124. [CrossRef] [PubMed]
44. ten Haaf, D.; van Dongen, E.; Nuijten, M.; Eijsvogels, T.; de Groot, L.; Hopman, M. Protein intake and distribution in relation to physical functioning and quality of life in community-dwelling elderly people: Acknowledging the role of physical activity. *Nutrients* **2018**, *10*, 506. [CrossRef] [PubMed]
45. Gingrich, A.; Spiegel, A.; Kob, R.; Schoene, D.; Skurk, T.; Hauner, H.; Sieber, C.C.; Volkert, D.; Kiesswetter, E. Amount, distribution, and quality of protein intake are not associated with muscle mass, strength, and power in healthy older adults without functional limitations-an enable study. *Nutrients* **2017**, *9*. [CrossRef] [PubMed]
46. Murphy, C.H.; Oikawa, S.Y.; Phillips, S.M. Dietary protein to maintain muscle mass in aging: A case for per-meal protein recommendations. *J. Frailty Aging* **2016**, *5*, 49–58. [CrossRef] [PubMed]
47. Mishra, S.; Goldman, J.D.; Sahyoun, N.R.; Moshfegh, A.J. Association between dietary protein intake and grip strength among adults aged 51 years and over: What we eat in america, national health and nutrition examination survey 2011–2014. *PLoS ONE* **2018**, *13*, e0191368. [CrossRef] [PubMed]
48. Loenneke, J.P.; Loprinzi, P.D.; Murphy, C.H.; Phillips, S.M. Per meal dose and frequency of protein consumption is associated with lean mass and muscle performance. *Clin. Nutr.* **2016**, *35*, 1506–1511. [CrossRef] [PubMed]
49. Anthony, J.C.; Yoshizawa, F.; Anthony, T.G.; Vary, T.C.; Jefferson, L.S.; Kimball, S.R. Leucine stimulates translation initiation in skeletal muscle of postabsorptive rats via a rapamycin-sensitive pathway. *J. Nutr.* **2000**, *130*, 2413–2419. [CrossRef] [PubMed]
50. Crozier, S.J.; Kimball, S.R.; Emmert, S.W.; Anthony, J.C.; Jefferson, L.S. Oral leucine administration stimulates protein synthesis in rat skeletal muscle. *J. Nutr.* **2005**, *135*, 376–382. [CrossRef] [PubMed]
51. Sancak, Y.; Peterson, T.R.; Shaul, Y.D.; Lindquist, R.A.; Thoreen, C.C.; Bar-Peled, L.; Sabatini, D.M. The rag gtpases bind raptor and mediate amino acid signaling to mTORC1. *Science* **2008**, *320*, 1496–1501. [CrossRef] [PubMed]
52. Jewell, J.L.; Russell, R.C.; Guan, K.L. Amino acid signalling upstream of mTOR. *Nat. Rev. Mol. Cell Biol.* **2013**, *14*, 133–139. [CrossRef] [PubMed]
53. Wilkinson, D.J.; Hossain, T.; Hill, D.S.; Phillips, B.E.; Crossland, H.; Williams, J.; Loughna, P.; Churchward-Venne, T.A.; Breen, L.; Phillips, S.M.; et al. Effects of leucine and its metabolite beta-hydroxy-beta-methylbutyrate on human skeletal muscle protein metabolism. *J. Physiol.* **2013**, *591*, 2911–2923. [CrossRef] [PubMed]
54. Katsanos, C.S.; Aarsland, A.; Cree, M.G.; Wolfe, R.R. Muscle protein synthesis and balance responsiveness to essential amino acids ingestion in the presence of elevated plasma free fatty acid concentrations. *J. Clin. Endocrinol. Metab.* **2009**, *94*, 2984–2990. [CrossRef] [PubMed]
55. Komar, B.; Schwingshackl, L.; Hoffmann, G. Effects of leucine-rich protein supplements on anthropometric parameter and muscle strength in the elderly: A systematic review and meta-analysis. *J. Nutr. Health Aging* **2015**, *19*, 437–446. [CrossRef] [PubMed]
56. Xu, Z.R.; Tan, Z.J.; Zhang, Q.; Gui, Q.F.; Yang, Y.M. The effectiveness of leucine on muscle protein synthesis, lean body mass and leg lean mass accretion in older people: A systematic review and meta-analysis. *Br. J. Nutr.* **2015**, *113*, 25–34. [CrossRef] [PubMed]

57. Devries, M.C.; McGlory, C.; Bolster, D.R.; Kamil, A.; Rahn, M.; Harkness, L.; Baker, S.K.; Phillips, S.M. Leucine, not total protein, content of a supplement is the primary determinant of muscle protein anabolic responses in healthy older women. *J. Nutr.* **2018**, *148*, 1088–1095. [CrossRef] [PubMed]
58. Devries, M.C.; McGlory, C.; Bolster, D.R.; Kamil, A.; Rahn, M.; Harkness, L.; Baker, S.K.; Phillips, S.M. Protein leucine content is a determinant of shorter- and longer-term muscle protein synthetic responses at rest and following resistance exercise in healthy older women: A randomized, controlled trial. *Am. J. Clin. Nutr.* **2018**, *107*, 217–226. [CrossRef] [PubMed]
59. Murphy, C.H.; Saddler, N.I.; Devries, M.C.; McGlory, C.; Baker, S.K.; Phillips, S.M. Leucine supplementation enhances integrative myofibrillar protein synthesis in free-living older men consuming lower- and higher-protein diets: A parallel-group crossover study. *Am. J. Clin. Nutr.* **2016**, *104*, 1594–1606. [CrossRef] [PubMed]
60. Holick, M.F. Vitamin D deficiency. *N. Engl. J. Med.* **2007**, *357*, 266–281. [CrossRef] [PubMed]
61. Holick, M.F. Sunlight and vitamin D for bone health and prevention of autoimmune diseases, cancers, and cardiovascular disease. *Am. J. Clin. Nutr.* **2004**, *80*, 1678S–1688S. [CrossRef] [PubMed]
62. van Schoor, N.M.; Lips, P. Worldwide vitamin D status. *Best Pract. Res. Clin. Endocrinol. Metab.* **2011**, *25*, 671–680. [CrossRef] [PubMed]
63. Simpson, R.U.; Thomas, G.A.; Arnold, A.J. Identification of 1,25-dihydroxyvitamin D3 receptors and activities in muscle. *J. Biol. Chem.* **1985**, *260*, 8882–8891. [PubMed]
64. Dirks-Naylor, A.J.; Lennon-Edwards, S. The effects of vitamin D on skeletal muscle function and cellular signaling. *J. Steroid Biochem. Mol. Biol.* **2011**, *125*, 159–168. [CrossRef] [PubMed]
65. Ross, A.C. The 2011 report on dietary reference intakes for calcium and vitamin D. *Public Health Nutr.* **2011**, *14*, 938–939. [CrossRef] [PubMed]
66. Houston, D.K.; Tooze, J.A.; Davis, C.C.; Chaves, P.H.; Hirsch, C.H.; Robbins, J.A.; Arnold, A.M.; Newman, A.B.; Kritchevsky, S.B. Serum 25-hydroxyvitamin D and physical function in older adults: The cardiovascular health study all stars. *J. Am. Geriatr. Soc.* **2011**, *59*, 1793–1801. [CrossRef] [PubMed]
67. Houston, D.K.; Cesari, M.; Ferrucci, L.; Cherubini, A.; Maggio, D.; Bartali, B.; Johnson, M.A.; Schwartz, G.G.; Kritchevsky, S.B. Association between vitamin D status and physical performance: The inCHIANTI study. *J. Gerontol. A Biol. Sci. Med. Sci.* **2007**, *62*, 440–446. [CrossRef] [PubMed]
68. Bischoff-Ferrari, H.A.; Dietrich, T.; Orav, E.J.; Hu, F.B.; Zhang, Y.; Karlson, E.W.; Dawson-Hughes, B. Higher 25-hydroxyvitamin D concentrations are associated with better lower-extremity function in both active and inactive persons aged > or =60 y. *Am. J. Clin. Nutr.* **2004**, *80*, 752–758. [CrossRef] [PubMed]
69. Houston, D.K.; Tooze, J.A.; Neiberg, R.H.; Hausman, D.B.; Johnson, M.A.; Cauley, J.A.; Bauer, D.C.; Cawthon, P.M.; Shea, M.K.; Schwartz, G.G.; et al. 25-hydroxyvitamin D status and change in physical performance and strength in older adults: The health, aging, and body composition study. *Am. J. Epidemiol.* **2012**, *176*, 1025–1034. [CrossRef] [PubMed]
70. Toffanello, E.D.; Perissinotto, E.; Sergi, G.; Zambon, S.; Musacchio, E.; Maggi, S.; Coin, A.; Sartori, L.; Corti, M.C.; Baggio, G.; et al. Vitamin D and physical performance in elderly subjects: The pro.V.A study. *PLoS ONE* **2012**, *7*, e34950. [CrossRef] [PubMed]
71. Dam, T.-T.L.; von Mühlen, D.; Barrett-Connor, E.L. Sex specific association of serum 25-hydroxyvitamin D levels with physical function in older adults. *Osteoporos. Int.* **2009**, *20*, 751–760. [CrossRef] [PubMed]
72. Mowe, M.; Haug, E.; Bohmer, T. Low serum calcidiol concentration in older adults with reduced muscular function. *J. Am. Geriatr. Soc.* **1999**, *47*, 220–226. [CrossRef] [PubMed]
73. Zamboni, M.; Zoico, E.; Tosoni, P.; Zivelonghi, A.; Bortolani, A.; Maggi, S.; Di Francesco, V.; Bosello, O. Relation between vitamin D, physical performance, and disability in elderly persons. *J. Gerontol. A Biol. Sci. Med. Sci.* **2002**, *57*, M7-11. [CrossRef] [PubMed]
74. Annweiler, C.; Beauchet, O.; Berrut, G.; Fantino, B.; Bonnefoy, M.; Herrmann, F.R.; Schott, A.M. Is there an association between serum 25-hydroxyvitamin D concentration and muscle strength among older women? Results from baseline assessment of the epidos study. *J. Nutr. Health Aging* **2009**, *13*, 90–95. [CrossRef] [PubMed]
75. Annweiler, C.; Henni, S.; Walrand, S.; Montero-Odasso, M.; Duque, G.; Duval, G.T. Vitamin D and walking speed in older adults: Systematic review and meta-analysis. *Maturitas* **2017**, *106*, 8–25. [CrossRef] [PubMed]

76. Vaes, A.M.M.; Brouwer-Brolsma, E.M.; Toussaint, N.; de Regt, M.; Tieland, M.; van Loon, L.J.C.; de Groot, L. The association between 25-hydroxyvitamin D concentration, physical performance and frailty status in older adults. *Eur. J. Nutr.* **2018**. [CrossRef] [PubMed]
77. Zhou, J.; Huang, P.; Liu, P.; Hao, Q.; Chen, S.; Dong, B.; Wang, J. Association of vitamin D deficiency and frailty: A systematic review and meta-analysis. *Maturitas* **2016**, *94*, 70–76. [CrossRef] [PubMed]
78. Sohl, E.; de Jongh, R.T.; Heijboer, A.C.; Swart, K.M.; Brouwer-Brolsma, E.M.; Enneman, A.W.; de Groot, C.P.; van der Velde, N.; Dhonukshe-Rutten, R.A.; Lips, P.; et al. Vitamin D status is associated with physical performance: The results of three independent cohorts. *Osteoporos. Int.* **2013**, *24*, 187–196. [CrossRef] [PubMed]
79. Houston, D.K.; Neiberg, R.H.; Tooze, J.A.; Hausman, D.B.; Johnson, M.A.; Cauley, J.A.; Bauer, D.C.; Shea, M.K.; Schwartz, G.G.; Williamson, J.D.; et al. Low 25-hydroxyvitamin D predicts the onset of mobility limitation and disability in community-dwelling older adults: The health abc study. *J. Gerontol. A Biol. Sci. Med. Sci* **2013**, *68*, 181–187. [CrossRef] [PubMed]
80. Wicherts, I.S.; van Schoor, N.M.; Boeke, A.J.; Visser, M.; Deeg, D.J.; Smit, J.; Knol, D.L.; Lips, P. Vitamin D status predicts physical performance and its decline in older persons. *J. Clin. Endocrinol. Metab.* **2007**, *92*, 2058–2065. [CrossRef] [PubMed]
81. Visser, M.; Deeg, D.J.; Lips, P.; Longitudinal Aging Study, A. Low vitamin D and high parathyroid hormone levels as determinants of loss of muscle strength and muscle mass (sarcopenia): The longitudinal aging study amsterdam. *J. Clin. Endocrinol. Metab.* **2003**, *88*, 5766–5772. [CrossRef] [PubMed]
82. Verreault, R.; Semba, R.D.; Volpato, S.; Ferrucci, L.; Fried, L.P.; Guralnik, J.M. Low serum vitamin D does not predict new disability or loss of muscle strength in older women. *J. Am. Geriatr. Soc.* **2002**, *50*, 912–917. [CrossRef] [PubMed]
83. Granic, A.; Hill, T.R.; Davies, K.; Jagger, C.; Adamson, A.; Siervo, M.; Kirkwood, T.B.; Mathers, J.C.; Sayer, A.A. Vitamin D status, muscle strength and physical performance decline in very old adults: A prospective study. *Nutrients* **2017**, *9*, 379. [CrossRef] [PubMed]
84. Annweiler, C.; Schott, A.M.; Berrut, G.; Fantino, B.; Beauchet, O. Vitamin D-related changes in physical performance: A systematic review. *J. Nutr. Health Aging* **2009**, *13*, 893–898. [CrossRef] [PubMed]
85. Muir, S.W.; Montero-Odasso, M. Effect of vitamin D supplementation on muscle strength, gait and balance in older adults: A systematic review and meta-analysis. *J. Am. Geriatr. Soc.* **2011**, *59*, 2291–2300. [CrossRef] [PubMed]
86. Rosendahl-Riise, H.; Spielau, U.; Ranhoff, A.H.; Gudbrandsen, O.A.; Dierkes, J. Vitamin D supplementation and its influence on muscle strength and mobility in community-dwelling older persons: A systematic review and meta-analysis. *J. Hum. Nutr. Diet.* **2017**, *30*, 3–15. [CrossRef] [PubMed]
87. Beaudart, C.; Buckinx, F.; Rabenda, V.; Gillain, S.; Cavalier, E.; Slomian, J.; Petermans, J.; Reginster, J.Y.; Bruyere, O. The effects of vitamin D on skeletal muscle strength, muscle mass, and muscle power: A systematic review and meta-analysis of randomized controlled trials. *J. Clin. Endocrinol. Metab.* **2014**, *99*, 4336–4345. [CrossRef] [PubMed]
88. Glendenning, P.; Zhu, K.; Inderjeeth, C.; Howat, P.; Lewis, J.R.; Prince, R.L. Effects of three-monthly oral 150,000 iu cholecalciferol supplementation on falls, mobility, and muscle strength in older postmenopausal women: A randomized controlled trial. *J. Bone Miner. Res.* **2012**, *27*, 170–176. [CrossRef] [PubMed]
89. Pirotta, S.; Kidgell, D.J.; Daly, R.M. Effects of vitamin D supplementation on neuroplasticity in older adults: A double-blinded, placebo-controlled randomised trial. *Osteoporos. Int.* **2015**, *26*, 131–140. [CrossRef] [PubMed]
90. Bischoff-Ferrari, H.A.; Dawson-Hughes, B.; Orav, E.; Staehelin, H.B.; Meyer, O.W.; Theiler, R.; Dick, W.; Willett, W.C.; Egli, A. Monthly high-dose vitamin D treatment for the prevention of functional decline: A randomized clinical trial. *JAMA Intern. Med.* **2016**, *176*, 175–183. [CrossRef] [PubMed]
91. Centers for Disease Control and Prevention. 10 Leading Causes of Injury Deaths by Age Group Highlighting Unintentional Injury Deaths, United States—2016. Available online: https://www.cdc.gov/injury/images/lc-charts/leading_causes_of_death_highlighting_unintentional_2016_1040w800h.gif (accessed on 8 August 2018).
92. Deandrea, S.; Lucenteforte, E.; Bravi, F.; Foschi, R.; La Vecchia, C.; Negri, E. Risk factors for falls in community-dwelling older people: A systematic review and meta-analysis. *Epidemiology* **2010**, *21*, 658–668. [CrossRef] [PubMed]

93. Bolland, M.J.; Grey, A.; Reid, I.R. Differences in overlapping meta-analyses of vitamin D supplements and falls. *J. Clin. Endocrinol. Metab.* **2014**, *99*, 4265–4272. [CrossRef] [PubMed]
94. Bolland, M.J.; Grey, A.; Reid, I.R. Vitamin D supplements and the risk of falls. *JAMA Intern. Med.* **2015**, *175*, 1723–1724. [CrossRef] [PubMed]
95. Bolland, M.J.; Grey, A.; Gamble, G.D.; Reid, I.R. Vitamin D supplementation and falls: A trial sequential meta-analysis. *Lancet Diabetes Endocrinol.* **2014**, *2*, 573–580. [CrossRef]
96. Guirguis-Blake, J.M.; Michael, Y.L.; Perdue, L.A.; Coppola, E.L.; Beil, T.L. Interventions to prevent falls in older adults: Updated evidence report and systematic review for the us preventive services task force. *JAMA* **2018**, *319*, 1705–1716. [CrossRef] [PubMed]
97. Sanders, K.M.; Stuart, A.L.; Williamson, E.J.; Simpson, J.A.; Kotowicz, M.A.; Young, D.; Nicholson, G.C. Annual high-dose oral vitamin D and falls and fractures in older women: A randomized controlled trial. *JAMA* **2010**, *303*, 1815–1822. [CrossRef] [PubMed]
98. U.S. Preventive Services Task Force. Interventions to prevent falls in community-dwelling older adults: Us preventive services task force recommendation statement. *JAMA* **2018**, *319*, 1696–1704. [CrossRef] [PubMed]
99. Burdge, G.C.; Jones, A.E.; Wootton, S.A. Eicosapentaenoic and docosapentaenoic acids are the principal products of alpha-linolenic acid metabolism in young men*. *Br. J. Nutr.* **2002**, *88*, 355–363. [CrossRef] [PubMed]
100. Burdge, G.C.; Wootton, S.A. Conversion of alpha-linolenic acid to eicosapentaenoic, docosapentaenoic and docosahexaenoic acids in young women. *Br. J. Nutr.* **2002**, *88*, 411–420. [CrossRef] [PubMed]
101. Simopoulos, A.P. Omega-3 fatty acids in inflammation and autoimmune diseases. *J. Am. Coll. Nutr.* **2002**, *21*, 495–505. [CrossRef] [PubMed]
102. Crupi, R.; Marino, A.; Cuzzocrea, S. N-3 fatty acids: Role in neurogenesis and neuroplasticity. *Curr. Med. Chem.* **2013**, *20*, 2953–2963. [CrossRef] [PubMed]
103. Tan, A.; Sullenbarger, B.; Prakash, R.; McDaniel, J.C. Supplementation with eicosapentaenoic acid and docosahexaenoic acid reduces high levels of circulating proinflammatory cytokines in aging adults: A randomized, controlled study. *Prostaglandins Leukot. Essent. Fatty Acids* **2018**, *132*, 23–29. [CrossRef] [PubMed]
104. Mozaffarian, D.; Lemaitre, R.N.; King, I.B.; Song, X.; Huang, H.; Sacks, F.M.; Rimm, E.B.; Wang, M.; Siscovick, D.S. Plasma phospholipid long-chain omega-3 fatty acids and total and cause-specific mortality in older adults: A cohort study. *Ann. Intern. Med.* **2013**, *158*, 515–525. [CrossRef] [PubMed]
105. Vannice, G.; Rasmussen, H. Position of the academy of nutrition and dietetics: Dietary fatty acids for healthy adults. *J. Acad. Nutr. Diet.* **2014**, *114*, 136–153. [CrossRef] [PubMed]
106. Papanikolaou, Y.; Brooks, J.; Reider, C.; Fulgoni, V.L., III. U.S. Adults are not meeting recommended levels for fish and omega-3 fatty acid intake: Results of an analysis using observational data from nhanes 2003–2008. *Nutr. J.* **2014**, *13*, 31. [CrossRef] [PubMed]
107. Ewaschuk, J.B.; Almasud, A.; Mazurak, V.C. Role of n-3 fatty acids in muscle loss and myosteatosis. *Appl. Physiol. Nutr. Metab.* **2014**, *39*, 654–662. [CrossRef] [PubMed]
108. Gray, S.R.; Mittendorfer, B. Fish oil-derived n-3 polyunsaturated fatty acids for the prevention and treatment of sarcopenia. *Curr. Opin. Clin. Nutr. Metab. Care* **2018**, *21*, 104–109. [CrossRef] [PubMed]
109. Lalia, A.Z.; Dasari, S.; Robinson, M.M.; Abid, H.; Morse, D.M.; Klaus, K.A.; Lanza, I.R. Influence of omega-3 fatty acids on skeletal muscle protein metabolism and mitochondrial bioenergetics in older adults. *Aging* **2017**, *9*, 1096–1129. [CrossRef] [PubMed]
110. Robinson, S.M.; Jameson, K.A.; Batelaan, S.F.; Martin, H.J.; Syddall, H.E.; Dennison, E.M.; Cooper, C.; Sayer, A.A.; Hertfordshire Cohort Study, G. Diet and its relationship with grip strength in community-dwelling older men and women: The hertfordshire cohort study. *J. Am. Geriatr. Soc.* **2008**, *56*, 84–90. [CrossRef] [PubMed]
111. Rousseau, J.H.; Kleppinger, A.; Kenny, A.M. Self-reported dietary intake of omega-3 fatty acids and association with bone and lower extremity function. *J. Am. Geriatr. Soc.* **2009**, *57*, 1781–1788. [CrossRef] [PubMed]
112. Brenna, J.T.; Plourde, M.; Stark, K.D.; Jones, P.J.; Lin, Y.H. Best practices for the design, laboratory analysis, and reporting of trials involving fatty acids. *Am. J. Clin. Nutr.* **2018**. [CrossRef] [PubMed]
113. Abbatecola, A.M.; Cherubini, A.; Guralnik, J.M.; Andres Lacueva, C.; Ruggiero, C.; Maggio, M.; Bandinelli, S.; Paolisso, G.; Ferrucci, L. Plasma polyunsaturated fatty acids and age-related physical performance decline. *Rejuvenation Res.* **2009**, *12*, 25–32. [CrossRef] [PubMed]

114. Frison, E.; Boirie, Y.; Peuchant, E.; Tabue-Teguo, M.; Barberger-Gateau, P.; Feart, C. Plasma fatty acid biomarkers are associated with gait speed in community-dwelling older adults: The three-city-bordeaux study. *Clin. Nutr.* **2015**. [CrossRef] [PubMed]
115. Fougere, B.; de Souto Barreto, P.; Goisser, S.; Soriano, G.; Guyonnet, S.; Andrieu, S.; Vellas, B.; Group, M.S. Red blood cell membrane omega-3 fatty acid levels and physical performance: Cross-sectional data from the mapt study. *Clin. Nutr.* **2018**, *37*, 1141–1144. [CrossRef] [PubMed]
116. Reinders, I.; Song, X.; Visser, M.; Eiriksdottir, G.; Gudnason, V.; Sigurdsson, S.; Aspelund, T.; Siggeirsdottir, K.; Brouwer, I.A.; Harris, T.B.; et al. Plasma phospholipid pufas are associated with greater muscle and knee extension strength but not with changes in muscle parameters in older adults. *J. Nutr.* **2015**, *145*, 105–112. [CrossRef] [PubMed]
117. Reinders, I.; Murphy, R.A.; Song, X.; Visser, M.; Cotch, M.F.; Lang, T.F.; Garcia, M.E.; Launer, L.J.; Siggeirsdottir, K.; Eiriksdottir, G.; et al. Polyunsaturated fatty acids in relation to incident mobility disability and decline in gait speed; the age, gene/environment susceptibility-reykjavik study. *Eur. J. Clin. Nutr.* **2015**, *69*, 489–493. [CrossRef] [PubMed]
118. Fougere, B.; Goisser, S.; Cantet, C.; Soriano, G.; Guyonnet, S.; De Souto Barreto, P.; Cesari, M.; Andrieu, S.; Vellas, B.; Group, M.S. Omega-3 fatty acid levels in red blood cell membranes and physical decline over 3 years: Longitudinal data from the mapt study. *Geroscience* **2017**. [CrossRef] [PubMed]
119. Hutchins-Wiese, H.L.; Kleppinger, A.; Annis, K.; Liva, E.; Lammi-Keefe, C.J.; Durham, H.A.; Kenny, A.M. The impact of supplemental n-3 long chain polyunsaturated fatty acids and dietary antioxidants on physical performance in postmenopausal women. *J. Nutr. Health Aging* **2013**, *17*, 76–80. [CrossRef] [PubMed]
120. Smith, G.I.; Julliand, S.; Reeds, D.N.; Sinacore, D.R.; Klein, S.; Mittendorfer, B. Fish oil-derived n-3 pufa therapy increases muscle mass and function in healthy older adults. *Am. J. Clin. Nutr.* **2015**, *102*, 115–122. [CrossRef] [PubMed]
121. Logan, S.L.; Spriet, L.L. Omega-3 fatty acid supplementation for 12 weeks increases resting and exercise metabolic rate in healthy community-dwelling older females. *PLoS ONE* **2015**, *10*, e0144828. [CrossRef] [PubMed]
122. Krzyminska-Siemaszko, R.; Czepulis, N.; Lewandowicz, M.; Zasadzka, E.; Suwalska, A.; Witowski, J.; Wieczorowska-Tobis, K. The effect of a 12-week omega-3 supplementation on body composition, muscle strength and physical performance in elderly individuals with decreased muscle mass. *Int J. Environ. Res. Public Health* **2015**, *12*, 10558–10574. [CrossRef] [PubMed]
123. Bo, Y.; Liu, C.; Ji, Z.; Yang, R.; An, Q.; Zhang, X.; You, J.; Duan, D.; Sun, Y.; Zhu, Y.; et al. A high whey protein, vitamin D and e supplement preserves muscle mass, strength, and quality of life in sarcopenic older adults: A double-blind randomized controlled trial. *Clin. Nutr.* **2018**. [CrossRef] [PubMed]
124. Chanet, A.; Verlaan, S.; Salles, J.; Giraudet, C.; Patrac, V.; Pidou, V.; Pouyet, C.; Hafnaoui, N.; Blot, A.; Cano, N.; et al. Supplementing breakfast with a vitamin D and leucine-enriched whey protein medical nutrition drink enhances postprandial muscle protein synthesis and muscle mass in healthy older men. *J. Nutr.* **2017**, *147*, 2262–2271. [CrossRef] [PubMed]
125. Bell, K.E.; Snijders, T.; Zulyniak, M.; Kumbhare, D.; Parise, G.; Chabowski, A.; Phillips, S.M. A whey protein-based multi-ingredient nutritional supplement stimulates gains in lean body mass and strength in healthy older men: A randomized controlled trial. *PLoS ONE* **2017**, *12*, e0181387. [CrossRef] [PubMed]
126. Bauer, J.M.; Verlaan, S.; Bautmans, I.; Brandt, K.; Donini, L.M.; Maggio, M.; McMurdo, M.E.; Mets, T.; Seal, C.; Wijers, S.L.; et al. Effects of a vitamin D and leucine-enriched whey protein nutritional supplement on measures of sarcopenia in older adults, the provide study: A randomized, double-blind, placebo-controlled trial. *J. Am. Med. Dir. Assoc.* **2015**, *16*, 740–747. [CrossRef] [PubMed]
127. Hangartner, T.N.; Warner, S.; Braillon, P.; Jankowski, L.; Shepherd, J. The official positions of the international society for clinical densitometry: Acquisition of dual-energy X-ray absorptiometry body composition and considerations regarding analysis and repeatability of measures. *J. Clin. Densitom.* **2013**, *16*, 520–536. [CrossRef] [PubMed]

5

Oxidative Stress, Telomere Shortening and Apoptosis Associated to Sarcopenia and Frailty in Patients with Multimorbidity

Máximo Bernabeu-Wittel [1,*], Raquel Gómez-Díaz [2], Álvaro González-Molina [1], Sofía Vidal-Serrano [3], Jesús Díez-Manglano [4], Fernando Salgado [5], María Soto-Martín [6], Manuel Ollero-Baturone [1]

1 Internal Medicine Department, Hospital Universitario Virgen del Rocío, 41013 Sevilla, Spain; aglezmolina@gmail.com (Á.G.-M.); m.ollero.baturone@gmail.com (M.O.-B.)
2 General and Multiple Use Laboratory, Instituto de Biomedicina de Sevilla, 41013 Sevilla, Spain; rgomez-ibis@us.es
3 Internal Medicine Department, Hospital San Juan de Dios del Aljarafe, 41930 Sevilla, Spain; sofiavidalserrano@gmail.com
4 Internal Medicine Department, Hospital Royo Villanova, 50015 Zaragoza, Spain; jdiez@aragon.es
5 Internal Medicine Department, Hospital Regional, 29010 Málaga, Spain; fersalord@gmail.com
6 Internal Medicine Department, Hospital Juan Ramón Jiménez, 21005 Huelva, Spain; msoto@hotmail.com
* Correspondence: wittel@cica.es.
† All researchers from the PROTEO project listed at Acknowledgments.

Abstract: Background: The presence of oxidative stress, telomere shortening, and apoptosis in polypathological patients (PP) with sarcopenia and frailty remains unknown. Methods: Multicentric prospective observational study in order to assess oxidative stress markers (catalase, glutathione reductase (GR), total antioxidant capacity to reactive oxygen species (TAC-ROS), and superoxide dismutase (SOD)), absolute telomere length (aTL), and apoptosis (DNA fragmentation) in peripheral blood samples of a hospital-based population of PP. Associations of these biomarkers to sarcopenia, frailty, functional status, and 12-month mortality were analyzed. Results: Of the 444 recruited patients, 97 (21.8%), 278 (62.6%), and 80 (18%) were sarcopenic, frail, or both, respectively. Oxidative stress markers (lower TAC-ROS and higher SOD) were significantly enhanced and aTL significantly shortened in patients with sarcopenia, frailty or both syndromes. No evidence of apoptosis was detected in blood leukocytes of any of the patients. Both oxidative stress markers (GR, $p = 0.04$) and telomere shortening ($p = 0.001$) were associated to death risk and to less survival days. Conclusions: Oxidative stress markers and telomere length were enhanced and shortened, respectively, in blood samples of polypathological patients with sarcopenia and/or frailty. Both were associated to decreased survival. They could be useful in the clinical practice to assess vulnerable populations with multimorbidity and of potential interest as therapeutic targets.

Keywords: multimorbidity; polypathological patients; sarcopenia; frailty; oxidative stress; telomere length; apoptosis

---

1. Introduction

As a result of populations' aging throughout the world, the prevalence of chronic conditions has drastically increased; these coexist frequently in the same patient, conditioning deleterious relationships, faster clinical and functional deterioration, poorer quality of life, and higher mortality. Taking multimorbidity seriously is of nuclear importance for the sustainability of all healthcare systems [1–3]. Multimorbidity is narrowly correlated to aging. As a matter of fact, there is a direct and strong correlation between the development of different chronic conditions and longevity. The easy explanation of this correlation is the longer exposure to different risk factors (environmental agents, unhealthy lifestyles, inherited risk factors, overuse deterioration), which impact in the development of diseases and failures of multiple organs and systems [3,4].

Sarcopenia and frailty are two major geriatric syndromes closely related to the aging process [5,6]. The development of one or both of them is linked to progressive functional disability, loss of quality of life and death. Their prevalence in elderly populations approximates 10% and 15%, respectively; however, in the presence of chronic conditions and multimorbidity, these prevalences can raise to 20% and 60%, respectively [7]. Both syndromes are narrowly interrelated; as a matter of fact, they have currently an identical therapeutic approach based on physical activity and optimal nutrition. In a recent study, both sarcopenia and frailty were present in the same patient in 18% of the studied cases; that is to say that most sarcopenic patients were frail, and about one third of frail patients were sarcopenic [7]. Nevertheless, these percentages are different in other studies, probably due to sample selection criteria [8].

Both syndromes have commonalities sharing a nuclear issue, which is the physical function impairment, usually assessed by different tools like walking speed and hand grip strength. Such impairment may be responsible for the concurrent existence of a disability in both phenotypes, but they also express differences; as a matter of fact, sarcopenia rather tends to assume the lineaments of cachexia and "muscle wasting", whereas frailty status is largely dominated by a low physical performance, homeostasis disruption to stressors, and disabling condition.

The deep and intimal relation between sarcopenia and frailty probably reflects that they share similar or identical pathophysiological routes and molecular mechanisms. In this field, many metabolic imbalances and other molecular factors have been studied and correlated in some ways to both geriatric syndromes. Sarcopenia has been associated to genetic expression of apoptosis and muscular autophagy, muscle androgenic and vitamin D receptors, chronic inflammation, oxidative stress, and telomere shortening [9–11]. On the other hand, frailty has been associated to inflammation pathways (demonstrated in the case of C-reactive protein, interleukin-1β, the IL-1 receptor antagonist, IL-18, and tumor necrosis factor alpha), unspecific immunological alterations linked to immunosenescence (mainly thymus involution and the corresponding decrease of T and B lymphocyte precursors and the reduction in the proliferative capacity of the T and B lymphocytes), and oxidative stress [12–14].

From these data, the narrow relation between frailty and sarcopenia can be extracted. This is more so in patients with multimorbidity, in which aging and chronic conditions may trigger more oxidative stress, telomere shortening, and apoptosis. In these patients, sarcopenia and frailty could be the results of a multisite "rusting" produced by chronic inflammation processes and their consequent imbalance between the production of reactive oxygen species (ROS) and cellular antioxidant defenses, present in chronic neurological, pulmonary, and cardiovascular diseases, along with atherosclerosis, diabetes, obesity, and arthritis. Nevertheless, the role and weight of any of these molecular alterations in sarcopenic and/or frail populations with multimorbidity remain unknown.

For all these reasons, we have explored the main oxidative stress markers, telomere length, and apoptosis parameters in a hospital-based multicenter cohort of multimorbidity patients. We hypothesized that all these biological markers have a deep impact and association to sarcopenia and frailty.

2. Patients and Methods

2.1. Development of the Study

This was a prospective observational, multi-institutional (6 centers) study carried out by researchers from the Polypathological Patient and Advanced Age Study Group of the Spanish Society of Internal Medicine (all participant centers are listed on the PROTEO Researchers list). The study was approved by the ethics committee of all participant centers. The study inclusion period ranged from January 2012 to March 2016.

All patients treated in the Internal Medicine and Geriatric areas who accomplished inclusion criteria (≥18 years old and fulfilling criteria of polypathological patient (PP)) were included, after providing their written informed consent. The patient's sample was collected by performing prevalence surveys every 14 days during the study period. A total of 155 surveys were performed (29 ± 19 surveys per hospital).

After receiving informed consent, a complete set of demographical, socio-familial, clinical, functional, biological, and pharmacological data were collected from all included patients.

Sarcopenia was defined following EWGSOP criteria [15]. This was established by the presence of a gait speed ≤ 0.8 m/seg, plus a skeletal muscle mass <6.76 Kg/m^2 in women, and <10.76 Kg/m^2 in men (for those patients able to walk) or a hand grip strength lower than 50 percentile of his/her age group and gender, and a skeletal muscle mass <6.76 Kg/m^2 in women and <10.76 Kg/m^2 in men (for those patents unable to walk). Frailty was defined when fulfilling 3 or more of Fried's criteria (slowness, weakness, weight loss, exhaustion, and low physical activity) [16].

All patients were clinically followed during a 12-month period in order to assess mortality, as previously described [7]. Time survival was assessed, and in case of death, chronology of the demise was incorporated. Therefore, we looked at mortality as a time-dependent outcome. For the dichotomous outcome, subjects were categorized depending on whether or not they survived 12 months from their initial interview date. For the continuous outcome, survival time was defined as the number of days between the baseline interview and the date of death. All these data were collected by clinicians in charge who were active members of the investigation team.

Ethics Committee Approval: The present study has been approved by the ethics committee of all participant centers (ethical approval code: CEI2012/PI242). Ethical Guidelines for Authorship and Publishing: The authors certify that they comply with the ethical guidelines for publishing in the Journal Clinical Medicine.

2.2. Biological Parameters Determination

We determined blood or plasma biological parameters of all included patients, including oxidative stress markers, apoptosis expression, and telomere length.

Oxidative stress markers: We determined activity/levels of catalase, glutathione reductase (GR), total antioxidant capacity to reactive oxygen species (TAC-ROS), and superoxide dismutase (SOD). Colorimetric studies were performed using a monochromator-based UV–VIS spectrophotometer (Multiskan® GO; Thermo Fisher Scientific Corporation, Carlsbad, CA, USA).

Catalase activity (nmol/min/mL) was measured in patients' plasma using the colorimetrical procedure provided by Cayman's Catalase Assay Kit, Item No. 707002 (Cayman Chemical, Ann Arbor, MI, USA). The method is based on the reaction of the enzyme wit methanol in the presence of an optimal concentration of H_2O_2. The formaldehyde produced is measured colorimetrically with Purpald as the chromogen. Purpald specifically forms a bicyclic heterocycle with aldehydes, which upon oxidation changes from colorless to purple color [17,18].

Glutathione reductase activity (U/mL; 1 Unit = the amount of enzyme that will cause the oxidation of 1.0 nmol of NADP to NADP+ per minute at 25 °C) was analyzed in patients' plasma by measuring the rate of NADPH oxidation, using for this purpose the Cayman's Glutathione reductase Assay Kit, Item No. 703202 (Cayman Chemical, Ann Arbor, MI, USA). The oxidation of NADPH is accompanied by a decrease in absorbance at 340 nm and is directly proportional to the GR activity in the sample [18,19].

Total antioxidant capacity to reactive oxygen species (mM Trolox equivalents) was analyzed measuring the ability of patients' plasma antioxidants to inhibit the oxidation of ABTS® (2,2′-Azino-di-3-ethylbenzthiazoline sulphonatel) to ABTS®+ by metmyoglobin. For this purpose, the Cayman's Antioxidant Assay Kit, Item No. 709001 (Cayman Chemical, Ann Arbor, MI, USA) was used. The antioxidants cause suppression of the absorbance at 750 nm or 405 nm to a degree that is proportional to their concentration. This capacity of the antioxidants is compared to that of Trolox, a water-soluble tocopherol analogue, and is quantified as millimolar Trolox equivalents [20,21].

Superoxide dismutase activity (U/mL) was measured in patients' plasma using the colorimetrical absorbance procedure provided by Cayman's Superoxide Dismutase Assay Kit, Item No. 706002 (Cayman Chemical, Ann Arbor, MI, USA). The method utilizes a tetrazolium salt for detection of superoxide radicals generated by xanthine oxidase and hypoxanthine. One unit of SOD is defined as the amount of enzyme needed to exhibit 50% dismutation of the superoxide radical. This assay measures all types of SOD (Cu/Zn-SOD, Mn-SOD, and Fe-SOD) [18].

Telomere length: We assessed telomere length following the procedure described by O'Callaghan and Fenech, in which the absolute telomere length (aTL) was measured [22]. For this purpose, we used Telomere standard Human/rodent (teloF and teloR) as primers for telomere length (TL) analysis and 36B4 standard human primers for single copy gene (SCG) determinations. All these were supplied by TaqMan™ Array Human Telomere Extension by Telomerase (Thermofisher Scientific, Waltham, MA, USA).

First standard curves were constructed for both experiments (TL and SCG). Then, all patients' samples were analyzed, and aTL was calculated dividing the absolute result of TL by the result of SCG. This result was again divided by 92 (each somatic human cell has 46 chromosomes, and each chromosome has 2 telomeres) in order to obtain the mean aTL per single telomere [22].

Apoptosis: In order to detect apoptosis, we evaluated possible DNA fragmentation in patients' leucocytes. For this purpose, we performed a DNA conventional constant field gel electrophoresis loading in a 0.8% agarose gel panel a total or 300 ng from a normalized purified DNA mixture with a DNA concentration of 30 ng/uL. DNA was purified by means of standard techniques already established [22]. When apoptosis is present, the result is fragmentation of DNA into multiples of 180 base-pair lengths; a characteristic "ladder" effect is obtained when these fragments are resolved in the agarose gel electrophoresis [23].

Statistical analysis: The dichotomous variables were described as whole numbers and percentages, and the continuous variables as mean and standard deviation (or median and interquartile rank (IQR) in those with no criteria of normal distribution). The distribution of all variables was analyzed with the Kolmorogov–Smirnov test. Possible biological parameters associated to the presence of sarcopenia and death were investigated performing the Student's *t* for normally distributed quantitative variables, and Mann–Whitney *U* test.

Finally, we also evaluated the association of these biological parameters with functional status (by means of basal Barthel index), death risk (by means of PROFUND index), and survival (considering death as a time-dependent variable), using linear regression models. Statistical significance was considered when obtained p values were ≤0.05. Statistics were performed using the SPSS 22.0 software (IBM, Armonk, NY, USA).

3. Results

We included 444 patients with a mean age of 77.3 ± 8.4 years. Fifty-five percent were male. The main clinical features and biological parameters of the recruited patients are detailed in Table 1. Sarcopenia was present in 97 (21.8%), frailty in 278 (62.6%), and the remaining 69 (15.6%) were robust. Eighty patients (18% of the whole cohort) out of those with sarcopenia or frailty had simultaneously both phenotypes.

And combined sarcopenia and frailty were present in 80 (18%) patients. Mortality in the 12-months follow-up period was 40% (N = 178). A detailed clinical description of the included patients has already been published [7]; briefly, sarcopenia was more frequent in men, and associated to chronic lung diseases, cancer, lower BMI, and previous hospital admissions, whereas frailty was more frequent in women and associated to a higher number of polypathology categories, chronic pain, anxiety, and pressure ulcers; both phenotypes shared association with age, asthenia, and lower BI scores.

Table 1. Main clinical and biological features of a multicenter sample of 444 polypathological patients recruited for sarcopenia and frailty assessment.

Clinical Features	Mean (SD)/Median -IQR-/*N* (%)
Number of defining categories (major diseases) per patient	2.5 (0.5)
Prevalence of defining categories (major diseases)	
Heart diseases	374 (84.6%)
Kidney/autoimmune diseases	202 (45.7%)
Lung diseases	183 (41.4%)
Neurological diseases	133 (30.1%)
Peripheral arterial disease/diabetes with neuropathy	80 (18.1%)
Neoplasia/chronic anemia	70 (15.8%)
Degenerative osteoarticular disease	43 (9.7%)
Liver disease	28 (6.3%)
Number of other comorbidities per patient	5.9 (2.3)
Most frequent comorbidities	
Hypertension	380 (86%)
Dyslipemia	232 (52.5%)
Diabetes with no visceral involvement	216 (49%)
Atrial fibrillation	178 (40%)
Obesity	159 (36%)
Anxiety and depressive disorders	74 (17%)
Benign prostate hyperplasia	64 (14.5%)
Frequent symptoms	
Fatigue	304 (70%)
Anorexia	212 (48%)
Insomnia	194 (44%)
Chronic pain	178 (40%)
Cough	158 (36%)
Patients with basal III-IV class of NYHA//III–IV class of mMRC	128 (29%)
PROFUND index	6 -6-
Basal Barthel's Index	66 (30)
BMI (Kg/m^2)	30 (6.6%)
Main biological parameters	
Hemoglobin (d/dL)	11.3 (2)
Creatinin (mg/dL)	1.26 (1)
Albumin (g/dL)	3.2 (0.9)
Cholesterol (mg/dL)	151 (42)
Triglicerydes (mg/dL)	116 -80-
Vitamin D (ng/mL)	11 -17-
Leucocytes (n°/µL)	8000 -4000-
Lymphocytes (n°/µL)	1200 -400-

SD: standard deviation; IQR: interquartile range; NYHA: New York Heart Association; mMRC: Medical Research Council. BMI: body mass index.

3.1. Oxidative Stress Markers

Median catalase and GR activity were 53 nmol/min/mL (IQR = 20–83), and 9.8 U/mL (IQR = 6.6–13.2), respectively. Total antioxidant activity against ROS was 2.4 mM Trolox equivalents (IQR = 1.8–3). Finally, median SOD activity was 4.6 U/mL (IQR = 2.8–6.6).

Differences of oxidative stress markers in patients with sarcopenia, frailty, or those with both conditions with respect to those without sarcopenia, robust, or those without both conditions are detailed in Table 2.

Table 2. Differences of oxidative stress markers, telomere length, and apoptosis markers in patients with multimorbidity according to their sarcopenia and frailty assessment.

Molecular Parameter	**Sarcopenia and Frailty Assessment**		*p*
Sarcopenia	**Not Sarcopenic**	**Sarcopenic**	
	Oxidative stress marker		
CAT	52 (12.6–82) *	58 (29.4–87.8)	0.16
GR	9.8 (6.8–13.4)	9.9 (5.5–13)	0.45
TAC-ROS	2.42 (1.8–3)	2.29 (1.75–2.8)	0.12
SOD	4.4 (2.7–6.5)	5.8 (3.7–6.9)	0.02
Absolute telomere length	4.96 (0.7–19)	1.65 (0.6–3.9)	0.001
Apoptosis (WBC DNA fragmentation)	No evidence	No evidence	-
Frailty	**Robust**	**Frail**	
	Oxidative stress marker		
CAT	55.6 (21.7–80)	51.4 (19–83.5)	0.6
GR	9.1 (5.3–9)	10.2 (6.9–13.5)	0.12
TAC-ROS	3.5 (1.6–9)	3.3 (1.9–3)	0.044
SOD	3.8 (2.3–6.2)	5.1 (3.2–7)	0.002
Absolute telomere length	5.7 (1.7–19)	1.5 (0.6–3.4)	<0.0001
Apoptosis (WBC DNA fragmentation)	No evidence	No evidence	-
Sarcopenia and Frailty	**Not Sarcopenic and Robust**	**Sarcopenic and Frail**	
	Oxidative stress marker		
CAT	46.4 (46.5–77.5)	51.5 (26.2–79)	0.2
GR	9.7 (6.7–13.2)	10.1 (5.9–14)	0.5
TAC-ROS	2.4 (1.8–3.1)	2.2 (1.8–2.8)	0.08
SOD	4.4 (2.8–6.4)	5.7 (4.1–6.4)	0.0012
Absolute telomere length	6.5 (0.7–20)	1.5 (0.6–3.8)	<0.0001
Apoptosis (WBC DNA fragmentation)	No evidence	No evidence	-

CAT: catalase (nmol/min/mL); GR: Glutathione reductase (U/mL); TAC-ROS: total antioxidant activity against reactive oxygen species (mM Trolox equivalents); SOD: superoxide dismutase (U/mL); absolute telomere length (kbases/telomere); * Interquartile range; WBC: white blood cells; DNA: deoxyribonucleic acid.

3.2. *Absolute Telomere Length Analysis*

Mean aTL was 2 kbases per telomere (IQR = 0.1–55). Differences of aTL in patients with sarcopenia, frailty, or those with both conditions with respect to those without sarcopenia, robust, or those without both conditions are also detailed in Table 2.

3.3. *Apoptosis*

Apoptosis by means of DNA fragmentation analysis was not present in any of the patients included in the study.

3.4. *Functional Parameters, Death Risk by PROFUND Index and Survival according to Different Molecular Parameters*

A worse functional status by means of lower Barthel's index score was associated to shorter telomere length (Beta = 1.25 (1.07–1.34)); $p = 0.001$), but not with any of the oxidative stress markers.

A higher death risk by means of PROFUND index was associated to shorter telomere length (Beta = 0.5 (0.14–0.65); $p = 0.001$) and to a higher GR activity (Beta = 1.7 (1.2–2); $p = 0.04$). On the other hand, a lower number of survival days was associated to shorter telomere length (Beta = 1.2 (1.01–1.32); $p = 0.003$) and to a higher GR activity (Beta = 0.3 (0.1–0.24)); $p = 0.02$).

4. Discussion

In the present study, we have detected enhanced oxidative stress and significant telomere shortening in PP with sarcopenia, frailty, or both syndromes combined. On the contrary, no evidence of apoptosis was detected.

Sarcopenia was prevalent in our cohort of polypathological patients and was associated to a significant higher SOD activity; other oxidative stress markers activity was also elevated, and the TAC-ROS decreased, but differences in these last were not significant. In the same way, we observed a significant telomere length shortening in these patients compared to other PP without sarcopenia. These results are highly concordant with the pathogenesis of sarcopenia in the elderly as already demonstrated by other authors [24–27]. Many authors have compared these markers among elderly and young people [28]; in the present study we have also detected important differences among elderly patients with chronic conditions with or without sarcopenia. These findings could have two major clinical applications: first, to use them as biological markers of sarcopenia in the elderly compared to persons of the same age; and second, to guide future treatments towards these targets in order to avoid or delay the development of sarcopenia. With respect to oxidative stress, SOD was the marker with the largest differences among PP with or without sarcopenia. As a matter of fact, SOD has been already strongly linked to muscular weakness, muscular wasting, and sarcopenia in clinical and experimental scenarios [29–31]; in this sense, among others, probably SOD could be the optimal oxidative stress marker in the evaluation of sarcopenia.

Frailty was also highly prevalent in the studied PP cohort and was associated to a significant increase in SOD activity and a decreased plasma TAC-ROS. It was also associated to a significant telomere length shortening compared to other PP without frailty. The deep relation between sarcopenia and frailty is already known; they share molecular and physiological pathways, symptoms, signs, and clinical phenotypes [32,33], so the presence of these molecular alterations in both of them is biologically coherent. In this case, we also observed a decreased antioxidant fitness of the plasma in frail PP. As main differences, frailty is more age related, whereas sarcopenia is also related to disease, starvation, and disuse [34]; additionally, despite criteria defining the two conditions overlap, frailty requires weight loss, whereas sarcopenia requires muscle loss [34,35].

In PP with sarcopenia and/or frailty we have observed the coexistence of telomere shortening and enhanced oxidative stress. There is accumulating evidence of the role of oxidative stress in DNA damage and telomere shortening with aging and chronic diseases [36]. These changes have been observed in humans, as well as in mouse models and cell cultures [36]. There are probably mixed mechanisms in this narrow relation of oxidative stress and telomere length. In aging and in many chronic conditions, processes associated to chronic inflammation play a nuclear role. Chronic inflammation is characterized by higher oxidative stress in affected tissues and circulating plasma. This may lead to direct cell DNA damage, including telomere regions. Additionally, inflammatory states are associated to enhanced necrosis and cellular regeneration cycles, and this increased cell turnover directly affects telomere length [37–42]. Many authors already point out that targeting oxidative stress could be of notable benefit in telomere length maintenance, especially in populations with chronic conditions like patients in the present study [39–42].

We did not detect any DNA fragmentation in our patients' leucocytes, so no apoptosis evidence could be detected in PP's blood samples by this technique. Apoptosis pathways have been classically associated to sarcopenia and frailty and nowadays are considered one of the main causes of these two syndromes [43,44]. As a matter of fact, there is multiple evidence of apoptosis presence in muscle tissue of experimental animal models, as well as in humans with sarcopenia [45–49]. Nevertheless, no information is available about the presence of apoptosis evidence in blood leukocytes of patients with sarcopenia and/or frailty. Some authors have described indirect apoptosis pathways data in blood leucocytes in elderly and in patients with dementia (like less resistance to experimental apoptosis inducers; senescence of CD8+ T-cells; and increased expression of HLA-DR, CD95, and Bcl-2 in CD3+ lymphocytes) [50]. Recently, increased ROS production and DNA fragmentation has been observed in blood monocytes of atherosclerotic mice, uprising again the interrelations of oxidative stress and apoptosis signaling [51]. Apoptosis will for sure be present in muscle tissues of patients with sarcopenia and frailty, like enhanced oxidative stress and telomere shortening. Nevertheless, according to our data, an easy detection of its presence in blood samples from these patients is probably not useful in the clinical setting, and demonstrating it in tissue specimens is not clinically justified.

A poorer functional status, higher mortality risk, and less survival days in the 12-month follow-up were associated to shorter telomere length; besides, mortality risk and survival days were also associated to enhanced GR activity. These data are in concordance with previous studies in which telomere shortening has been associated to poorer survival in cancer, diabetes, cardiovascular diseases, and even to higher all-cause mortality [52–56]; additionally, oxidative stress has also been related to poor health outcomes in many clinical scenarios, and to all-cause mortality [57–60]. Our data confirm this deleterious relationships with sarcopenia and frailty in patients with multimorbidity, as well as the association to poorer functional status. Some authors have already claimed the clinical usefulness of biomarkers' panels including aTL, if we want to accurately assess and predict outcomes in vulnerable aged populations [61]. We suggest including also oxidative stress markers in these panels, mainly GR, TAC-ROS, and SOD.

This study has some limitations that should be noted. The results could be limited by the number of patients, but on the other hand, the cohort was recruited in various centers, was homogeneous, and probably represents adequately hospital-based populations with moderate–severe multimorbidity. Additionally, the studied biomarkers are also associated to some of the chronic conditions of the included patients and could raise the question of their real correlation to sarcopenia and frailty; this issue always underlies the frailty and sarcopenia phenotypes, since they have multiple concurrent causes, with a prominent role of debilitating chronic diseases; in our opinion, they behave as parts of the same clinical-molecular syndrome; as a matter of fact, the term "inflamm-aging" is already established, and probably in the future, it will be necessary to add chronic conditions and call it "inflamm-chronic-aging".

In conclusion, oxidative stress and telomere shortening, but not apoptosis markers, were enhanced in blood samples of polypathological patients with sarcopenia and/or frailty with respect to those patients without these two geriatric syndromes. Telomere shortening was associated to functional decline, and both, oxidative stress markers and telomere shortening, were associated to higher mortality risks and decreased survival. Both of these biomarkers could be useful in the clinical evaluation of vulnerable patients prone to sarcopenia and frailty and of potential interest as therapeutic targets.

Author Contributions: Conceptualization, M.B.-W. and M.O.-B.; Formal analysis, M.B.-W.; Investigation, M.B.-W., R.G.-D., Á.G.-M., S.V.-S., J.D.-M., F.S. and M.S.-M.; Methodology, M.B.-W., R.G.-D. and J.D.-M.; Supervision, M.O.-B.; Visualization, M.O.-B.; Writing–original draft, M.B.-W.; Writing–review & editing, Á.G.-M. and M.O.-B. All authors have contributed substantially to the work. All authors have read and agreed to the published version of the manuscript.

Acknowledgments: Special thanks to all researchers from the proteo project listed below. Máximo Bernabeu-Wittel (1), Álvaro González-Molina (1), Rocío Fernández-Ojeda (2), Jesús Díez-Manglano (3), Fernando Salgado-Ordóñez (4), María Soto-Martín (5), Marta Muniesa (6), Manuel Ollero-Baturone (1), Juan Gómez-Salgado (7), Sofía Vidal-Serrano (2), Adriana Rivera-Sequeiros (2), Antonio Fernández-Moyano (2), Lourdes Moreno-Gaviño (1), Dolores Nieto-Martín (1), Nieves Ramírez-Duque (1), Esther del Corral-Beamonte (3), Pablo Martínez-Rodés (3), María Sevil-Puras (3), Rosa Bernal-López (4), Ricardo Gómez-Huelgas (4), Bosco Barón-Franco (5). Hospitals: (1) Hospital Universitario Virgen del Rocío, Sevilla, Spain; (2) Hospital San Juan de Dios del Aljarafe, Sevilla, Spain; (3) Hospital Royo Villanova, Zaragoza, Spain; (4) Hospital Regional, Málaga, Spain; (5) Hospital Juan Ramón Jiménez, Huelva, Spain; (6) Hospital San Juan de Dios de Pamplona, Pamplona, Spain; (7) School of Nursery, University of Huelva, Spain.

References

1. Colombo, F.; García-Goñi, M.; Schwierz, C. Addressing multimorbidity to improve healthcare and economic sustainability. *J. Comorb.* **2016**, *6*, 21–27. [CrossRef] [PubMed]
2. Yarnall, A.J.; Sayer, A.A.; Clegg, A.; Rockwood, K.; Parker, S.; Hindle, J.V. New horizons in multimorbidity in older adults. *Age Ageing* **2017**, *46*, 882–888. [CrossRef] [PubMed]
3. Puth, M.T.; Weckbecker, K.; Schmid, M.; Münster, E. Prevalence of multimorbidity in Germany: Impact of age and educational level in a cross-sectional study on 19,294 adults. *BMC Public Health* **2017**, *17*, 826. [CrossRef] [PubMed]
4. Fabbri, E.; Zoli, M.; Gonzalez-Freire, M.; Salive, M.E.; Studenski, S.A.; Ferrucci, L. Aging and multimorbidity: New tasks, priorities, and frontiers for integrated gerontological and clinical research. *J. Am. Med. Dir. Assoc.* **2015**, *16*, 640–647. [CrossRef]
5. Von Haehling, S.; Morley, J.E.; Anker, S.D. An overview of sarcopenia: Facts and numbers on prevalence and clinical impact. *J. Cachex Sarcopenia Muscle* **2010**, *1*, 129–133. [CrossRef]
6. Ligthart-Melis, G.C.; Luiking, Y.C.; Kakourou, A.; Cederholm, T.; Maier, A.B.; de van der Schueren, M.A.E. Frailty, Sarcopenia, and Malnutrition Frequently (Co-)occur in Hospitalized Older Adults: A Systematic Review and Meta-analysis. *J. Am. Med. Dir. Assoc.* **2020**. online ahead of print. [CrossRef]
7. Bernabeu-Wittel, M.; González-Molina, Á.; Fernández-Ojeda, R.; Díez-Manglano, J.; Salgado, F.; Soto-Martín, M.; Muniesa, M.; Ollero-Baturone, M.; Gómez-Salgado, J. Impact of sarcopenia and frailty in a multicenter cohort of polypathological patients. *J. Clin. Med.* **2019**, *8*, 535. [CrossRef]
8. Davies, B.; García, F.; Ara, I.; Artalejo, F.R.; Rodriguez-Mañas, L.; Walter, S. Relationship between sarcopenia and frailty in the toledo study of healthy aging: A population based cross-sectional study. *J. Am. Med. Dir. Assoc.* **2018**, *19*, 282–286. [CrossRef]
9. Shafiee, G.; Keshtkar, A.; Soltani, A.; Ahadi, Z.; Larijani, B.; Heshmat, R. Prevalence of sarcopenia in the world: A systematic review and meta-analysis of general population studies. *J. Diabetes Metab. Disord.* **2017**, *16*, 21. [CrossRef]
10. Marty, E.; Liu, Y.; Samuel, A.; Or, O.; Lane, J. A review of sarcopenia: Enhancing awareness of an increasingly prevalent disease. *Bone* **2017**, *105*, 276–286. [CrossRef]
11. Tournadre, A.; Vial, G.; Capel, F.; Soubrier, M.; Boirie, Y. Sarcopenia. *Jt. Bone Spine* **2019**, *86*, 309–314. [CrossRef]
12. Xue, Q.L. The frailty syndrome: Definition and natural history. *Clin. Geriatr. Med.* **2011**, *27*, 1–15. [CrossRef] [PubMed]
13. Wou, F.; Conroy, S. The frailty syndrome. *Medicine* **2013**, *41*, 13–15. [CrossRef]
14. Wang, J.; Maxwell, C.A.; Yu, F. Biological processes and biomarkers related to frailty in older adults: A state-of-the-science literature review. *Biol. Res. Nurs.* **2019**, *21*, 80–106. [CrossRef] [PubMed]
15. Cruz-Jentoft, A.J.; Baeyens, J.P.; Bauer, J.M.; Boirie, Y.; Cederholm, T.; Landi, F.; Martin, F.C.; Michel, J.-P.; Rolland, Y.; Schneider, S.M.; et al. Sarcopenia: European consensus on definition and diagnosis. Report of the European Working Group on Sarcopenia in Older People. *Age Ageing* **2010**, *39*, 412–423. [CrossRef]
16. Fried, L.P.; Tangen, C.M.; Walston, J.; Newman, A.B.; Hirsch, C.; Gottdiener, J.; Seeman, T.; Tracy, R.; Kop, W.J.; Burke, G.; et al. Frailty in older adults: Evidence for a phenotype. *J. Gerontol. Ser. A Boil. Sci. Med. Sci.* **2001**, *56*, M146–M157. [CrossRef]
17. Johansson, L.H.; Borgh, L.A.H. A spectrophotometric method for determination of catalase activity in small tissue samples. *Anal. Biochem.* **1988**, *174*, 331–336. [CrossRef]
18. Wheeler, C.R.; Salzman, J.A.; Elsayed, N.M.; Omaye, S.T.; Korte, D.W. Automated assays for superoxide dismutase, catalase, glutathione peroxidase, and glutathione reductase activity. *Anal. Biochem.* **1990**, *184*, 193–199. [CrossRef]
19. Carlberg, I.; Mannervik, B. Glutathione reductase. *Met. Enzymol.* **1985**, *113*, 484–490.
20. Miller, N.; Rice-Evans, C. Factors influencing the antioxidant activity detemirned by the $ABTS^+$ radical cation assay. *Free Radic. Res.* **1997**, *26*, 195–199. [CrossRef]
21. Koracevic, D.; Harris, G.; Rayner, A.; Blair, J.; Watt, B.; Koracevic, G.; Djordjevic, V.; Andrejevic, S.; Cosic, V. Method for the measurement of antioxidant activity in human fluids. *J. Clin. Pathol.* **2001**, *54*, 356–361. [CrossRef] [PubMed]

22. O'Callaghan, N.J.; Fenech, M. A quantitative PCR method for measuring absolute telomere length. *Biol. Proc. Online* **2011**, *13*, 3–13. [CrossRef] [PubMed]
23. Allen, P.D.; Newland, A.C. Electrophoretic DNA analysis for the detection of apoptosis. *Mol. Biotechnol.* **1998**, *9*, 247–251. [CrossRef] [PubMed]
24. Liguori, I.; Russo, G.; Curcio, F.; Bulli, G.; Aran, L.; Della-Morte, D.; Gargiulo, G.; Testa, G.; Francesco, C.; Domenico, B.; et al. Oxidative stress, aging, and diseases. *Clin. Interv. Aging* **2018**, *13*, 757–772. [CrossRef] [PubMed]
25. Marzetti, E.; Calvani, R.; Cesari, M.; Buford, T.W.; Lorenzi, M.; Behnke, B.J.; Leeuwenburgh, C. Mitochondrial dysfunction and sarcopenia of aging: From signaling pathways to clinical trials. *Int. J. Biochem. Cell Biol.* **2013**, *45*, 2288–2301. [CrossRef]
26. Kameda, M.; Teruya, T.; Yanagida, M.; Kondoh, H. Frailty markers comprise blood metabolites involved in antioxidation, cognition, and mobility. *Proc. Natl. Acad. Sci. USA* **2020**, *117*, 9483–9489. [CrossRef]
27. Marzetti, E.; Lorenzi, M.; Antocicco, M.; Bonassi, S.; Celi, M.; Mastropaolo, S.; Settanni, S.; Valdiglesias, V.; Landi, F.; Bernabei, R.; et al. Shorter telomeres in peripheral blood mononuclear cells from older persons with sarcopenia: Results from an exploratory study. *Front. Aging Neurosci.* **2014**, *6*, 233. [CrossRef]
28. Fasching, C.L. Telomere length measurement as a clinical biomarker of aging and disease. *Crit. Rev. Clin. Lab. Sci.* **2018**, *55*, 443–465. [CrossRef]
29. Muller, F.L.; Song, W.; Liu, Y.; Chaudhuri, A.; Pieke-Dahl, S.; Strong, R.; Huang, T.T.; Epstein, C.J.; Roberts, L.J., 2nd; Csete, M.; et al. Absence of CuZn superoxide dismutase leads to elevated oxidative stress and acceleration of age-dependent skeletal muscle atrophy. *Free Radic. Biol. Med.* **2006**, *40*, 1993–2004. [CrossRef]
30. Barreiro, E.; Coronell, C.; Laviña, B.; Ramírez-Sarmiento, A.; Orozco-Levi, M.; Gea, J. PENAM Project. Aging, sex differences, and oxidative stress in human respiratory and limb muscles. *Free Radic. Biol. Med.* **2006**, *41*, 797–809. [CrossRef]
31. Belenguer-Varea, Á.; Tarazona-Santabalbina, F.J.; Avellana-Zaragoza, J.A.; Martínez-Reig, M.; Mas-Bargues, C.; Inglés, M. Oxidative stress and exceptional human longevity: Systematic review. *Free Radic. Biol. Med.* **2019**. [CrossRef] [PubMed]
32. Reijnierse, E.M.; Trappenburg, M.C.; Blauw, G.J.; Verlaan, S.; de van der Schueren, M.A.; Meskers, C.G.; Maier, A.B. Common ground? The concordance of sarcopenia and frailty definitions. *J. Am. Med. Dir. Assoc.* **2015**, *17*, 371. [CrossRef] [PubMed]
33. Carmeli, E. Frailty and primary sarcopenia: A review. *Adv. Exp. Med. Biol.* **2017**, *1020*, 53–68. [PubMed]
34. Cederholm, T. Overlaps between frailty and sarcopenia definitions. *Nestle Nutr. Inst. Workshop Ser.* **2015**, *83*, 65–69. [PubMed]
35. Cruz-Jentoft, A.J.; Kiesswetter, E.; Drey, M.; Sieber, C.C. Nutrition, frailty, and sarcopenia. *Aging Clin. Exp. Res.* **2017**, *29*, 43–48. [CrossRef]
36. Barnes, R.P.; Fouquerel, R.P.; Opresko, P.L. The impact of oxidative DNA damage and stress on telomere homeostasis. *Mech. Ageing Dev.* **2019**, *177*, 37–45. [CrossRef]
37. Richter, T.; von Zglinicki, T. A continuous correlation between oxidative stress and telomere shortening in fibroblasts. *Exp. Gerontol.* **2007**, *42*, 1039–1042. [CrossRef]
38. Reichert, S.; Stier, A. Does oxidative stress shorten telomeres in vivo? A review. *Biol. Lett.* **2017**, *13*, 20170463. [CrossRef]
39. Markkanen, E. Not breathing is not an option: How to deal with oxidative DNA damage. *DNA Repair* **2017**, *59*, 82–105. [CrossRef]
40. Martens, D.S.; Nawrot, T.S. Air pollution stress and the aging phenotype: The telomere connection. *Curr. Environ. Health Rep.* **2016**, *3*, 258–269. [CrossRef]
41. Von Zglinicki, T. Oxidative stress shortens telomeres. *Trends Biochem. Sci.* **2002**, *27*, 339–344. [CrossRef]
42. Sfeir, A.; Kosiyatrakul, S.T.; Hockemeyer, D.; MacRae, S.L.; Karlseder, J.; Schildkraut, C.L.; de Lange, T. Mammalian telomeres resemble fragile sites and require TRF1 for efficient replication. *Cell* **2009**, *138*, 90–103. [CrossRef] [PubMed]
43. Marzetti, E.; Calvani, R.; Bernabei, R.; Leeuwenburgh, C. Apoptosis in skeletal myocytes: A potential target for interventions against sarcopenia and physical frailty—A mini-review. *Gerontology* **2012**, *58*, 99–106. [CrossRef] [PubMed]

44. Marzetti, E.; Leeuwenburgh, C. Skeletal muscle apoptosis, sarcopenia and frailty at old age. *Exp. Gerontol.* **2006**, *41*, 1234–1238. [CrossRef]
45. Du, J.; Wang, X.; Miereles, C.; Bailey, J.L.; Debigare, R.; Zheng, B.; Price, S.R.; Mitch, W.E. Activation of caspase-3 is an initial step triggering accelerated muscle proteolysis in catabolic conditions. *J. Clin. Investig.* **2004**, *113*, 115–123. [CrossRef]
46. Argiles, J.M.; Lopez-Soriano, F.J.; Busquets, S. Apoptosis signalling is essential and precedes protein degradation in wasting skeletal muscle during catabolic conditions. *Int. J. Biochem. Cell Biol.* **2008**, *40*, 1674–1678. [CrossRef]
47. Schindowski, K.; Leutner, S.; Müller, W.E.; Eckert, A. Age-related changes of apoptotic cell death in human lymphocytes. *Neurobiol. Aging* **2000**, *21*, 661–670. [CrossRef]
48. Effros, R.B. Replicative senescence of CD8 T cells: Effect on human ageing. *Exp. Gerontol.* **2004**, *39*, 517–524. [CrossRef]
49. Hodkinson, C.F.; O'Connor, J.M.; Alexander, H.D.; Bradbury, I.; Bonham, M.P.; Hannigan, B.M.; Gilmore, W.S.; Strain, J.J.; Wallace, J.M. Whole blood analysis of phagocytosis, apoptosis, cytokine production, and leukocyte subsets in healthy older men and women: The ZENITH study. *J. Gerontol. A Biol. Sci. Med. Sci.* **2006**, *61*, 907–917. [CrossRef]
50. Leuner, K.; Schulz, K.; Schütt, T.; Pantel, J.; Prvulovic, D.; Rhein, V.; Savaskan, E.; Czech, C.; Eckert, A.; Müller, W.E. Peripheral mitochondrial dysfunction in Alzheimer's disease: Focus on lymphocytes. *Mol. Neurobiol.* **2012**, *46*, 194–204. [CrossRef]
51. Jacinto, T.A.; Meireles, G.S.; Dias, A.T.; Aires, R.; Porto, M.L.; Gava, A.L.; Gava, A.L.; Meyrelles, S.S. Increased ROS production and DNA damage in monocytes are biomarkers of aging and atherosclerosis. *Biol. Res.* **2018**, *51*, 33. [CrossRef] [PubMed]
52. Pusceddu, I.; Kleber, M.; Delgado, G.; Herrmann, W.; März, W.; Herrmann, M. Telomere length and mortality in the Ludwigshafen Risk and Cardiovascular Health study. *PLoS ONE* **2018**, *13*, e0198373. [CrossRef] [PubMed]
53. Bonfigli, A.R.; Spazzafumo, L.; Prattichizzo, F.; Bonafè, M.; Mensà, E.; Micolucci, L.; Giuliani, A.; Fabbietti, P.; Testa, R.; Boemi, M.; et al. Leukocyte telomere length and mortality risk in patients with type 2 diabetes. *Oncotarget* **2016**, *7*, 50835–50844. [CrossRef] [PubMed]
54. Bendix, L.; Thinggaard, M.; Fenger, M.; Kolvraa, S.; Avlund, K.; Linneberg, A.; Osler, M. Longitudinal changes in leukocyte telomere length and mortality in humans. *J. Gerontol. A Biol. Sci. Med. Sci.* **2014**, *69*, 231–239. [CrossRef] [PubMed]
55. Weischer, M.; Nordestgaard, B.G.; Cawthon, R.M.; Freiberg, J.J.; Tybjærg-Hansen, A.; Bojesen, S.E. Short telomere length, cancer survival, and cancer risk in 47102 individuals. *J. Natl. Cancer Instig.* **2013**, *105*, 459–468. [CrossRef]
56. Wang, Q.; Zhan, Y.; Pedersen, N.L.; Fang, F.; Hägg, S. Telomere length and all-cause mortality: A meta-analysis. *Ageing Res. Rev.* **2018**, *48*, 11–20. [CrossRef]
57. Schöttker, B.; Saum, K.U.; Jansen, E.H.; Boffetta, P.; Trichopoulou, A.; Holleczek, B.; Dieffenbach, A.K.; Brenner, H. Oxidative stress markers and all-cause mortality at older age: A population-based cohort study. *J. Gerontol. A Biol. Sci. Med. Sci.* **2015**, *70*, 518–524. [CrossRef]
58. Xuan, Y.; Gào, X.; Anusruti, A.; Holleczek, B.; Jansen, E.H.J.M.; Muhlack, D.C.; Brenner, H.; Schöttker, B. Association of serum markers of oxidative stress with incident major cardiovascular events, cancer incidence, and all-cause mortality in type 2 diabetes patients: Pooled results from two cohort studies. *Diabetes Care* **2019**, *42*, 1436–1445. [CrossRef]
59. Gao, X.; Gào, X.; Zhang, Y.; Holleczek, B.; Schöttker, B.; Brenner, H. Oxidative stress and epigenetic mortality risk score: Associations with all-cause mortality among elderly people. *Eur. J. Epidemiol.* **2019**, *34*, 451–462. [CrossRef]
60. Xuan, Y.; Bobak, M.; Anusruti, A.; Jansen, E.H.J.M.; Pająk, A.; Tamosiunas, A.; Saum, K.-U.; Holleczek, B.; Gao, X.; Brenner, H.; et al. Association of serum markers of oxidative stress with myocardial infarction and stroke: Pooled results from four large European cohort studies. *Eur. J. Epidemiol.* **2019**, *34*, 471–481. [CrossRef]
61. Lorenzi, M.; Bonassi, S.; Lorenzi, T.; Giovannini, S.; Bernabei, R.; Onder, G. A review of telomere length in sarcopenia and frailty. *Biogerontology* **2018**, *19*, 209–221. [CrossRef] [PubMed]

Low Physical Activity in Patients with Complicated Type 2 Diabetes Mellitus is Associated with Low Muscle Mass and Low Protein Intake

Ilse J. M. Hagedoorn [1,*], Niala den Braber [1,2], Milou M. Oosterwijk [1], Christina M. Gant [3,4], Gerjan Navis [3], Miriam M. R. Vollenbroek-Hutten [1,2], Bert-Jan F. van Beijnum [2], Stephan J. L. Bakker [3] and Gozewijn D. Laverman [1]

1 Division of Nephrology, Department of Internal Medicine, Ziekenhuisgroep Twente, 7609 PP Almelo, The Netherlands; n.braber@zgt.nl (N.d.B); Mi.oosterwijk@zgt.nl (M.M.O.); m.vollenbroek@zgt.nl (M.M.R.V.-H.); g.laverman@zgt.nl (G.D.L.)
2 Faculty of Electrical Engineering, Mathematics and Computer Science, University of Twente, 7522 NB Enschede, The Netherlands; b.j.f.vanbeijnum@utwente.nl
3 Division of Nephrology, Department of Internal Medicine, University of Groningen, University Medical Center Groningen, 9713 GZ Groningen, The Netherlands; cm.gant@meandermc.nl (C.M.G.); g.j.navis@umcg.nl (G.N); s.j.l.bakker@umcg.nl (S.J.L.B.)
4 Department of Internal Medicine, Meander Medisch Centrum, 3813 TZ Amersfoort, The Netherlands
* Correspondence: ilse_hagedoorn10@hotmail.com.

Abstract: Objective: In order to promote physical activity (PA) in patients with complicated type 2 diabetes, a better understanding of daily movement is required. We (1) objectively assessed PA in patients with type 2 diabetes, and (2) studied the association between muscle mass, dietary protein intake, and PA. Methods: We performed cross-sectional analyses in all patients included in the Diabetes and Lifestyle Cohort Twente (DIALECT) between November 2016 and November 2018. Patients were divided into four groups: <5000, 5000–6999, 7000–9999, ≥ 10,000 steps/day. We studied the association between muscle mass (24 h urinary creatinine excretion rate, CER) and protein intake (by Maroni formula), and the main outcome variable PA (steps/day, Fitbit Flex device) using multivariate linear regression analyses. Results: In the 217 included patients, the median steps/day were 6118 (4115–8638). Of these patients, 48 patients (22%) took 7000–9999 steps/day, 37 patients (17%) took ≥ 10,000 steps/day, and 78 patients (36%) took <5000 steps/day. Patients with <5000 steps/day had, in comparison to patients who took ≥10,000 steps/day, a higher body mass index (BMI) (33 ± 6 vs. 30 ± 5 kg/m^2, $p = 0.009$), lower CER (11.7 ± 4.8 vs. 14.8 ± 3.8 mmol/24 h, $p = 0.001$), and lower protein intake (0.84 ± 0.29 vs. 1.08 ± 0.22 g/kg/day, $p < 0.001$). Both creatinine excretion ($\beta = 0.26$, $p < 0.001$) and dietary protein intake ($\beta = 0.31$, $p < 0.001$) were strongly associated with PA, which remained unchanged after adjustment for potential confounders. Conclusions: Prevalent insufficient protein intake and low muscle mass co-exist in obese patients with low physical activity. Dedicated intervention studies are needed to study the role of sufficient protein intake and physical activity in increasing or maintaining muscle mass in patients with type 2 diabetes.

Keywords: type 2 diabetes; physical activity; muscle mass; protein intake; accelerometer

1. Introduction

Type 2 diabetes is a predominately lifestyle-related disease and has become one of the major global public health concerns, with highest prevalence in older adults [1]. Sufficient physical activity (PA) is a main focus of treatment, in addition to improving diet quality. There are two different aspects of PA: aerobic training and resistance exercise. While guidelines first mainly recommended moderate to vigorous PA, contemporary public health guidelines state that 'some physical activity is better than none' by suggest reducing the time spent in sedentary behaviour [2]. Total steps per day is a good indicator of the overall volume of physical activity [3].

However, the vast majority of patients with type 2 diabetes do not adhere to the American Diabetes Association (ADA) guidelines of >150 min per week of moderate to vigorous PA, which is comparable with 7000 steps per day [3–5]. Traditionally, a goal of 10,000 steps per day has been advocated by popular media, although this goal is under debate in scientific literature [6,7]. In order to promote PA and reduce sedentary behaviour, a better understanding of total daily movement is required, especially in patients with complicated type 2 diabetes.

In regard to PA, sufficient muscle mass is mandatory to perform PA, and conversely, PA promotes an increase in muscle mass. Compared with non-diabetic subjects, patients with type 2 diabetes show decreased muscle strength and mass [8,9]. In type 2 diabetes, reduced muscle mass and muscle function, defined as sarcopenia, have been implicated both as a cause and as a consequence of increased insulin resistance [8–10]. Furthermore, it is known that low muscle mass in obese individuals is associated with frailty, disability, and increased morbidity and mortality [11].

However, dietary counselling (such as is performed in the geriatric population) consists mainly of caloric restriction, and not the preservation of muscle mass. Adequate protein intake is an important requirement for sustaining, and especially increasing, muscle mass, which has been confirmed by several observational and intervention studies [12–17]. Moreover, combining physical exercise with protein intake has a positive synergistic effect on muscle protein synthesis [16,17]. Therefore, adequate protein intake might be a current blind spot in the treatment of type 2 diabetes.

We hypothesize that in patients with complicated type 2 diabetes, low protein intake and low muscle mass are associated with low PA, and the former could be an important actionable item to improve PA. Therefore, here we (1) objectively measure PA (in steps/day) in patients with complicated type 2 diabetes, and (2) investigate the association between protein intake and muscle mass and PA.

2. Materials and Methods

2.1. Patient Inclusion

This study was performed in the DIAbetes and LifEstyle Cohort Twente (DIALECT), an observational cohort study in patients with complicated type 2 diabetes mellitus, treated in the secondary healthcare level in the outpatient clinic of the Ziekenhuisgroep Twente (ZGT), Almelo and Hengelo, the Netherlands. The study consists of two sub-cohorts: DIALECT-1 and DIALECT-2. The general procedures have been described extensively previously [18]. In DIALECT-2, the data collection at baseline is more extensive, including a one-week PA registration.

The study was performed in accordance with the Helsinki agreement and the guidelines of good clinical practice, has been approved by the local institutional review boards (METC-registration numbers NL57219.044.16 and 1009.68020) and is registered in the Netherlands Trial Register (NTR trial code 5855). Prior to participation, all patients signed an informed consent form. All adult patients with type 2 diabetes treated in the secondary healthcare level in the outpatient clinic of internal medicine in ZGT Hospital were eligible for participation. The patients were treated in the secondary healthcare level because the diabetes care became complex for primary healthcare services (for example, in the presence of complications such as nephropathy or because of a complex insulin schedule). Exclusion criteria were renal replacement therapy, inability to understand the informed consent procedure, and inability to walk. We report here on all patients included in DIALECT-2 between November 2016 and November 2018.

2.2. Data Collection

Participation in DIALECT-2 consisted of at least two hospital visits with one week in between. Information on medical condition and medication was obtained from electronic patient files and verified with the patient during the baseline visit. Smoking habits were collected through questionnaires. Anthropometric measurements, leg length, and presence of diabetic polyneuropathy were obtained from physical examination at baseline. Leg length was measured using a tape measure from the anterior superior iliac spine to the ground. Polyneuropathy was assessed by touch test (Semmes Weinstein monofilament) and vibration (Vibratip) by the on–off method; both tests have been validated as screening methods for polyneuropathy [19]. Polyneuropathy was present if at least one of the two tests was positive. Body composition parameters were determined by Bio impedance using a TANITA device (type BC-418MA, Tokyo, Japan), which calculates segmental body composition, including fat percentage and predicted muscle mass. Blood samples were taken from a single non-fasting venapunction, and patients collected 24 h urine to provide objective data on nutritional intake, including protein intake. We used the 24 h urinary creatinine excretion rate (CER) as a measure of muscle mass [11,20,21]. The estimated daily protein intake (g/kg/day) was calculated using the universally adopted formula of Maroni, ((24 h urea excretion $\times$ 0.18) + 15 + 24 h protein excretion)/weight (kg) [22]. Blood pressure was measured in supine position by an automated device for 15 min with one-minute intervals (Dinamap®; GE Medical systems, Milwaukee, WI, USA). The mean systolic and diastolic pressure of the last three measurements was used for further analysis.

2.3. Main Outcome: Physical Activity

During 8 consecutive days, daily movement was measured by a triaxial Fitbit accelerometer worn around the wrist on the non-dominant side. The devices used were either a Fitbit Flex (Fitbit Inc., Boston, MA, USA), a Fitbit charge HR (Fitbit, San Francisco, CA, USA), or Fitbit Charge 2 (Fitbit Inc., San Francisco, CA, USA). These Fitbit devices share the same recording mechanisms and record the number of steps taken on a minute-to-minute basis. Patients were asked to adhere to their daily activities as normal and were blinded from the online activity data. Also, the Fitbit screens showed no results. Only during swimming or showering was the Fitbit removed. At visit 2 (day 8), the patients returned the Fitbit and data were transferred to a hospital server for further analysis. Patients were asked to write down information regarding non-wearing time in a lifestyle diary. Valid days were defined as days without significant non-wearing time (i.e., >2 h non-wearing time during waking hours). Patients with more than two days of significant non-wearing time were excluded. To indicate the total daily movement, we used the average of the total steps per day, excluding day 1 and 8 from the average because of non-wearing time.

2.4. Statistical Analysis

Statistical procedures were performed by using SPSS statistics (IBM Statistics for Windows, Version 23.0, Armonk, NY, USA). Normality of data was determined by visual inspection of histograms. Data were presented as mean ± standard deviation (normal distribution), as median and interquartile range (IQR 25th–75th percentiles, skewed data), or as number and percentage (dichotomous and categorical data). To compare the characteristics of total steps per day, the population was divided into four different groups based on reference values from current literature (i.e., <5000, 5000–6999, 7000–9999, ≥10,000 steps per day) [3]. Differences between the groups were analysed using One-Way ANOVA, Kruskal–Wallis, or Chi-square test when appropriate. A two-sided $p < 0.05$ was considered statistically significant. The estimated daily protein intake was divided into three groups (i.e., <0.8 g/kg/day, 0.8–1.2 g/kg/day, and >1.2 g/kg/day). The recommended dietary protein intake is ≥0.8 g/kg/day [12,23].

To investigate whether 24 h CER and protein intake were associated with total steps/day, we performed multivariate linear regression analyses. First, we identified possible confounders using univariate analyses. Model 2, adjusted for age and gender, was the main basis for confounder selection. Parameters with a $p < 0.15$ were considered contenders for the multivariate model. For each group of closely associated variables (for example, body mass index (BMI), waist circumference, and hip circumference as measures of body size), we included the variable with the highest β for the multivariate model. Potential interaction of protein intake and CER with total steps/day was evaluated by inclusion of the product term in the linear regression analysis. We considered a $p < 0.10$ to be statistically significant for the product term. To graphically represent the interaction between protein intake, CER, and total steps per day, we created nine groups based on the tertiles of protein intake and tertiles of muscle mass. Low, medium, and high represent respectively the lowest, middle, and highest tertiles of protein intake and muscle mass.

3. Results

3.1. Baseline Characteristics and Total Steps per Day

Of 231 eligible participants, 217 patients were included in the study. The reasons for exclusion were: hardware malfunction ($n = 6$), non-fitting wristband ($n = 4$), patient dropped out during participation ($n = 2$), and patient not able to walk ($n = 2$) (Figure S1). Patient characteristics stratified by total steps per day are shown in Table 1.

Median total steps per day was 6118 (4115–8638, data not shown). Of the total study population, 85 patients (39%) took ≥7000 steps/day, of whom 37 patients (17%) reached ≥10,000 steps/day (Table 1).

The mean age of the total study population was 65 ± 12 years, two-thirds were men, and the mean BMI was 32 ± 6 kg/m^2. Of all patients, 64% used insulin, and the mean HbA1c was 60 ± 13 mmol/mol (7.6% ± 3.3%). The prevalence of micro- (74%) and macrovascular (35%) complications was high. Compliance with wearing of the Fitbit sensor was good; 22 patients reported significant non-wearing time (>2 h/day) at any day during day 2 until day 7, however, no patient had more than two days of non-wearing time (compliance data not shown).

The mean age was highest (69 ± 11 years) in the group of patients with <5000 steps per day ($p < 0.001$). There were no differences in gender between the groups ($p = 0.99$). Patients with <5000 steps/day had the highest BMI (33 ± 6 kg/m^2, $p = 0.009$) and the highest waist- and hip circumference (waist: 116 ± 14 cm, $p = 0.001$; hip: 115 ± 14 cm, $p = 0.009$). Both measurements of muscle mass (i.e., 24 h CER and percentage of predicted muscle mass (PMM) using bio-impedance) were lowest in patients with 5000 steps/day ($p = 0.001$ and $p = 0.06$, respectively).

No significant differences were observed in HbA1c, insulin use, and years of diabetes between the groups. Patients with <5000 steps per day had the most pack-years of smoking ($p = 0.005$), the lowest diastolic blood pressure (0.02), and the lowest HDL-cholesterol ($p = 0.03$). The prevalence of micro- and macrovascular complications was consistently and progressively lower in each group of increasing number of steps/day, especially for diabetic kidney disease ($p = 0.004$), polyneuropathy ($p = 0.008$), and cerebrovascular disease ($p = 0.008$). Protein intake was also lowest in patients with <5000 steps/day (0.84 g/kg/day, $p < 0.001$, Figure 1). Almost half of all patients with <5000 steps per day had a protein intake <0.8 g/kg/day.

Table 1. Patient characteristics stratified by total steps per day.

Characteristics	*n*	Total Population (*n* = 217)	<5000 steps/day (*n* = 78)	5000–6999 steps/day (*n* = 54)	7000–9999 steps/day (*n* = 48)	≥10,000 steps/day (*n* = 37)	*p*-Value
Age, years	217	65 ± 12	69 ± 11	64 ± 10	62 ± 13 [a]	60 ± 10 [a]	<0.001
Gender, men *n* (%)	217	144 (66)	51 (65)	36 (67)	32 (67)	25 (68)	0.99
BMI, kg/m^2	217	32 ± 6	33 ± 6	31 ± 5	31 ± 5	30 ± 5 [a]	0.009
Education level, *n* (%) [b]							
Low	185	65 (35)	31 (44)	16 (36)	11 (28)	7 (23)	0.10
Medium		81 (44)	29 (41)	17 (38)	16 (41)	19 (63)	
High		39 (21)	11 (16)	12 (27)	12 (31)	4 (13)	
Waist circumference, cm	216	112 ± 13	116 ± 14	109 ± 12 [a]	111 ± 13	107 ± 10 [a]	0.001
Hip circumference, cm	216	111 ± 13	115 ± 14	109 ± 12	110 ± 11	108 ± 9 [a]	0.009
Leg length, cm	120	98 ± 7	96 ± 8	97 ± 6	100 ± 8	99 ± 7	0.11
Fat percentage, %	206	33 ± 9	34 ± 8	33 ± 9	32 ± 10	30 ± 8	0.10
Predicted muscle mass, % [c]	206	64 ± 8	62 ± 8	63 ± 8	65 ± 8	67 ± 8	0.06
Creatinine excretion, mmol/24 h	215	13.2 ± 5	11.7 ± 4.8	13.6 ± 4.3	14.3 ± 5.1 [a]	14.8 ± 3.8 [a]	0.001
Systolic blood pressure, mmHg	211	130 ± 15	132 ± 16	127 ± 14	131 ± 16	133 ± 13	0.26
Diastolic blood pressure, mmHg	211	74 ± 9	72 ± 9	76 ± 9	73 ± 8	77 ± 12[a]	0.02
Pulse rate, bpm	211	71 ± 12	71 ± 13	73 ± 11	69 ± 10	70 ± 13	0.44
Diabetes duration, years	217	13 (8–19)	14 (8–20)	14 (8–19)	13 (5–20)	11 (7–18)	0.65
Insulin use, yes *n* (%)	215	138 (64)	56 (73)	32 (59)	25 (52)	25 (70)	0.09
Units of insulin	135	62 (34–101)	66 (40–118)	78 (38–114)	53 (26–105)	50 (35–77)	0.53
Alcohol intake units/month	213	3 (0–25)	0 (0–24)	5 (0–26)	2 (0–11)	8 (0–30)	0.27
Smoking, pack-years	199	8 (0–24)	14 (1–32)	7 (0–28)	1 (0–19) [a]	1 (0–21) [a]	0.005
Hba1c, mmol/mol (%)	215	60 ± 13 (7.6 ± 3.3)	60 ± 13 (7.6 ± 3.3)	60 ± 11 (7.6 ± 3.1)	62 ± 14 (7.8 ± 3.4)	59 ± 11 (7.5 ± 3.1)	0.69
Total cholesterol, mmol/L	215	4.2 ± 1.0	4.2 ± 1.1	4.2 ± 1.0	4.4 ± 0.9	4.2 ± 0.8	0.85
HDL-cholesterol, mmol/L	214	1.13 ± 0.3	1.10 ± 0.3	1.16 ± 0.3	1.15 ± 0.4	1.24 ± 0.3[a]	0.03
LDL-cholesterol, mmol/L	200	2.04 ± 0.8	2.0 ± 0.9	2.03 ± 0.9	2.16 ± 0.8	1.97 ± 0.6	0.67
Microvascular complications, *n* (%)	217	160 (74)	66 (85)	37 (69)	27 (56)	16 (43)	<0.001
Diabetic kidney disease, *n* (%)	211	106 (50)	48 (66)	27 (50)	19 (40)	12 (33)	0.004
eGFR < 60 mL/min/1.73 m^2, *n* (%)	217	70 (32)	38 (59)	17 (32)	10 (21)	5 (14)	<0.001
Micro-albuminuria, *n* (%)	211	83 (39)	40 (55)	20 (37)	14 (29)	9 (25)	0.006
Polyneuropathy, *n* (%)	217	97 (45)	46 (59)	24 (44)	17 (36)	10 (28)	0.008
Retinopathy, *n* (%)	210	41 (20)	18 (24)	10 (19)	6 (13)	7 (19)	0.532
Macrovascular complications, *n* (%)	217	75 (35)	33 (42)	22 (41)	12 (25)	8 (22)	0.05
Peripheral arterial diseases, *n* (%)	217	8 (4)	4 (5)	1 (2)	2 (4)	1 (3)	0.78
Coronary artery diseases, *n* (%)	216	54 (25)	23 (30)	18 (34)	8 (17)	5 (14)	0.06
Cerebrovascular accident or TIA, *n* (%)	217	27 (12)	17 (22)	6 (11)	1 (2)	3 (8)	0.008
Amputation, *n* (%)	217	3 (2)	3 (4)	0 (0)	0 (0)	0 (0)	0.14
Urea excretion, mmol/24 h	206	387 (291–510)	342 (242–448)	402 (274–505)	432 (327–508) [a]	465 (331–528) [a]	0.02
Protein intake, g/day	202	88 ± 28	79 ± 27	90 ± 31	93 ± 24 [a]	96 ± 24 [a]	0.004
Protein intake, g/kg/day	202	0.95 ± 0.30	0.84 ± 0.29	0.99 ± 0.33[a]	0.99 ± 0.27 [a]	1.08 ± 0.22 [a]	<0.001
<0.8 g/kg /day, *n* (%)		64 (31)	35 (46)	15 (28)	10 (24)	4 (11)	
0.8–1.2 g/kg/day, *n* (%)		102 (50)	32 (42)	28 (53)	22 (54)	20 (56)	0.006
>1.2 g/kg/day, *n* (%)		40 (19)	9 (12)	10 (19)	9 (22)	12 (33)	

[a] Significant difference from <5000 steps/day. [b] Education level according to the International Standard Classification of Education (ISCED), as follows: Low: ISCED 1–2; Medium: ISCED 3; High ISCED 4–8: [c] Predicted Muscle Mass %: TANITA predicted muscle mass (kg) divided by total body weight (kg). Data presented as mean ± standard deviation, as median and interquartile range (IQR 25th–75th), or in number and (percentage). eGFR: estimated glomerular filtration rate. TIA: transient ischemic attack.

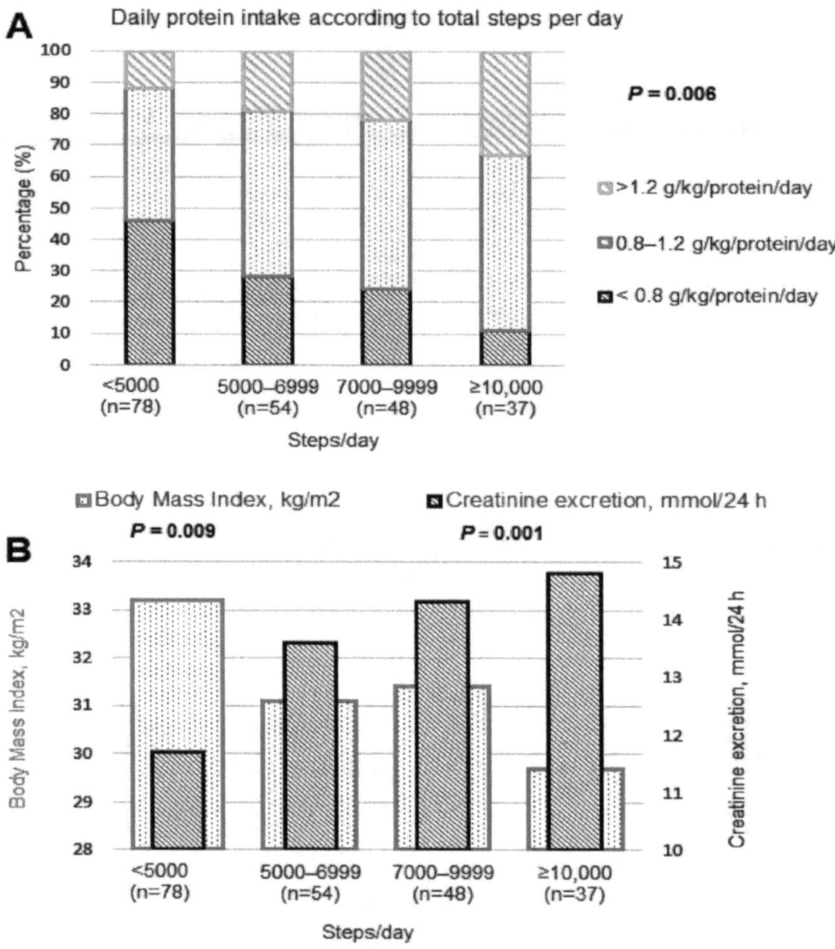

Figure 1. Protein intake, body mass index (BMI), and 24 h urinary creatinine excretion according to total steps per day. Distribution of total protein intake (**A**) and urinary creatinine excretion and body mass index (**B**) in four groups of total steps per day. (**A**) demonstrates that insufficient protein intake is significantly more prevalent in patients with <5000 steps/day. (**B**) shows higher body mass index and lower creatinine excretion in patients with <5000 steps/day, demonstrating a more unfavourable body composition.

3.2. Association between Urinary Creatinine Excretion, Total Protein Intake, and Total Steps per Day

To analyse the association between total steps per day, muscle mass (24 h CER), and daily dietary protein intake, we performed linear regression analyses. Unadjusted, both CER ($\beta = 0.28$, $p = 0.03$) and dietary protein intake ($\beta = 0.29$, $p = 0.004$) (Model 1) were positively associated with steps/day. When adjusting for possible confounders (Table S1), both for CER and protein intake, the association with total steps/day did not markedly change (Table 2). It should be noted that the predicted variance of both models remained low (0.23 and 0.24, respectively). There was a significant interaction between CER and protein intake on total steps per day, where higher CER combined with higher protein was associated with more steps/day ($p = 0.096$, Figure 2). As there was a very strong correlation between CER and dietary protein intake ($R = 0.57$), both variables could not be inserted simultaneously in the analysis.

Table 2. Multivariate linear regression analyses on the associations between CER, protein intake and total steps/day (dependent variable)

Independent Variables		Total Steps per day (Dependent)			Independent Variables	Total Steps per day (Dependent)		
		Standardized Beta	p-Value	R^2		Standardized Beta	p-Value	R^2
Model 1	CER	0.28	0.003	0.08	Protein intake	0.29	0.004	0.08
Model 2	CER	0.23	0.03	0.10	Protein intake	0.28	0.004	0.13
Model 3	CER	0.23	0.04	0.19	Protein intake	0.18	0.10	0.19
Model 4	CER	0.26	0.04	0.21	Protein intake	0.23	0.04	0.22
Model 5	CER	0.26	0.02	0.23	Protein intake	0.23	0.04	0.24

CER: creatinine excretion rate. Model 1 is unadjusted; Model 2 is adjusted for model 1 and age and gender; Model 3 is adjusted for model 2 and BMI and leg length; Model 4 is adjusted for model 3 and pack-years; Model 5 is adjusted for model 4 and eGFR < 60 mL/min/1.73 m^2, polyneuropathy, and presence of macrovascular disease.

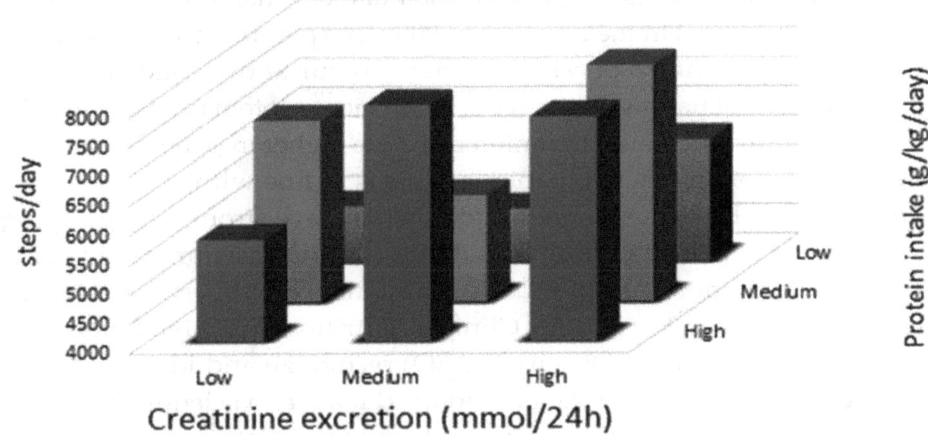

Figure 2. Low, medium, and high represent the lowest, middle, and highest tertiles of protein intake and creatinine excretion. The figure shows the interaction between urinary creatinine excretion (CER) and protein intake on total steps per day. Both high CER and high protein intake were associated with more steps/day, and total steps per day was highest in those with both high CER and high protein intake.

4. Discussion

We investigated the total daily physical activity (PA) of patients with complicated type 2 diabetes. We found that more than one-third of the study participants had limited activity (less than 5000 steps per day). On the other hand, 39% of participants took ≥7000 steps per day, which has been advocated as the movement target for adults ≥ 65 years and/or patients with chronic diseases [3], demonstrating that sufficient PA in a complicated type 2 diabetes population is indeed a reachable goal.

Our main finding was that low muscle mass was an important determinant of low PA. Additionally, protein intake was significantly and relevantly lower in patients with both low PA and low muscle mass. It is tempting to speculate on a downward spiral of reduced protein intake, lower muscle mass, and reduced PA, against the background of a sedentary lifestyle. The insight that insufficient protein intake is associated with low muscle mass and physical inactivity may provide an important actionable item to improve physical fitness in patients with type 2 diabetes: namely, increase protein intake.

Low muscle mass is increasingly recognized as an important health concern in patients with chronic disease, diminishing physical fitness and PA. In contrast to previous beliefs, declining muscle mass is not only due to ageing and physical inactivity, but has many other contributing causes, such as mitochondrial dysfunction [11,24,25]. This is especially important in patients with type 2 diabetes, as data suggest skeletal muscle lipid content is associated with systemic insulin resistance [11]. Damage to the skeletal muscles, with pronounced and accelerated decline in muscle quality, has been described as a new complication of diabetic patients attributed to their longer survival [8]. Insulin resistance and oxidative stress are components of the pathophysiological basis of sarcopenia, which would be related to characteristic components of diabetes, such as vascular alterations, chronic inflammation, and lipid infiltration in muscles [8,11]. In regard to our population, 24 h CER in the group with ≤5000 steps per day (11.7 ± 4.8 mmol/24 h) was significantly lower compared to the total study population (13.2 ± 5 mmol/24 h), and also lower when compared to the general Dutch population (13.3 ± 4.1 mmol/24 h, based on data from the Lifelines cohort study) [12]. However, it should be noted that no diagnostic methods or definitive cut-off points exist to identify patients who might benefit from muscle-boosting therapy.

Adequate protein intake is an important requirement for sustaining, and especially increasing, muscle mass, which has been confirmed by several observational and intervention studies [12–17]. Moreover, combining physical exercise with protein intake has a positive synergistic effect on muscle protein synthesis [16,17].

The recommended dietary allowance (RDA) and the Netherlands Nutrition Centre [12,23] recommend a dietary protein intake of ≥0.8 g/kg/day. However, for elderly adults, the Dutch guideline suggests a higher protein intake (1.2–2.0 g/kg/day) to maintain optimal muscle health [26,27]. We found that almost half of all patients (46%) in the group of <5000 steps per day had a daily protein intake < 0.8 g/kg/day, and only 12% had an intake of >1.2 g/kg/day. To our knowledge, this is the first study in patients with type 2 diabetes that has highlighted the insufficient protein intake of inactive patients with type 2 diabetes. However, BMI and waist circumference were higher in patients with low PA, consistent with altered body composition in inactive patients. This is in line with previous studies in patients with type 2 diabetes [4,28,29]. Low muscle mass and function have strong negative prognostic impacts in obese individuals, which may lead to frailty disability and increased morbidity and mortality [11]. However, awareness of the importance of muscle maintenance in obesity is low among clinicians and scientists [11]. The European Society for Clinical Nutrition and Metabolism (ESPEN) and the European Association for the study of Obesity (EASO) recognize and identify obesity with altered body composition due to low skeletal muscle function and mass as a scientific and clinical priority for researchers and clinicians. ESPEN and EASO therefore call for action in particular regard to optimal nutritional therapy. Generally, the first step in treating obese patients with type 2 diabetes is weight loss interventions by following a caloric restricted diet, which, however, might increase the risk for undesirable decreases in muscle mass.

To our knowledge, this is the first study to objectively measure daily PA by using steps/day in complicated type 2 diabetes. Most of the previous studies in type 2 diabetes used metabolic equivalent (MET) or counts per minute (CPM) to measure daily movement, which makes it somewhat difficult to compare previous results with our findings [4,24,25,28–34]. However, in a study population with older patients (≥55 years) with type 2 diabetes, the average total steps per day was similar to our results [34]. In contrast to this previous study, which showed that older women had fewer steps per day, we found no difference in steps/day between genders.

Additionally, we found that the presence of micro- and macrovascular complications was higher in patients with physical inactivity. This is in line with a recent review on diabetic polyneuropathy and nephropathy [35]. Interestingly, diabetic polyneuropathy is associated with lower muscle strength measured by knee extension force [25,32,35], providing an alternative cause of muscle mass decline in addition to reduced dietary protein intake. Additionally, in patients with chronic kidney disease, uremic muscle mass decline has been suggested by a significant inverse association between uremic toxin indoxyl sulphate and skeletal muscle mass [33,35]. Of note, in our study, a third of the patients with ≥10,000 steps per day had polyneuropathy and nephropathy (28% and 33%, respectively), suggesting that sufficient PA is indeed possible in spite of the presence of these complications. However, in contrast to other studies in patients with type 2 diabetes, we found associations between HDL-cholesterol, diastolic blood pressure, macrovascular complications, and physical activity [4,28,29].

Strengths of our study included the objective measurements of daily movement by the Fitbit Flex, a light and simple wristband, well applicable in daily life clinical practice that hardly interferes with daily activities. We chose to present steps/day, which is easily interpretable by clinicians and patients. Another strength of our study was muscle mass estimation by 24 h CER, which is well accepted for estimation of total body skeletal muscle mass, even in patients with advanced renal failure [12,21]. Additionally, we objectively determined protein intake by 24 h urinary urea excretion. In the future, we plan to extend our analysis to also include muscle quality using gait speed, as well as quality of life questionnaires. An important limitation of our study is the cross-sectional design, which allows only research of associations and not causality. Additional prospective studies are warranted to confirm our findings. Another limitation is that one-week record of the Fitbit may not be sufficiently representative of PA, as certain activities, such as swimming, and seasonal variations were not taken into account. However, only 8 patients of the total 217 patients (4%) recorded swimming in their lifestyle diary. Secondly, we had the sampling periods of our population distributed over the seasons. Making these effect negligible.

Our study has important clinical implications. We found clear associations between low protein intake, loss of muscle mass, and low PA in patients with complicated type 2 diabetes. Our study suggests that optimizing protein intake might be a first step to improving physical fitness in patients with type 2 diabetes. As current dietary guidelines focus on reducing overall caloric intake, and carbohydrate intake in particular, adequate protein intake might be an important blind spot in current nutritional management. This has also been advocated in previous studies, which suggest that dietary protein should be prescribed together with physical exercise in order to optimize muscle health [12,16,17,36]. The review by Scot and colleagues also emphasizes that lifestyle modification programs for older adults with type 2 diabetes, particularly for those with sarcopenia, should incorporate progressive resistance training, along with adequate intakes of protein and vitamin D, which may improve both functional and metabolic health and prevent undesirable decreases in muscle mass associated with weight loss intervention [9]. In the future, we want to include data from the Food Frequency Questionnaire (FFQ) in the analyses in order to investigate how intakes of total energy, carbohydrate, fat, and vitamin D may contribute to muscle mass and physical activity. It is important to note that the source of dietary protein (animal or vegetable) should also be taken into account, as we have previously shown that higher vegetable protein intake is associated with lower prevalence of renal function impairment [37].

5. Conclusions

In conclusion, our study shows that prevalent low protein intake and low muscle mass co-exist in patients with complicated type 2 diabetes with low physical activity. Dedicated intervention studies are needed to study the role of sufficient protein intake and PA in increasing or maintaining muscle mass in patients with type 2 diabetes.

Supplementary Materials: The following are available online at Figure S1: flow chart of patient inclusion, Table S1: linear regression analyses for total steps per day.

Author Contributions: I.J.M.H. researched data and wrote the manuscript. N.d.B. analyzed the Fitbit data and reviewed/edited the manuscript. C.M.G., G.D.L., G.N., S.J.L.B. and M.M.R.V.-H. researched data and reviewed/edited the manuscript. M.M.O. and B.-J.F.v.B. reviewed/edited the manuscript. G.D.L. is the principal investigator of DIALECT and the guarantor. All authors have read and agreed to the published version of the manuscript.

Acknowledgments: The authors would like to thank Nicole Oosterom, Annis Jalving, Roos Nijboer, and all of the students who have participated in DIALECT 1 and 2, Ziekenhuisgroep Twente, for their general contributions to DIALECT, including patient inclusion.

References

1. Wild, S.; Roglic, G.; Green, A.; Sicree, R.; King, H. Global prevalence of diabetes: Estimates for the year 2000 and projections for 2030. *Diabetes Care* **2004**, *27*, 1047–1053. [CrossRef] [PubMed]
2. Weggemans, R.M.; Backx, F.J.G.; Borghouts, L.; Chinapaw, M.; Hopman, M.T.E.; Koster, A.; Kremers, S.; van Loon, L.J.C.; May, A.; Mosterd, A.; et al. The 2017 Dutch Physical Activity Guidelines. *Int. J. Behav. Nutr. Phys. Act.* **2018**, *15*, 58. [CrossRef] [PubMed]

3. Tudor-Locke, C.; Craig, C.L.; Aoyagi, Y.; Bell, R.C.; Croteau, K.A.; De Bourdeaudhuij, I.; Ewald, B.; Gardner, A.W.; Hatano, Y.; Lutes, L.D.; et al. How many steps/day are enough? For older adults and special populations. *Int. J. Behav. Nutr. Phys. Act.* **2011**, *8*, 1–19.
4. Jakicic, J.M.; Greg, E.; Knowler, W.; Kelley, D.E.; Lang, W.; Miller, G.D.; Pi-Sunyer, F.X.; Regensteiner, J.G.; Rejeski, W.J.; Ribisl, P.; et al. Activity patterns of obese adults with Type 2 Diabetes in the look AHEAD study. *Med. Sci. Sports. Exerc.* **2010**, *42*, 1995–2005. [CrossRef] [PubMed]
5. Oosterom, N.; Gant, C.M.; Ruiterkamp, N.; van Beijnum, B.J.F.; Hermens, H.; Bakker, S.J.L.; Navis, G.; Vollenbroek-Hutten, M.M.R.; Laverman, G.D. Physical activity in patients with type 2 diabetes: The case for objective measurement in routine clinical care. *Diabetes Care* **2018**, *41*, e50–e51. [CrossRef]
6. Min Lee, L.; Shiroma, E.J.; Kamada, M.; Basset, D.R.; Matthews, C.E.; Buring, J. E Association of Step Volume and Intensity with All-Cause Mortality in Older Women. *JAMA Intern. Med.* **2019**, *179*, 1105–1112.
7. Saint-Maurice, P.F.; Troiano, R.P.; Bassett, D.R.; Graubard, B.I.; Carlson, S.A.; Shirom, E.J.; Fulton, J.E.; Matthews, C.E. Association of Daily Step Count and Step Intensity with Mortality Among US Adults. *J. Am. Med. Assoc.* **2020**, *323*, 1151–1160. [CrossRef]
8. Trierweiler, H.; Kisielewicz, G.; Hoffmann Jonasson, T.; Rasmussen Petterle, R.; Aguiar Moreira, C.; Cochenski Borba, V.Z. Sarcopenia: A chronic complication of type 2 diabetes mellitus. *Diabetol. Metab. Syndr.* **2018**, *10*, 1–9. [CrossRef]
9. Scot, D.; Courten de, B.; Ebeling, P.R. Sarcopenia: A potential cause and consequence of type 2 diabetes in Australia's ageing population? *Med. J. Aust.* **2016**, *205*, 329–333. [CrossRef]
10. Mesinovic, J.; Zengin, A.; Courten, B.; Ebeling, P.R.; Scott, D. Sarcopenia and type 2 diabetes mellitus: A bidirectional relationship. *Diabetes Metab. Syndr. Obes. Targets Ther.* **2019**, *2*, 1057–1072. [CrossRef]
11. Barazzoni, R.; Bischoff, S.C.; Boiirie, Y.; Busetto, L.; Cederholm, T.; Dicker, D.; Toplak, H.; Van Gossum, A.; Yumuk, V.; Vettor, R. Sarcopenic obesity: Time to meet the challenge. *Clin. Nutr.* **2018**, *37*, 1787–1793. [CrossRef] [PubMed]
12. Alexandrov, N.V.; Eelderink, C.; Singh-Povel, C.M.; Navis, G.J.; Bakker, S.J.L.; Corpeleijn, E. Dietary protein sources and muscle mass over the life course: The Lifelines Cohort study. *Nutrients* **2018**, *10*, 1471. [CrossRef] [PubMed]
13. Housten, D.K.; Nicklas, B.J.; Ding, J.; Harris, T.B.; Tylavsky, F.A.; Newman, A.B.; Lee, J.S.; Sahyoun, N.R.; Visser, M.; Kritchevsky, S.B.; et al. Dietary protein intake is Associated with Lean Mass Change in Older, Community-Dwelling Adults: The Health, Aging, and Body Composition (Health ABC) study. *Am. J. Clin. Nutr.* **2008**, *87*, 150–155. [CrossRef]
14. Huang, R.Y.; Yang, K.C.; Chang, H.H.; Lee, L.T.; Lu, C.W.; Huang, K.C. The association between total protein and vegetable protein intake and low muscle mass among the community-dwelling elderly population in Northern Taiwan. *Nutrients* **2016**, *8*, 373. [CrossRef] [PubMed]
15. Sahni, S.; Mangano, K.M.; Hannan, M.T.; Kiel, D.P.; McLean, R.R. Higher Protein Intake is Associated with Higher Lean Mass and Quadriceps Muscle Strength in Adults Men and Women. *J. Nutr.* **2015**, *145*, 1569–1575. [CrossRef]
16. Tieland, M.; Borgonjen-Van den Berg, K.J.; van Loon, L.J.; de Groot, L.C. Dietary Protein Intake in Community-Dwelling, Frail, and Institutionalized Elderly People: Scope for Improvement. *Eur. J. Nutr.* **2012**, *51*, 173–179. [CrossRef]
17. Liao, C.D.; Tsauo, J.Y.; Wu, Y.T.; Cheng, C.-P.; Chen, H.-C.; Huang, Y.C.; Liou, T.-H. Effects of protein supplementation combined with resistance exercise on body composition and physical function in older adults: A systematic review and meta-analysis. *Am. J. Clin. Nutr.* **2017**, *106*, 1078–1091. [CrossRef]
18. Gant, C.M.; Binnenmars, S.H.; Berg, E.V.D.; Bakker, S.J.L.; Navis, G.; Laverman, G.D. Integrated assessment of pharmocological and nutritional cardiovascular risk management: Blood pressure control in the DIAbetes and LifEstyle Cohort Twente (DIALECT). *Nutrients* **2017**, *9*, 709. [CrossRef]
19. Olaleye, D.; Perkins, B.A.; Bril, V. Evaluation of three screening tests and a risk assessment model for diagnosing peripheral neuropathy in the diabetes clinic. *Diabetes Res. Clin. Pract.* **2015**, *4*, 115–128.
20. Proctor, D.N.; O'Brien, P.C.; Atkinson, E.J.; Nair, K.S. Comparison of techniques to estimate total body skeletal muscle mass in people of different age groups. *Am. J. Physiol.* **1999**, *277*, 489. [CrossRef]
21. Heymsfield, S.B.; Arteaga, C.; McManus, C.; Smith, J.; Moffitt, S. Measurement of muscle mass in humans: Validity of the 24-hour urinary creatinine method. *Am. J. Clin. Nutr.* **1983**, *37*, 478–494. [CrossRef] [PubMed]

22. Maroni, B.J.; Steinman, T.I.; Mitch, W.E. A method for estimating nitrogen intake of patients with chronic renal failure. *Kidney Int.* **1985**, *27*, 58–65. [CrossRef] [PubMed]
23. Trumbo, P.; Schlicker, S.; Yates, A.A.; Poos, M.; Food and nutrition board of the institute of medicine; The National Academies. Dietary references intakes for Energy, Carbohydrate, Fiber, fat, fatty acids, cholesterol, protein and amino acids. *J. Am. Diet. Assoc.* **2002**, *102*, 1621–1630. [CrossRef]
24. Cruz-Jentoft, A.J.; Bahat, G.; Bauer, J.; Boirie, Y.; Bruyère, O.; Cederholm, T.; Cooper, C.; Landi, F.; Rolland, Y.; Sayer, A.A.; et al. Guidelines. Sarcopenia: Revised European consensus on definition and diagnosis. *Age Aging* **2019**, *48*, 16–31. [CrossRef]
25. Nomura, T.; Ishiguro, T.; Ohira, M.; Ikeda, Y. Diabetic polyneuropathy is a risk factor for decline of lower extremity strength in patients with type 2 diabetes. *J. Diabetes Investig.* **2018**, *91*, 86–192. [CrossRef]
26. Baum, J.I.; Kim, I.Y.; Wolfe, R.R. Protein consumption and the Elderly: What is the optimal level of intake? *Nutrients* **2016**, *8*, 359. [CrossRef]
27. Nowson, C.; Connell, S. Protein requirements and recommendations for older people: A review. *Nutrients* **2015**, *7*, 6574–6599. [CrossRef]
28. Healy, G.N.; Winkler, E.A.H.; Brakenridge, C.L.; Reeves, M.M.; Eakin, E.G. Accelerometer-Derived sedentary and physical activitiy time in overweight/obese adults with type 2 diabetes; Cross-sectional associations with cardiometabolic biomarkers. *PLoS ONE* **2015**, *10*, e0119140. [CrossRef]
29. Balducci, S.; D'Errico, V.; Haxhi, J.; Sacchetti, M.; Orlando, G.; Cardelli, P.; Di Biase, N.; Bollanti, L.; Conti, F.; Zanuso, S. Level and correlates of physical activity and sedentary behavior in patients with type 2 diabetes: A cross-sectional analysis of the Italian Diabetes and Exercise Study_2. *PLoS ONE* **2017**, *12*, e0173337. [CrossRef]
30. Cooper, A.R.; Sebire, S. Sedentary time, breaks in sedentary time and metabolic variables in people with newly diagnosed type 2 diabetes. *Diabetologia* **2012**, *55*, 589–599. [CrossRef]
31. Cichosz, S.L.; Fleischer, J.; Hoeyem, P.; Laugesen, E.; Poulsen, P.L.; Christinansen, J.S.; Ejskjær, N.; Hansen, T.K. Objective measurements of activity patterns in people with newly diagnosed Type 2 diabetes demonstrate a sedentary lifestyle. *Diabet. Med.* **2013**, *30*, 1063–1066. [CrossRef] [PubMed]
32. Andersen, H.; Nielsen, S.; Mogensen, C.E.; Jakobsen, J. Muscle strenght in type 2 diabetes. *Diabetes* **2004**, *53*, 1543–1548. [PubMed]
33. Sato, E.; Mori, T.; Mishima, E.; Suzuki, A.; Sugawara, S.; Saigusa, D.; Miura, D.; Morikawa-Ichinose, T.; Saito, R.; Saito, R.; et al. Metabolic alterations by indoxyl sulfate in skeletal muscle induce uremic sarcopenia in chronic kidney disease. *Sci. Rep.* **2016**, *6*, 36618. [PubMed]
34. Joan, J.K.; Edney, K.; Moran, C.; Strikanth, V.; Calisaya, M. Gender differences in physical activity levels of older people with type 2 diabetes mellitus. *J. Phys. Act. Health* **2016**, *13*, 409–415.
35. Nomura, T.; Kawae, T.; Kataoka, H.; Ikeda, Y. Aging, physical activity and diabetic complications related to loss of muscle strength in patients with type 2 diabetes. *Phys. Ther. Res.* **2018**, *21*, 33–38. [PubMed]
36. Landi, F.; Calvani, R.; Tosato, M.; Martone, A.M.; Ortolani, E.; Savera, G.; D'Angelo, E.; Sisto, A.; Marzetti, E. Protein intake and muscle health in old age: From biological plausibility to clinical evidence. *Nutrients* **2016**, *8*, 295.
37. Oosterwijk, M.M.; Soedamah-Muthu, S.; Geleijnse, J.M.; Bakker, S.J.L.; Navis, G.; Binnenmars, S.H.; Gant, C.M.; Laverman, G.D. High Dietary intake of vegetable protein is associated with lower prevalence of renal function impairment: Results of the Dutch DIALECT-1 Cohort. *Kidney Int. Rep.* **2019**, *4*, 710–719.

7

Correlations between the Quality of Life Domains and Clinical Variables in Sarcopenic Osteoporotic Postmenopausal Women

Mariana Cevei [1], Roxana Ramona Onofrei [2,*], Felicia Cioara [1] and Dorina Stoicanescu [3]

1 Psychoneuro Sciences and Rehabilitation Department, Faculty of Medicine & Pharmacy, University of Oradea, 410087 Oradea, Romania; cevei_mariana@yahoo.com (M.C.); felicia_cioara@yahoo.com (F.C.)
2 Department of Rehabilitation, Physical Medicine and Rheumatology, "Victor Babeş" University of Medicine and Pharmacy Timişoara, 300041 Timişoara, Romania
3 Microscopic Morphology Department, "Victor Babeş" University of Medicine and Pharmacy Timişoara, 300041 Timişoara, Romania; dstoicanescu@yahoo.com
* Correspondence: onofrei.roxana@umft.ro

Abstract: (1) Background: both sarcopenia and osteoporosis are major health problems in postmenopausal women. The aim of the study was to evaluate the quality of life (QoL) and the associated factors for sarcopenia in osteoporotic postmenopausal women, diagnosed according to EWGSOP2 criteria. (2) Methods: the study sample comprised 122 osteoporotic postmenopausal women with low hand grip strength and was divided into two groups: group 1 (probable sarcopenia) and group 2 (sarcopenia). QoL was assessed using the validated Romanian version of SarQol questionnaire. (3) Results: the D1, D4, D5, D7 and total SarQoL scores were significantly lower in women from group 2 compared to group 1. In group 2, women older than 70 years had significant lower values for D1, D3, D4, D6 and total SarQoL scores. Age, history of falls and the presence of confirmed and severe sarcopenia were predictors for overall QoL. (4) Conclusions: the frequency of sarcopenia was relatively high in our sample, with body mass index and history of falls as predictors for sarcopenia. Older osteoporotic postmenopausal women, with previous falls and an established sarcopenia diagnosis (low muscle strength and low muscle mass), were more likely to have a decreased quality of life.

Keywords: sarcopenia; quality of life; osteoporosis; postmenopausal women

1. Introduction

Sarcopenia is characterized by decreased muscle strength, loss of muscle mass and poor physical performance [1]. The condition is associated with aging. Aging is a complex process, involving many variables that interact with each other and include, besides genetic factors, lifestyle and chronic diseases. Even if sarcopenia is more common among older individuals, it can also occur earlier in life. It typically begins in the fourth decade of life, but the decline is accelerated after the sixth decade [2,3].

The decrease in muscle strength and muscle mass contributes to the loss of the ability to live independently and thus becomes an important public health problem. Sarcopenia is associated with physical disability, poor physical performance, functional decline, falls, and hospitalization [4]. Multimorbidity is frequent in older individuals and some diseases, such as heart failure or chronic obstructive pulmonary disease, accelerate the loss of muscle strength and mass, creating a vicious cycle [5]. All these have a major impact on the patient's quality of life [6]. Sarcopenia also increases the risk of falls. There is a high risk for hip fractures, as loss of muscle mass is frequently associated with loss of bone [5]. The high risk of falls in sarcopenic patients was found to be regardless of age, gender and other confounding factors [7]. In turn, falls are associated with functional deterioration, physical disability, impairment in activities of daily living, increased morbidity and mortality [8]. In a meta-analysis that included 17 studies, a significant association between sarcopenia and fractures was found, independent of study design, study population, gender, sarcopenia definition, geographical area or study quality [9].

Considering the specificities of older individuals, a sarcopenia-specific quality of life questionnaire (SarQoL) has been developed [10,11] and validated [12]. The Romanian version of the SarQoL® was validated in 2017 [13]. Previous studies have reported the associated factors and the effects on the quality of life in adults with sarcopenia, using different diagnostic criteria. Only a few studies used the revised criteria of the European Working Group on Sarcopenia in Older People (EWGSOP2) [14–16]. The purpose of the present study was to evaluate the quality of life and the associated factors for sarcopenia in Romanian osteoporotic postmenopausal women, using the EWGSOP2 diagnostic criteria.

2. Materials and Methods

2.1. Study Design and Participants

Participants for this observational study were recruited from the postmenopausal women admitted to Medical Rehabilitation Clinical Hospital Băile Felix, România. To be selected, participants had to be previously diagnosed with primary osteoporosis (T-score ≤ -2.5, evaluated by DXA) and to have low hand grip strength. Low hand grip strength was defined according to the EWGSOP2 recommended cut-off of < 16 kg for women and was used to quantify the loss of muscle strength [1]. Criteria for exclusion were: (1) severe mobility disorders of the weight-bearing joints and cases with neurological conditions that affect balance and gait; (2) inability to walk for at least 10 min without a walking aid; (3) history of hip or knee arthroplasty; (4) inflammatory musculoskeletal conditions; (5) malignancies; (6) infectious diseases, (7) diabetic neuropathy; (8) cognitive impairments.

All participants provided written informed consent. The study complied with the Declaration of Helsinki and was approved by the Local Ethics Commission for Scientific Research of Medical Rehabilitation Clinical Hospital Băile Felix, România (4016/30.04.2018).

2.2. Assessments

Socio-demographic and clinical data (age, weight, height, body mass index, marital status, occupational status, years of menopause, history of and tendency towards falls, history of osteoporotic fractures, clinical conditions) were collected by interview and from medical documents. From the medical documents, the appendicular lean muscle mass determined by dual-energy X-ray absorptiometry was recorded for each participant in the study. Based on these results, and according to the recommended EWGSOP2 cut-off points for skeletal muscle mass index (appendicular lean mass/height^2), the participants were categorized as having low muscle mass (<5.5 kg/m^2) and normal muscle mass [1].

2.2.1. Physical Performance

Physical performance was examined by the Timed Up&Go test, with the G-Walk system (BTS Bioengineering, Milan, Italy). It uses a validated wireless inertial sensor, made up of four inertial platforms, each composed of a tri-axial accelerometer, a tri-axial gyroscope and a magnetometer [17]. The G-sensor was attached to the participants fifth lumbar vertebra. The subjects were asked to stand up from a chair, to walk along a 3 m pathway at a self-selected speed, turn around and walk back to the chair and sit down. The recorded data were transmitted to the PC through a Bluetooth connection and processed by the BTS G-studio software (BTS Bioengineering, Milan, Italy). Women who scored ≥ 20 s were considered to have low physical performance.

Cases with low muscle strength were classified as having probable sarcopenia. We considered all participants that met the two EWGSOP2 diagnostic criteria-low muscle strength and low muscle mass—to have confirmed sarcopenia. Women with confirmed sarcopenia and low physical performance were categorized as having severe sarcopenia, according to the EWGSOP2 revised criteria [1]. We divided the study sample in two groups: group 1 comprised participants with probable sarcopenia ($n = 58$) and group 2, those with an established sarcopenia diagnosis, which included participants with confirmed and severe sarcopenia, according to EWGSOP2 ($n = 64$).

2.2.2. Quality of Life

The quality of life was assessed using the validated Romanian version of SarQol questionnaire (Sarcopenia Quality of Life). This is a multidimensional questionnaire, evaluating seven domains of health-related quality of life—physical and mental health (D1), locomotion (D2), body composition (D3), functionality (D4), activities of daily living (D5), leisure activities (D6) and fears (D7) [10]. The 22 questions are rated on a 4-point Likert scale. Each domain is scored from 0 to 100 and an overall score is calculated. A higher score reflects a higher quality of life [12]. The SarQol questionnaire has good internal consistency and construct validity, good discriminative power and good responsiveness [12–14,18].

2.3. Statistical Analysis

The statistical analysis was performed using the Medcalc Statistical Software version 19.1 (MedCalc Software bv, Ostend, Belgium). All data were tested for normality with the Shapiro–Wilk's test. Descriptive statistics were calculated for all socio-demographics' characteristics (frequencies, means and standard deviation), SarQoL scores and TUG (median and interquartile range (IQR)). Between-groups differences were assessed using the independent t-test and Mann–Whitney test, respectively. Categorical data were compared using Chi-squared test. Logistic regression analysis was used to identify the factors associated with sarcopenia. Odds ratios (OR), 95% confidence intervals (CI) and p values were reported. Spearman rank correlation coefficient was used to assess the relationship between socio-demographic and clinical factors and the SarQoL scores. Variables that demonstrated significance were then entered into a stepwise multiple linear regression analysis to assess the predictors of quality of life, with SarQoL domains and total scores as a dependent variable. The significance level was set at $p < 0.05$ for all tests.

3. Results

The study sample comprised 122 women (mean age 67.02 ± 8.3 years) (ranging between 48 and 83 years) that met the inclusion criteria and agreed to participate in the study. More than half of the participants (52.46%) were diagnosed with confirmed and severe sarcopenia.

Table 1 summarizes the characteristics of the participants. There were no significant differences between the two groups in participants' characteristics, except for weight, BMI and fall history. There was a higher percent of overweight and obese women in group 1 compared to group 2 ($p < 0.0001$). The proportion of overweight or obese women in our sample was 69.67%. A total of 93.10% of participants with probable sarcopenia and 48.43% of those with sarcopenia were overweight or obese. Women with sarcopenia had a higher frequency of history of falls than those with probable sarcopenia ($p = 0.03$).

Table 1. Socio-Demographic and Clinical Characteristics.

	All (n = 122)	Group 1 (n = 58)	Group 2 (n = 64)	p
Age, years	67.02 ± 8.03	66.48 ± 7.76	67.5 ± 8.79	NS
<60 years	26 (21.31)	10 (17.24)	16 (25)	
60–69 years	49 (40.16)	29 (50)	20 (31.25)	NS
>70 years	47 (38.53)	19 (32.76)	28 (43.75)	
Weight, kg	67.82 ± 11.02	72.34 ± 9.56	63.72 ± 10.69	<0.0001
Height, cm	157.93 ± 6.19	158 ± 6.18	157.9 ± 6.25	NS
BMI, kg/m^2	27.22 ± 4.28	29.07 ± 3.71	25.55 ± 4.1	<0.0001
Underweigth (<18.5 kg/m^2)	3 (2.46)	1 (1.72)	2 (3.13)	
Normal (18.5–24.9 kg/m^2)	34 (27.87)	3 (5.17)	31 (48.44)	<0.0001
Overweight (25–29.9 kg/m^2)	55 (45.08)	33 (56.9)	22 (34.37)	
Obese (>30 kg/m^2)	30 (24.59)	21 (36.21)	9 (14.06)	
Years of menopause	19.66 ± 9.1	19.21 ± 8.25	20.08 ± 9.85	NS
Tendency to fall	55 (45.08)	24 (41.38)	31 (48.44)	NS
Fall history	28 (22.95)	8 (13.79)	20 (31.25)	0.02
Osteoporotic fractures history	30 (24.59)	18 (31.03)	12 (18.75)	NS
Number of comorbitites	5.85 ± 2.07	6 ± 1.97	5.72 ± 2.17	NS
Education				NS
Primary education (<8 classes)	52 (42.63)	23 (39.66)	29 (45.31)	
High school	50 (40.98)	27 (46.55)	23 (35.94)	
University	20 (16.39)	8 (13.79)	12 (18.75)	
Marital status				NS
Married	73 (59.84)	39 (67.24)	34 (53.13)	
Single	49 (40.16)	19 (32.76)	30 (46.88)	
Occupational status				NS
Working	46 (37.7)	23 (39.66)	23 (35.94)	
Retired	76 (62.3)	35 (60.34)	41 (64.06)	
Physical performance				
TUG (s)	19.6 (15.17–25.5)	19.45 (14.75–25.13)	19.65 (15.65–26.74)	NS
TUG>20s	61 (50)	28 (48.27)	33 (51.56)	NS

Data are presented as mean ± SD, number (percentage) or median [IQR]

The associations between the socio-demographic and clinical factors and the presence of sarcopenia were analysed by logistic regression. The factors significantly associated with sarcopenia were BMI (OR 0.79, 95%CI 0.71–0.88, $p < 0.0001$) and the history of falls (OR 2.84, 95%CI 1.13–7.09, $p = 0.003$). After adjusting for covariates (age, marital status, number of comorbidities and years since menopause), multiple logistic regression showed that BMI (OR 0.77, 95%CI 0.69–0.87, $p < 0.0001$) and the history of falls (OR 3.95, 95%CI 1.38–11.29, $p = 0.01$) together can predict the sarcopenic status. A lower BMI associated with at least one fall in the past would predispose osteoporotic postmenopausal women to sarcopenia.

Table 2 presents the total scores, as well as each domain scores of the SarQoL questionnaire. The D1, D4, D5, D7 and total SarQoL scores were significantly lower in women from group 2 compared to group 1.

In the whole study sample, significant lower scores were observed for D1, D4, D5, D7 and total SarQoL scores in the > 70 years group compared to the other two age groups, and for D2 and D3 in the > 70 years compared to the < 60 years group. In the probable sarcopenia group, no significant differences in all the SarQoL scores were observed between age groups. In group 2, women older than 70 years had significantly lower values for D1, D3, D4, D6 and total SarQoL scores than those from the other two age groups. For the D5 and D7 domains, women from group 2, older than 70 years, had significantly lower scores than those younger than 60 years ($p < 0.05$). When comparing the SarQoL scores between the two groups based on age, significantly lower scores were recorded only in the >70 years old group for D3, D4, D5 and total scores.

Table 2. Results of the SarQol Questionnaire in the Three Age Groups.

SarQoL Domains	All (n = 122)	Group 1 (n = 58)	Group 2 (n = 64)	p [a]
D1	52.20 (45.50–65.50)	56.65 (48.90–72.20)	54.10 (49.45–62.20)	0.01
<60 years	58.30 (51.38–75.50)	66.65 (54.68–79.13)	53.85 (48.9–69.73)	NS
60–69	57.80 (48.90–67.20)	58.90 (52.20–71.1)	55.50 (42.25–65.60)	NS
>70 years	47.80 (37.80–55.50) [b,c]	52.20 (45.50–58.9)	47.80 (35.25–51.93) [b,c]	NS
D2	55.60 (47.20–66.70)	56.95 (50–70.10)	55.60 (42.38–63.90)	NS
<60 years	59.70 (55.60–70.10)	68.05 (54.85–73.60)	58.30 (55.60–66)	NS
60–69	55.60 (50–68.05)	55.60 (50–72.20)	53.50 (47.20–63.90)	NS
>70 years	50 (38.90–61.10) [c]	55.60 (50–63.90)	47.20 (31.28–61.10)	NS
D3	54.20 (45.80–66.70)	58.3 (48.95–66.07)	54.20 (41.70–65.65)	NS
<60 years	60.40 (53.15–70.80)	64.6 (50–68.78)	58.30 (54.20–70.80)	NS
60–69	58.30 (45.8–70.80)	58.30 (45.80–68.75)	58.30 (46.85–73.95)	NS
>70 years	50 (37.50–62.50) [c]	50 (50–66.7)	45.80 (37.50–57.28) [b,c]	<0.05
D4	63.50 (53.32–75)	67.3 (57.7–78.6)	59.60 (50–70.80)	0.01
<60 years	69.60 (66.35–78.65)	73.10 (67.3–80.38)	68.75 (62.75–77.85)	NS
60–69	63.50 (56.45–78.7)	63.50 (57.70–78.80)	63 (52.78–75.98)	NS
>70 years	55.80 (48.10–69.20) [b,c]	65.40 (55.80–71.20)	50 (45.18–55.80) [b,c]	<0.05
D5	48.25 (37.30–60.17)	53.30 (43.30–66.25)	43.30 (33.30–55.60)	0.001
<60 years	56.70 (44.58–66.65)	59.15 (56.28–80.53)	51.65 (43–63.65)	NS
60–69	48.30 (41.70–63.80)	51.70 (42.50–66.30)	48.30 (34.20–61.45)	NS
>70 years	40 (33.30–50) [b,c]	46.70 (38.30–60.70)	35.85 (30.83–45.45) [c]	<0.05
D6	33.30 (16.60–33.3)	33.30 (16.60–52.85)	33.3 (16.6–33.3)	NS
<60 years	33.30 (16.60–37.45)	33.30 (12.45–41.60)	33.30 (33.30–45.75)	NS
60–69	33.30 (33.30–55.80)	33.30 (16.60–66.50)	33.30 (33.30–33.30)	NS
>70 years	33.30 (0–33.30) [b]	33.30 (16.60–33.30)	24.95 (0–33.30) [b,c]	NS
D7	87.50 (75–87.50)	87.5 (84.38–100)	87.50 (75–87.50)	0.006
<60 years	87.50 (87.50–100)	87.5 (87.50–100)	87.50 (77.08–96.88)	NS
60–69	87.5 (75–100)	87.5 (81.25–100)	87.50 (75–87.50)	NS
>70 years	75 (62.50–87.50) [b,c]	87.5 (75–87.50)	75 (62.50–87.50) [c]	NS
Total	55.45 (46.57–65.10)	57.90 (51.23–67.23)	53.33 (44.23–59.20)	0.003
<60 years	60.75 (54.30–68.05)	65.30 (59.33–76.2)	59 (54.30–66.98)	NS
60–69	56.30 (49.85–66.45)	59.90 (51.45–67.85)	56.30 (46.15–64.60)	NS
>70 years	48.10 (39.60–57.80) [b,c]	56.10 (48.10–59.90)	45.25 (38.75–52.75) [b,c]	<0.05

Data are presented as median and (IQR); p [a] relates to group 1–group 2 comparison ($p < 0.05$); [b] relates to the > 70 years and 60–69 years comparison ($p < 0.05$); [c] relates to the >70 years and <60 years ($p < 0.05$).

Physical performance did not differ significantly between the two groups. Low physical performance assessed with TUG (TUG > 20 s) was observed in 28 women from group 1 (48.27%) and in 34 women from group 2 (53.12%). According to the EWGSOP2 criteria, 53.12% women from group 2 were classified as having severe sarcopenia when using TUG performance. No age differences were observed between those with confirmed sarcopenia and those with severe sarcopenia.

In the whole study sample and in the probable sarcopenia group, significant greater TUG scores were observed in women older than 70 years compared to those younger than 60 years (21.8(17.9–30.6) vs. 16.3(13.3–21.38) s, $p = 0.001$ for the whole sample; 25.10(19.06–33.3) vs. 13.90(9.54–17.18) s, $p < 0.001$ for the probable sarcopenia group).

Significant negative correlations were found between SarQoL domains and total scores and some of the socio-anthropometric data for the whole study sample (Table 3). The history of falls and the number of comorbidities were negatively correlated with all SarQoL scores, except the D6 domains.

Table 3. Correlations between Sarqol Domaines and Clinical Variables.

	SarQoL D1	SarQoL D2	SarQoL D3	SarQoL D4	SarQoL D5	SarQoL D6	SarQoL D7	SarQoL Total
Age	−0.339 *	−0.238	−0.141	−0.318 *	−0.339 *	−0.062	−0.392 *	−0.392 *
BMI	−0.374 *	−0.171	−0.196	−0.302 *	−0.207	−0.184	−0.214	−0.297 *
Years of menopause	−0.379 *	−0.205	−0.153	−0.264 *	−0.303 *	0.017	−0.323 *	−0.314 *
No of comorbidities	−0.455 *	−0.312 *	−0.425 *	−0.396 *	−0.305 *	−0.204	−0.307 *	−0.381 *
Tendency to fall	−0.110	−0.113	−0.092	−0.077	−0.006	−0.059	−0.197	−0.086
Falls history	−0.406 *	−0.315 *	−0.344 *	−0.330 *	−0.263 *	−0.148	−0.361 *	−0.372 *
Osteoporotic fractures history	−0.061	0.08	−0.008	−0.059	−0.057	−0.150	0.005	−0.03
TUG	−0.206	−0.19	−0.137	−0.217	−0.236	0.053	−0.307 *	−0.244

Data represents the Spearman correlation coefficient; * $p < 0.05$

The stepwise multiple linear regression analysis with SarQoL total score as a dependent variable revealed a negative association with age, history of falls and being sarcopenic (adjusted $R^2 = 0.238$; $F_{3,118} = 13.59, p < 0.0001$). Being older, sarcopenic with at least one fall in the past would negatively affect the quality of life of osteoporotic postmenopausal women. Table 4 shows the results of the regression analysis for all the SarQoL scores. In all regression models, history of falls was negatively correlated with all quality of life questionnaire domains, indicating that osteoporotic postmenopausal women with low muscle strength and falls in the past will have a poorer quality of life.

Table 4. Multiple Linear Regression Analysis with the Total and the Seven Domain Scores of SarQoL as Dependent Variables.

Independent Variable	B	SE	Beta	T	*p*	R^2	Adjusted R^2	Model Significance
SarQoL Total Score								
1. Age	−0.443	0.149	−0.268	−3.023	0.003	0.256	0.238	$F_{3,118} = 13.59$ $p < 0.0001$
2. Fall history	−10.318	2.946	−0.306	−3.502	0.0001			
3. Sarcopenia (confirmed and severe)	−5.140	2.365	−0.196	0.031	0.03			
SarQoL D1								
1. Age	−0.425	0.17	−0.222	−2.483	0.01	0.248	0.228	$F_{3.118} = 12.97$ $p < 0.0001$
2. Number of comorbidities	−1.454	0.66	−0.198	−2.202	0.02			
3. Fall history	−11.562	3.262	−0.310	−3.544	0.0006			
SarQoL D2								
1. Fall history	−15.035	3.608	−0.355	−4.167	0.0001	0.126	0.119	$F_{1,120} = 17.3$ $p = 0.0001$
SarQoL D3								
1. Number of comorbidities	−1.628	0.653	−0.222	−2.491	0.01	0.135	0.116	$F_{2,119} = 9$ $p = 0.0002$
2. Fall history	−9.679	3.208	−2.66	−3.017	0.003			
SarQoL D4								
1. Age	−0.474	0.145	−0.286	−3.259	0.001	0.261	0.249	$F_{2,119} = 21.07$ $p < 0.0001$
2. Fall history	−12.440	2.865	−0.369	−4.341	<0.0001			
SarQoL D5								
1. Age	−0.540	0.190	−0.252	−2.838	0.006	0.189	0.168	$F_{3,118} = 9.186$ $p < 0.0001$
2. Fall history	−7.976	3.820	−0.188	−2.088	0.01			
3. Sarcopenia (confirmed and severe)	−7.522	3.066	−0.220	−2.453	0.01			
SarQoL D6								
1. Fall history	−12.402	4.671	−0.235	−2.655	0.009	0.055	0.047	$F_{1,120} = 7.04$ $p = 0.009$
SarQoL D7								
1. Years of menopause	−0.458	0.137	−0.293	−3.344	0.001	0.187	0.174	$F_{2,119} = 13.75$ $p < 0.0001$
2. Fall history	−8.802	2.954	−0.263	−2.980	0.003			

4. Discussion

The main aim of this study was to assess the relationship between sarcopenia and the quality of life in osteoporotic postmenopausal women. Both sarcopenia and osteoporosis are major health problems in postmenopausal women, negatively affecting the quality of life [19–21], the incidence of falls, and mortality [22–25]. To the best of our knowledge, there are no studies investigating the quality of life in Romanian postmenopausal osteoporotic women diagnosed with sarcopenia according to the updated EWGSOP diagnostic criteria.

There are several definitions, diagnostic criteria and cut-offs used for the diagnosis of sarcopenia [1,26–31]. In our study, we used the revised EWGSOP2 criteria. The percentage of confirmed and severe sarcopenia in osteoporotic postmenopausal women aged between 48 and 83 years at the time of assessment was 52.46%. Similar results were also found in other studies, showing the association of sarcopenia and osteoporosis [32–37]. Walsh et al., reported a similar prevalence of sarcopenia of 50% in osteoporotic postmenopausal women, using the loss of muscle mass for the sarcopenia diagnosis [38]. Hamad et al. found that sarcopenia was present in 74.6% of postmenopausal women with osteoporosis, supporting the results of Yoshimura that osteoporosis increases the risk of sarcopenia [39,40]. Studies indicate that the prevalence of sarcopenia increases with age [41,42]. In our study, the percentage of osteoporotic postmenopausal women diagnosed with sarcopenia increased with age, with 43.75% of women being older than 70 years. The true prevalence of sarcopenia cannot be correctly estimated, since various definitions, cut-offs or populations were used across studies.

History of falls and BMI were significantly associated with the presence of sarcopenia in osteoporotic postmenopausal women. Our results showed that osteoporotic postmenopausal women with at least one fall in the past had a significantly higher risk of developing sarcopenia. Similar results were presented by Clynes et al., who reported an association of falls in the last year and sarcopenia, diagnosed using the IWGS (International Working Group of Sarcopenia) definition, but not the EWGSOP one [43]. In their meta-analysis, Yeung et al. also reported a positive association between sarcopenia and falls [9]. Sepulveda-Loyola et al. found a strong association between osteosarcopenia (defined as the concomitant presence of osteoporosis/osteopenia with sarcopenia [44]) and falls and fractures history in community-dwelling older adults [45]. Other prospective studies have reported the association between sarcopenia and the incidence and risk of falls [7,46–48].

We found that BMI was lower in sarcopenic women than in those with probable sarcopenia from group 1. There was a higher percent of overweight and obese women with probable sarcopenia compared to those with an established sarcopenia diagnosis. In the sarcopenic group, we identified 14.06% cases of sarcopenic obesity. In recent years, the prevalence of obesity combined with sarcopenia had increased, resulting in a high-risk geriatric syndrome. Affected individuals are at risk of synergistic complications from both sarcopenia and obesity [49].

The logistic regression results in our study showed that osteoporotic postmenopausal women with a higher body mass index had a significantly reduced risk of developing sarcopenia. Similar results were found in previous studies [50–52], although in these studies the comparisons were made with non-sarcopenic subjects. Other studies also reported the protective effect of high body mass against sarcopenia in Asian population [53–55]. Moreno-Aguilar et al. found that a higher BMI represents a protective factor against the presence of osteosarcopenia [56]. Despite these findings, in a recent meta-analysis Shen et al. suggested, as well as Gonzales et al. in 2017, that BMI should not be used for making clinically important decisions at the individual patient level, since it could not differentiate between body weight components (body fat and lean mass) [57,58].

The SarQoL questionnaire is a specific health-related quality of life questionnaire for sarcopenia and muscle impairments [59]. Previous studies have demonstrated the ability of SarQoL to discriminate sarcopenic individuals with regard to their quality of life, as long as for the diagnosis of sarcopenia both muscle mass and muscle strength criteria were used [12,13,59–61]. The present study showed that osteoporotic postmenopausal women with probable and established sarcopenia had a reduced quality of life, as assessed with the SarQoL questionnaire. Our results were slightly lower than those obtained in previous studies by the sarcopenic participants [12,14,59–62]. We have to mention that, in previous studies, the EWGSOP criteria were used for establishing the diagnosis of sarcopenia, with a few exceptions where the revised EWGSOP2 criteria were used [14,62,63]. We found that the domains of physical and mental health (D1), functionality (D4), activities of daily living (D5), fears (D7) and total SarQoL scores were significantly lower in women with sarcopenia than those with probable sarcopenia. For locomotion (D2), body composition (D3) and leisure activities (D6) domains we have not found significant differences between sarcopenic groups. Similar results were found for the D6 domain in the study of Gasparik et al., with no significant differences between sarcopenic and non-sarcopenic participants when using the Romanian version of the SarQoL, as well as in the study of Konstantynowicz et al., who used the Polish version of the SarQoL [13,60]. The reason could be due to the fact that Romanian and Polish older people are not involved in many leisure activities [60].

In our study, osteoporotic postmenopausal women with sarcopenia who were older than 70 years had significantly lower values for physical and mental health (D1), body composition (D3), functionality (D4), leisure (D6) and total SarQoL scores than the younger ones. In the probable sarcopenia cases, the SarQoL scores were not influenced by age.

The negative impact of sarcopenia on quality of life has been largely investigated, although different criteria and questionnaires were used. The physical function domain of the quality of life has been proved to be impaired in sarcopenic patients, as assessed by the SF-36 questionnaire [52,64–67].

The multiple regression analysis in the present study showed a significant impact of age, history of falls and the presence of sarcopenia on the overall quality of life of postmenopausal osteoporotic women, as assessed with the SarQoL questionnaire. Older osteoporotic postmenopausal women with previous falls were more likely to have lower scores on physical and mental health (D1), functionality (D4) and activities of daily living (D5) domains. In association with the history of falls, the number of comorbidities was found to be a predictor only in the physical and mental health domain (D1) and body composition domain scores, respectively. Years since menopause, along with the history of falls, negatively influenced the fear domain (D7) score.

Several limitations of this study should be addressed. The study sample comprised only osteoporotic postmenopausal women with low grip strength, and no control group (premenopausal, non-sarcopenic) was included. Another issue that has to be mentioned is that the number of comorbidities was quite high and could influence the quality of life. The sample could have also been biased compared to the normal population, since the subjects were recruited from a rehabilitation clinic.

5. Conclusions

In summary, in our sample of osteoporotic postmenopausal women, the frequency of sarcopenia, as defined with the EWGSOP2 criteria, was relatively high. The body mass index and the history of falls could predict, together, sarcopenia in osteoporotic postmenopausal women. Our results showed that osteoporotic postmenopausal women with at least one fall in the past and a lower body mass index had a significantly higher risk of developing sarcopenia. History of falls and the number of comorbidities were negatively correlated with all quality of life questionnaire domains, indicating that postmenopausal women with low muscle strength and falls in the past will have a poorer quality of life. Older osteoporotic postmenopausal women, with previous falls and a confirmed sarcopenia diagnosis (low muscle strength and low muscle mass) were more likely to have a decreased quality of life. Future studies are required to identify women at risk, in order to reduce the prevalence of sarcopenia and its negative effects.

Author Contributions: Conceptualization, M.C., D.S. and R.R.O.; methodology, M.C., D.S., F.C. and R.R.O.; formal analysis, M.C., D.S., F.C. and R.R.O.; investigation, M.C. and F.C.; data curation, D.S. and R.R.O.; writing—original draft preparation, M.C., D.S., F.C. and R.R.O.; writing—review and editing, M.C., D.S. and R.R.O.; visualization, M.C., D.S., F.C. and R.R.O.; supervision, M.C. All authors have read and agreed to the published version of the manuscript.

References

1. Cruz-Jentoft, A.J.; Bahat, G.; Bauer, J.; Boirie, Y.; Bruyère, O.; Cederholm, T.; Cooper, C.; Landi, F.; Rolland, Y.; Sayer, A.A.; et al. Sarcopenia: Revised European consensus on definition and diagnosis. *Age Ageing* **2019**, *48*, 16–31. [CrossRef] [PubMed]
2. Han, A.; Bokshan, S.; Marcaccio, S.; DePasse, J.; Daniels, A. Diagnostic Criteria and Clinical Outcomes in Sarcopenia Research: A Literature Review. *J. Clin. Med.* **2018**, *7*, 70. [CrossRef] [PubMed]
3. Roubenoff, R.; Hughes, V.A. Sarcopenia: Current concepts. *J. Gerontol. Ser. A Biol. Sci. Med. Sci.* **2000**, *55*, M716–M724. [CrossRef] [PubMed]
4. Beaudart, C.; Rizzoli, R.; Bruyère, O.; Reginster, J.Y.; Biver, E. Sarcopenia: Burden and challenges for public health. *Arch. Public Health* **2014**, *72*, 45. [CrossRef]
5. Morley, J.E.; Anker, S.D.; von Haehling, S. Prevalence, incidence, and clinical impact of sarcopenia: Facts, numbers, and epidemiology—Update 2014. *J. Cachexia. Sarcopenia Muscle* **2014**, *5*, 253–259. [CrossRef]
6. Rizzoli, R.; Reginster, J.Y.; Arnal, J.F.; Bautmans, I.; Beaudart, C.; Bischoff-Ferrari, H.; Biver, E.; Boonen, S.; Brandi, M.L.; Chines, A.; et al. Quality of life in sarcopenia and frailty. *Calcif. Tissue Int.* **2013**, *93*, 101–120. [CrossRef]
7. Landi, F.; Liperoti, R.; Russo, A.; Giovannini, S.; Tosato, M.; Capoluongo, E.; Bernabei, R.; Onder, G. Sarcopenia as a risk factor for falls in elderly individuals: Results from the ilSIRENTE study. *Clin. Nutr.* **2012**, *31*, 652–658. [CrossRef]
8. Terroso, M.; Rosa, N.; Torres Marques, A.; Simoes, R. Physical consequences of falls in the elderly: A literature review from 1995 to 2010. *Eur. Rev. Aging Phys. Act.* **2014**, *11*, 51–59. [CrossRef]
9. Yeung, S.S.Y.; Reijnierse, E.M.; Pham, V.K.; Trappenburg, M.C.; Lim, W.K.; Meskers, C.G.M.; Maier, A.B. Sarcopenia and its association with falls and fractures in older adults: A systematic review and meta-analysis. *J. Cachexia. Sarcopenia Muscle* **2019**, *10*, 485–500. [CrossRef]
10. Beaudart, C.; Biver, E.; Reginster, J.Y.; Rizzoli, R.; Rolland, Y.; Bautmans, I.; Petermans, J.; Gillain, S.; Buckinx, F.; Van Beveren, J.; et al. Development of a self-administrated quality of life questionnaire for sarcopenia in elderly subjects: The SarQoL. *Age Ageing* **2015**, *44*, 960–966. [CrossRef]
11. Beaudart, C.; Reginster, J.Y.; Geerinck, A.; Locquet, M.; Bruyère, O. Current review of the SarQoL®: A health-related quality of life questionnaire specific to sarcopenia. *Expert Rev. Pharm. Outcomes Res.* **2017**, *17*, 335–341. [CrossRef] [PubMed]
12. Beaudart, C.; Biver, E.; Reginster, J.Y.; Rizzoli, R.; Rolland, Y.; Bautmans, I.; Petermans, J.; Gillain, S.; Buckinx, F.; Dardenne, N.; et al. Validation of the SarQoL®, a specific health-related quality of life questionnaire for Sarcopenia. *J. Cachexia. Sarcopenia Muscle* **2017**, *8*, 238–244. [CrossRef] [PubMed]
13. Ildiko, G.A.; Gabriela, M.; Charlotte, B.; Olivier, B.; Raluca-Monica, P.; Jean-Yves, R.; Maria, P.I. Psychometric performance of the Romanian version of the SarQoL®, a health-related quality of life questionnaire for sarcopenia. *Arch. Osteoporos.* **2017**, *12*. [CrossRef] [PubMed]
14. Alekna, V.; Kilaite, J.; Tamulaitiene, M.; Geerinck, A.; Mastaviciute, A.; Bruyère, O.; Reginster, J.Y.; Beaudart, C. Validation of the Lithuanian version of sarcopenia-specific quality of life questionnaire (SarQoL®). *Eur. Geriatr. Med.* **2019**. [CrossRef]
15. Franzon, K.; Zethelius, B.; Cederholm, T.; Kilander, L. The impact of muscle function, muscle mass and sarcopenia on independent ageing in very old Swedish men. *BMC Geriatr.* **2019**, *19*, 153. [CrossRef]
16. Su, Y.; Hirayama, K.; Han, T.; Izutsu, M.; Yuki, M. Sarcopenia Prevalence and Risk Factors among Japanese Community Dwelling Older Adults Living in a Snow-Covered City According to EWGSOP2. *J. Clin. Med.* **2019**, *8*, 291. [CrossRef]
17. Available online: https://www.btsbioengineering.com/products/g-walk-inertial-motion-system. (accessed on 7 October 2019).
18. Geerinck, A.; Bruyère, O.; Locquet, M.; Reginster, J.Y.; Beaudart, C. Evaluation of the Responsiveness of the SarQoL® Questionnaire, a Patient-Reported Outcome Measure Specific to Sarcopenia. *Adv. Ther.* **2018**, *35*, 1842–1858. [CrossRef]
19. Stoicanescu, D.L.; Cevei, M.L.; Guler, N. Physical function limitation in osteoporotic cases. *Osteoporos. Int.* **2018**, *29*, 416–417.
20. Cevei, M.; Stoicanescu, D.; Suciu, R.; Cioara, F. Immobilization osteoporosis and sarcopenia in patients with vertebromedullary trauma. *Osteoporos. Int.* **2019**, *30*, 444.

21. Go, S.W.; Cha, Y.H.; Lee, J.A.; Park, H.S. Association between sarcopenia, bone density, and health-related quality of life in korean men. *Korean J. Fam. Med.* **2013**, *34*, 281–288. [CrossRef]
22. Beaudart, C.; Zaaria, M.; Pasleau, F.; Reginster, J.Y.; Bruyère, O. Health outcomes of sarcopenia: A systematic review and meta-analysis. *PLoS ONE* **2017**, *12*, e0169548. [CrossRef] [PubMed]
23. Lang, T.; Streeper, T.; Cawthon, P.; Baldwin, K.; Taaffe, D.R.; Harris, T.B. Sarcopenia: Etiology, clinical consequences, intervention, and assessment. *Osteoporos. Int.* **2010**, *21*, 543–559. [CrossRef] [PubMed]
24. Sim, M.; Prince, R.L.; Scott, D.; Daly, R.M.; Duque, G.; Inderjeeth, C.A.; Zhu, K.; Woodman, R.J.; Hodgson, J.M.; Lewis, J.R. Sarcopenia Definitions and Their Associations With Mortality in Older Australian Women. *J. Am. Med. Dir. Assoc.* **2019**, *20*, 76–82. [CrossRef] [PubMed]
25. Greco, E.A.; Pietschmann, P.; Migliaccio, S. Osteoporosis and sarcopenia increase frailty syndrome in the elderly. *Front. Endocrinol. (Lausanne)* **2019**, *10*, 255. [CrossRef]
26. Cruz-Jentoft, A.J.; Baeyens, J.P.; Bauer, J.M.; Boirie, Y.; Cederholm, T.; Landi, F.; Martin, F.C.; Michel, J.-P.; Rolland, Y.; Schneider, S.M.; et al. Sarcopenia: European consensus on definition and diagnosis: Report of the European Working Group on Sarcopenia in Older People. *Age Ageing* **2010**, *39*, 412–423. [CrossRef]
27. Fielding, R.A.; Vellas, B.; Evans, W.J.; Bhasin, S.; Morley, J.E.; Newman, A.B.; Abellan van Kan, G.; Andrieu, S.; Bauer, J.; Breuille, D.; et al. Sarcopenia: An Undiagnosed Condition in Older Adults. Current Consensus Definition: Prevalence, Etiology, and Consequences. International Working Group on Sarcopenia. *J. Am. Med. Dir. Assoc.* **2011**, *12*, 249–256. [CrossRef]
28. Morley, J.E.; Abbatecola, A.M.; Argiles, J.M.; Baracos, V.; Bauer, J.; Bhasin, S.; Cederholm, T.; Stewart Coats, A.J.; Cummings, S.R.; Evans, W.J.; et al. Sarcopenia With Limited Mobility: An International Consensus. *J. Am. Med. Dir. Assoc.* **2011**, *12*, 403–409. [CrossRef]
29. Delmonico, M.J.; Harris, T.B.; Lee, J.S.; Visser, M.; Nevitt, M.; Kritchevsky, S.B.; Tylavsky, F.A.; Newman, A.B. Alternative definitions of sarcopenia, lower extremity performance, and functional impairment with aging in older men and women. *J. Am. Geriatr. Soc.* **2007**, *55*, 769–774. [CrossRef]
30. Muscaritoli, M.; Anker, S.D.; Argilés, J.; Aversa, Z.; Bauer, J.M.; Biolo, G.; Boirie, Y.; Bosaeus, I.; Cederholm, T.; Costelli, P.; et al. Consensus definition of sarcopenia, cachexia and pre-cachexia: Joint document elaborated by Special Interest Groups (SIG) cachexia-anorexia in chronic wasting diseases and nutrition in geriatrics. *Clin. Nutr.* **2010**, *29*, 154–159. [CrossRef]
31. Studenski, S.A.; Peters, K.W.; Alley, D.E.; Cawthon, P.M.; McLean, R.R.; Harris, T.B.; Ferrucci, L.; Guralnik, J.M.; Fragala, M.S.; Kenny, A.M.; et al. The FNIH Sarcopenia Project: Rationale, Study Description, Conference Recommendations, and Final Estimates. *J. Gerontol. Ser. A* **2014**, *69*, 547–558. [CrossRef]
32. Sjöblom, S.; Suuronen, J.; Rikkonen, T.; Honkanen, R.; Kröger, H.; Sirola, J. Relationship between postmenopausal osteoporosis and the components of clinical sarcopenia. *Maturitas* **2013**, *75*, 175–180. [CrossRef] [PubMed]
33. Miyakoshi, N.; Hongo, M.; Mizutani, Y.; Shimada, Y. Prevalence of sarcopenia in Japanese women with osteopenia and osteoporosis. *J. Bone Miner. Metab.* **2013**, *31*, 556–561. [CrossRef] [PubMed]
34. He, H.; Liu, Y.; Tian, Q.; Papasian, C.J.; Hu, T.; Deng, H.-W. Relationship of sarcopenia and body composition with osteoporosis. *Osteoporos. Int.* **2016**, *27*, 473–482. [CrossRef] [PubMed]
35. Nielsen, B.R.; Abdulla, J.; Andersen, H.E.; Schwarz, P.; Suetta, C. Sarcopenia and osteoporosis in older people: A systematic review and meta-analysis. *Eur. Geriatr. Med.* **2018**, *9*, 419–434. [CrossRef]
36. Tarantino, U.; Baldi, J.; Celi, M.; Rao, C.; Liuni, F.M.; Iundusi, R.; Gasbarra, E. Osteoporosis and sarcopenia: The connections. *Aging Clin. Exp. Res.* **2013**, *25*, 93–95. [CrossRef]
37. Reiss, J.; Iglseder, B.; Alzner, R.; Mayr-Pirker, B.; Pirich, C.; Kässmann, H.; Kreutzer, M.; Dovjak, P.; Reiter, R. Sarcopenia and osteoporosis are interrelated in geriatric inpatients. *Z. Gerontol. Geriatr.* **2019**, *52*, 688–693. [CrossRef]
38. Walsh, M.C.; Hunter, G.R.; Livingstone, M.B. Sarcopenia in premenopausal and postmenopausal women with osteopenia, osteoporosis and normal bone mineral density. *Osteoporos. Int.* **2006**, *17*, 61–67. [CrossRef]
39. Hamad, B.; Basaran, S.; Coskun Benlidayi, I. Osteosarcopenia among postmenopausal women and handgrip strength as a practical method for predicting the risk. *Aging Clin. Exp. Res.* **2019**. [CrossRef]
40. Yoshimura, N.; Muraki, S.; Oka, H.; Iidaka, T.; Kodama, R.; Kawaguchi, H.; Nakamura, K.; Tanaka, S.; Akune, T. Is osteoporosis a predictor for future sarcopenia or vice versa? Four-year observations between the second and third ROAD study surveys. *Osteoporos. Int.* **2017**, *28*, 189–199. [CrossRef]

41. Volpato, S.; Bianchi, L.; Cherubini, A.; Landi, F.; Maggio, M.; Savino, E.; Bandinelli, S.; Ceda, G.P.; Guralnik, J.M.; Zuliani, G.; et al. Prevalence and Clinical Correlates of Sarcopenia in Community-Dwelling Older People: Application of the EWGSOP Definition and Diagnostic Algorithm. *J. Gerontol. Ser. A* **2013**, *69*, 438–446. [CrossRef]
42. Cruz-Jentoft, A.J.; Landi, F.; Schneider, S.M.; Zúñiga, C.; Arai, H.; Boirie, Y.; Chen, L.-K.; Fielding, R.A.; Martin, F.C.; Michel, J.-P.; et al. Prevalence of and interventions for sarcopenia in ageing adults: A systematic review. Report of the International Sarcopenia Initiative (EWGSOP and IWGS). *Age Ageing* **2014**, *43*, 748–759. [CrossRef] [PubMed]
43. Clynes, M.A.; Edwards, M.H.; Buehring, B.; Dennison, E.M.; Binkley, N.; Cooper, C. Definitions of Sarcopenia: Associations with Previous Falls and Fracture in a Population Sample. *Calcif. Tissue Int.* **2015**, *97*, 445–452. [CrossRef] [PubMed]
44. Huo, Y.R.; Suriyaarachchi, P.; Gomez, F.; Curcio, C.L.; Boersma, D.; Muir, S.W.; Montero-Odasso, M.; Gunawardene, P.; Demontiero, O.; Duque, G. Phenotype of Osteosarcopenia in Older Individuals With a History of Falling. *J. Am. Med. Dir. Assoc.* **2015**, *16*, 290–295. [CrossRef] [PubMed]
45. Sepúlveda-Loyola, W.; Phu, S.; Bani Hassan, E.; Brennan-Olsen, S.L.; Zanker, J.; Vogrin, S.; Conzade, R.; Kirk, B.; Al Saedi, A.; Probst, V.; et al. The Joint Occurrence of Osteoporosis and Sarcopenia (Osteosarcopenia): Definitions and Characteristics. *J. Am. Med. Dir. Assoc.* **2019**. [CrossRef] [PubMed]
46. Bischoff-Ferrari, H.A.; Orav, J.E.; Kanis, J.A.; Rizzoli, R.; Schlögl, M.; Staehelin, H.B.; Willett, W.C.; Dawson-Hughes, B. Comparative performance of current definitions of sarcopenia against the prospective incidence of falls among community-dwelling seniors age 65 and older. *Osteoporos. Int.* **2015**, *26*, 2793–2802. [CrossRef] [PubMed]
47. Mori, H.; Tokuda, Y. Differences and overlap between sarcopenia and physical frailty in older community-dwelling Japanese. *Asia Pac. J. Clin. Nutr.* **2019**, *28*, 157–165.
48. Gadelha, A.B.; Neri, S.G.R.; Oliveira RJ, d.e.; Bottaro, M.; David AC, d.e.; Vainshelboim, B.; Lima, R.M. Severity of sarcopenia is associated with postural balance and risk of falls in community-dwelling older women. *Exp. Aging Res.* **2018**, *44*, 258–269. [CrossRef]
49. Batsis, J.A.; Villareal, D.T. Sarcopenic obesity in older adults: Aetiology, epidemiology and treatment strategies. *Nat. Rev. Endocrinol.* **2018**, *14*, 513–537. [CrossRef]
50. Akune, T.; Muraki, S.; Oka, H.; Tanaka, S.; Kawaguchi, H.; Nakamura, K.; Yoshimura, N. Exercise habits during middle age are associated with lower prevalence of sarcopenia: The ROAD study. *Osteoporos. Int.* **2014**, *25*, 1081–1088. [CrossRef]
51. Fukuoka, Y.; Narita, T.; Fujita, H.; Morii, T.; Sato, T.; Sassa, M.H.; Yamada, Y. Importance of physical evaluation using skeletal muscle mass index and body fat percentage to prevent sarcopenia in elderly Japanese diabetes patients. *J. Diabetes Investig.* **2019**, *10*, 322–330. [CrossRef]
52. Beaudart, C.; Reginster, J.Y.; Petermans, J.; Gillain, S.; Quabron, A.; Locquet, M.; Slomian, J.; Buckinx, F.; Bruyère, O. Quality of life and physical components linked to sarcopenia: The SarcoPhAge study. *Exp. Gerontol.* **2015**, *69*, 103–110. [CrossRef] [PubMed]
53. Yu, R.; Wong, M.; Leung, J.; Lee, J.; Auyeung, T.W.; Woo, J. Incidence, reversibility, risk factors and the protective effect of high body mass index against sarcopenia in community-dwelling older Chinese adults. *Geriatr. Gerontol. Int.* **2014**, *14*, 15–28. [CrossRef] [PubMed]
54. Han, P.; Zhao, J.; Guo, Q.; Wang, J.; Zhang, W.; Shen, S.; Wang, X.; Dong, R.; Ma, Y.; Kang, L.; et al. Incidence, risk factors, and the protective effect of high body mass index against sarcopenia in suburb-dwelling elderly Chinese populations. *J. Nutr. Health Aging* **2016**, *20*, 1056–1060. [CrossRef] [PubMed]
55. Kim, H.; Suzuki, T.; Kim, M.; Kojima, N.; Yoshida, Y.; Hirano, H.; Saito, K.; Iwasa, H.; Shimada, H.; Hosoi, E.; et al. Incidence and predictors of sarcopenia onset in community-dwelling elderly japanese women: 4-Year follow-up study. *J. Am. Med. Dir. Assoc.* **2015**, *16*, e1–e85. [CrossRef]
56. Moreno-Aguilar, M.; Molina, M.M.; Hernandez, M.F.H. Inverse Association Between Body Mass Index and Osteosarcopenia in Community Dwelling Elderly. *Surg. Obes. Relat. Dis.* **2017**, *13*, 190. [CrossRef]
57. Shen, Y.; Chen, J.; Chen, X.; Hou, L.S.; Lin, X.; Yang, M. Prevalence and Associated Factors of Sarcopenia in Nursing Home Residents: A Systematic Review and Meta-analysis. *J. Am. Med. Dir. Assoc.* **2019**, *20*, 5–13. [CrossRef]
58. Gonzalez, M.C.; Correia, M.I.T.D.; Heymsfield, S.B. A requiem for BMI in the clinical setting. *Curr. Opin. Clin. Nutr. Metab. Care* **2017**, *20*, 314–321. [CrossRef]

59. Beaudart, C.; Locquet, M.; Reginster, J.Y.; Delandsheere, L.; Petermans, J.; Bruyère, O. Quality of life in sarcopenia measured with the SarQoL®: Impact of the use of different diagnosis definitions. *Aging Clin. Exp. Res.* **2018**, *30*, 307–313. [CrossRef]
60. Konstantynowicz, J.; Abramowicz, P.; Glinkowski, W.; Taranta, E.; Marcinowicz, L.; Dymitrowicz, M.; Reginster, J.-Y.; Bruyere, O.; Beaudart, C. Polish Validation of the SarQoL®, a Quality of Life Questionnaire Specific to Sarcopenia. *J. Clin. Med.* **2018**, *7*, 323. [CrossRef]
61. Geerinck, A.; Scheppers, A.; Beaudart, C.; Bruyère, O.; Vandenbussche, W.; Bautmans, R.; Delye, S.; Bautmans, I. Translation and validation of the dutch sarqol®, a quality of life questionnaire specific to sarcopenia. *J. Musculoskelet. Neuronal Interact.* **2018**, *18*, 463–472.
62. Geerinck, A.; Alekna, V.; Beaudart, C.; Bautmans, I.; Cooper, C.; De Souza Orlandi, F.; Konstantynowicz, J.; Montero-Errasquín, B.; Topinková, E.; Tsekoura, M.; et al. Standard error of measurement and smallest detectable change of the Sarcopenia Quality of Life (SarQoL) questionnaire: An analysis of subjects from 9 validation studies. *PLoS ONE* **2019**, *14*. [CrossRef] [PubMed]
63. Fábrega-Cuadros, R.; Martínez-Amat, A.; Cruz-Díaz, D.; Aibar-Almazán, A.; Hita-Contreras, F. Psychometric Properties of the Spanish Version of the Sarcopenia and Quality of Life, a Quality of Life Questionnaire Specific for Sarcopenia. *Calcif. Tissue Int.* **2019**. [CrossRef] [PubMed]
64. Patel, H.P.; Syddall, H.E.; Jameson, K.; Robinson, S.; Denison, H.; Roberts, H.C.; Edwards, M.; Dennison, E.; Cooper, C.; Aihie Sayer, A. Prevalence of sarcopenia in community-dwelling older people in the UK using the European Working Group on Sarcopenia in Older People (EWGSOP) definition: Findings from the Hertfordshire Cohort Study (HCS). *Age Ageing* **2013**, *42*, 378–384. [CrossRef] [PubMed]
65. Manrique-Espinoza, B.; Salinas-Rodríguez, A.; Rosas-Carrasco, O.; Gutiérrez-Robledo, L.M.; Avila-Funes, J.A. Sarcopenia Is Associated With Physical and Mental Components of Health-Related Quality of Life in Older Adults. *J. Am. Med. Dir. Assoc.* **2017**, *18*, e1–e636. [CrossRef]
66. Kull, M.; Kallikorm, R.; Lember, M. Impact of a New Sarco-Osteopenia Definition on Health-related Quality of Life in a Population-Based Cohort in Northern Europe. *J. Clin. Densitom.* **2012**, *15*, 32–38. [CrossRef]
67. Trombetti, A.; Reid, K.F.; Hars, M.; Herrmann, F.R.; Pasha, E.; Phillips, E.M.; Fielding, R.A. Age-associated declines in muscle mass, strength, power, and physical performance: Impact on fear of falling and quality of life. *Osteoporos. Int.* **2016**, *27*, 463–471. [CrossRef]

Effect of Sleep Quality on the Prevalence of Sarcopenia in Older Adults

Jacobo Á. Rubio-Arias [1,*], Raquel Rodríguez-Fernández [2], Luis Andreu [3,4], Luis M. Martínez-Aranda [4,5], Alejandro Martínez-Rodriguez [6] and Domingo J. Ramos-Campo [4]

1 LFE Research Group, Department of Health and Human Performance, Faculty of Physical Activity and Sport Science-INEF, Universidad Politécnica de Madrid, 28040 Madrid, Spain
2 Department of Methodology of Behavioral Sciences, Faculty of Psychology, Universidad Nacional de Educación a Distancia (UNED), 28040 Madrid, Spain; rrodriguez@psi.uned.es
3 International Chair of Sports Medicine, Universidad Católica San Antonio de Murcia (UCAM), 30107 Murcia, Spain; landreu@ucam.edu
4 Faculty of Sports, Universidad Católica San Antonio de Murcia (UCAM), 30107 Murcia, Spain; lmmartinez2@ucam.edu (L.M.M.-A.); Djramos@ucam.edu (D.J.R.-C.)
5 Neuroscience of Human Movement Research Group (Neuromove), Universidad Católica San Antonio de Murcia (UCAM), 30107 Murcia, Spain
6 Department of Analytical Chemistry, Nutrition and Food Science, Faculty of Science, Alicante University, 03690 Alicante, Spain; amartinezrodriguez@ua.es
* Correspondence: ja.rubio@upm.es or jacobo.rubio2@gmail.com

Abstract: Sarcopenia is an age-related condition. However, the prevalence of sarcopenia may increase due to a range of other factors, such as sleep quality/duration. Therefore, the aim of the study is to conduct a systematic review with meta-analysis to determine the prevalence of sarcopenia in older adults based on their self-reported sleep duration. Methods: Three electronic databases were used—PubMed-Medline, Web of Science, and Cochrane Library. We included studies that measured the prevalence of sarcopenia, divided according to sleep quality and excluded studies (a) involving populations with neuromuscular pathologies, (b) not showing prevalence values (cases/control) on sarcopenia, and (c) not including classificatory models to determine sleep quality. Results: high prevalence values in older adults with both long and short sleep duration were shown. However, prevalence values were higher in those with inadequate sleep (<6–8 h or low efficiency) (OR 0.76; 95% CI (0.70–0.83); Q = 1.446; $p = 0.695$; test for overall effect, Z = 6.01, $p < 0.00001$). Likewise, higher prevalence levels were shown in men (OR 1.61; 95% CI (0.82–3.16); Q = 11.80; $p = 0.0189$) compared to women (OR 0.77; 95% CI (0.29–2.03); Q = 21.35; $p = 0.0003$). Therefore, the prevalence of sarcopenia appears to be associated with sleep quality, with higher prevalence values in older adults who have inadequate sleep.

Keywords: muscle-mass; sleep efficiency; sleep duration; insomnia

---

1. Introduction

Together with the increment of the world population and life span over the years, a parallel increase in chronic diseases [1] has been observed, such as sarcopenia. This pathology has become a serious global public health problem [2] since it can lead to a considerable increase in costs due to the frequency and duration of hospitalization, as well as an increase in the number of falls as a consequence of muscle weakness [3,4]. In addition, people who suffer a high loss of muscle mass have an increased risk of other health problems, such as heart failure, chronic obstructive pulmonary diseases, kidney failure [5] or osteoporosis [6] and, therefore, a greater risk of bone fracture, turning sarcopenia into a major health problem that should be addressed in order to determine the possible factors associated with sarcopenia.

Sarcopenia has been defined as a decrease and deterioration of muscle mass associated with aging [7]. Thus, the skeletal muscle mass is progressively lost during aging and is partially replaced by fat and connective tissue due to a reduction and leakage of type II fibers generated by a slow degenerative neurological process [8]. This decrease in muscle mass due to aging also generates a decrease in muscle strength and, therefore, a physical disability generating a functional limitation (activities of the daily life) as well as a decrease in the life quality [9,10] with an associated increase in the risk of mortality [11,12]. In addition, this muscle mass loss has a greater impact on women during menopause as a consequence of the decrease in the estrogen levels after the fifth decade of life [13]. Sex differences in body composition are well known [14], with men having a higher cross-sectional area in skeletal muscle than women and greater muscle in the upper body [15]. Additionally, women are at higher risk of developing sarcopenic obesity due to increased fat and lower muscle mass [14]. Nevertheless, the results of prevalence related to sex are inconsistent [2]. In these circumstances, efforts are required to identify the factors associated with sarcopenia and to implement interventions for the prevention or the incidence reduction of this pathology among the elderly population [16], considering sex as a modifying variable.

However, the loss of muscle mass (sarcopenia) is not only related to age and sex but also depends on a number of endogenous and exogenous factors that influence the prevalence values of sarcopenia. The most studied and validated factors that can generate an effect on the sarcopenia are age (main moderating variable), genetic factors, birth weight, early growth, diet, physical activity, other chronic diseases, and hormonal changes (secondary variables) [17,18]. In line with this, a recent systematic review with meta-analysis on the general population [2] concludes that the prevalence of sarcopenia can be modified by other factors such as race, nutrition, quality of life, and sex among others.

Nonetheless, the scientific literature shows a gap between the role that sleep quality could play and the effects on the prevalence of sarcopenia. As Buchmann et al. (2016) [19] suggest, sleep is associated with a biological and mental regeneration process. Moreover, Vitale et al. (2019) [20] reported that the maintenance of circadian rhythms can be altered by aging and the development of many chronic diseases, including sarcopenia. The preservation of circadian rhythm is very important for the sustainment of cellular physiology, metabolism, and function in the skeletal muscle. Therefore, people who have an inadequate sleeping time could have an increased risk of mortality compared to those who sleep the recommended daily hours [21]. In addition, under low sleep conditions, the cognitive abilities might be affected and can be an increment in the risk of mortality and falling in older adults [22]. In this way, sex may also play a significant role in sleep quality, due to the fact that women have a greater predisposition of insomnia found among different criteria, frequencies, and duration [23]. Nevertheless, the association between muscle mass, sleep quality, and sex is not clear yet and no studies have been found to support such affirmation.

Certainly, the lack of sleep not only leads to a deterioration of cognitive abilities but can also have a negative effect at the cellular level on muscle physiology. It impairs muscle recovery due to increased stimulation of protein degradation, which is detrimental for protein synthesis and promotes muscle atrophy [24]. In addition to the negative effect on muscle mass, it has been associated with cardiovascular disease [25], type II diabetes [26], hypertension [25], obesity [27], and colorectal cancer [28]. In this regard, public health should include sleep duration/quality as one of the risk factors associated with a large number of diseases.

Some correlational studies have determined the effect of sleep duration on muscle mass, showing that less sleep duration or quality leads to a loss of muscle mass [29]. However, no meta-analyses addressing the effect of sleep duration or quality on the prevalence of sarcopenia have been found. Therefore, the objectives of this systematic review with meta-analysis are (1) to analyze the overall prevalence of sarcopenia in people with optimal sleep duration/quality compared to those with inadequate sleep quality, (2) to analyze whether the prevalence of sarcopenia is correlated to the sex of the participants. Our starting hypothesis is that people with poor rest show a higher prevalence of sarcopenia than those who rest in better conditions and, in addition, men will have a lower prevalence compared to women.

2. Experimental Section

2.1. Study Design

A systematic review with meta-analysis was performed following the recommendations of PRISMA (preferred reporting items for systematic review and meta-analysis) [30]. All the analyses were performed in duplicate (J.A.R.A. and L.A.), all disagreements on inclusion/exclusion were discussed and resolved by consensus. The extrinsic characteristics of the publications and the substantive characteristics—population, sex, associated pathology, habits of alcohol, tobacco, physical activity, age, and BMI—were extracted from the studies that were finally included in the quantitative analysis. Finally, the methodological characteristics—duration of sleep, quality of sleep, muscular mass and presence or not of sarcopenia—were also considered. All subjects included in the analysis were classified as cases or control differentiating sleep and sex.

2.2. Search and Data Sources

Three electronic databases were used: PubMed-Medline, Web of Science, and Cochrane Library. The search was conducted without search date restriction and ended on 28 July 2019. The key search words and strategy were "Sleep Disorders" OR "Sleep Deprivation" OR "Sleep Hygiene" OR "Sleep duration" OR insomnia OR sleep* and "muscle mass" OR "muscular atrophy" OR sarcopenia.

2.3. Data extraction and Inclusion/Exclusion Criteria

The following inclusion criteria were considered: prevalence studies analyzing the effect of sleep on sarcopenia and conducted in adults (>40). Studies were excluded if they included (a) populations with neuromuscular pathologies, (b) studies that did not show prevalence values (cases/control) on sarcopenia, and (c) studies that did not include classificatory models that allowed sleep quality to be determined.

2.4. Outcomes

The variables to determine the prevalence of sarcopenia as a function of sleep were (1) the presence or absence of sarcopenia, and (2) sleep quality. Sleep can be assessed to estimate adequate or inadequate sleep in terms of quality or duration in different ways. For the questionnaires, adequate-sleep (sleep well) for those who obtained between very good or quite good in the percentage of quality and not-adequate-sleep (sleep bad), rather bad or very bad were considered [19]. Regarding the hours of sleep, they were considered inadequate (<6–8) and adequate (≥8), following the recommendations of the National Sleep Foundation [21].

2.5. Assessment of Risk of Bias

The Q-index was used to assess the methodological quality, a scale that allows us to quantify the bias, obtaining a final score between 0 (minimum quality) and 1 (maximum quality). This rescaled quality range (called Qi in MetaXL) has a monotonic relationship to ICC bias, defined as the variance of the study bias divided by the sum of the variance of bias within and between studies [31,32]. Quality analysis was performed on each study based on the method of assessing sleep quality and sarcopenia, giving higher preference to the studies that measured the sleep with instruments previously validated for this purpose, as well as sarcopenia with DXA or BIA. Therefore, the studies using both DXA and a validated questionnaire to analyze sleep quality were scored with 1. The following criteria were conducted:

(Q1) Were the target population and the observation period well defined?: yes = 1 and no = 0;

(Q2) Diagnostic criteria, use of diagnostic system reported: sarcopenia = DXA or BIA and sleep quality = instruments validated = 1 and own system/symptoms described/no system/not specified = 0;

(Q3) Method of case ascertainment: community survey/multiple institutions = 2, inpatient/ inpatients and outpatients/case registers = 1, and not specified = 0;

(Q4) Administration of measurement protocol: administered interview = 3, systematic case-note review = 2, chart diagnosis/case records = 1 and not specified = 0;

(Q5) Catchment area: broadly representative (national or multi-site survey) = 2, small area/not representative (single community, single university) = 1, and convenience sampling/other (primary care sample/treatment group) = 0; and

(Q6) Prevalence measure: point prevalence (e.g., one month) = 2, 12-month prevalence = 1 and lifetime prevalence = 0.

In addition, the overall publication bias of the studies was analyzed using the funnel plot, dividing between older adults who slept well and those who had inadequate sleep.

2.6. Data Synthesis and Statistical Analysis

Meta-analysis and statistical analysis were performed using MetaXL software version 2.0 (Sunrise Beach, Queensland, Australia). The prevalence of sarcopenia (cases vs. control) was initially calculated in the included studies for random-effects model analysis (no transformation methods) and then recalculated under a rescaled quality of bias effects model. For the analysis, the sleep category was considered (sleep well and sleep poorly) for the calculation of the overall prevalence of sarcopenia, and this method was applied under the random-effects model and effects in quality of the rescaled bias using three possible transformations (None, Logit, and Arcsine) [31,32] to contrast the effects of the prevalence of sarcopenia. In all cases, pooled prevalence values were shown, 95% CI, heterogeneity I^2, Cochran's Q, chi^2, p, tau^2. On the other hand, the grouped odds ratios (OR) and their IC95% were also calculated following a model of "quality effects" [31,33] to analyze the association between those who sleep well (control) and those who sleep poorly (effect). In addition, OR and sleep category analysis were estimated, excluding studies that did not report participants' total hours of sleep and only showed sleep quality [19,34]. Heterogeneity between studies was conducted using the I^2 statistic, and the variation between studies was calculated using the tau^2 statistic (τ^2) [35]. I^2 values between 30–60% were considered as moderate levels of heterogeneity, while a value of $\tau^2 > 1$ suggested the presence of substantial statistical heterogeneity. The minimum level of significance was set as $p \leq 0.05$.

3. Results

3.1. General Characteristics of the Studies

A total of 551 items were identified from the selected databases, and 0/0 items were included from other sources. After the removal of duplicated articles from the different databases, 361 titles and abstracts, as well as 106 articles, were reviewed, and 255 were removed. Finally, statistical analysis was performed on a total of 6 studies [19,34,36–39] (5 were performed in Asia and only 1 in Europe; Figure 1), with a mean age of 68.7 years (range = 44–80 years). Table 1 shows the descriptive characteristics of the studies included in our analysis. The selected studies included 6405 (990 cases and 5415 controls) older adults with adequate sleep and 12,708 (1762 cases and 10,946 controls) adults with inadequate sleep. However, only four studies contained data divided by sex (1232 men) including 142 cases with adequate sleep and 95 cases with inadequate sleep. In addition, 1381 women were enrolled in the four studies, with 109 cases in the adequate sleep group and 118 cases in the inadequate sleep group.

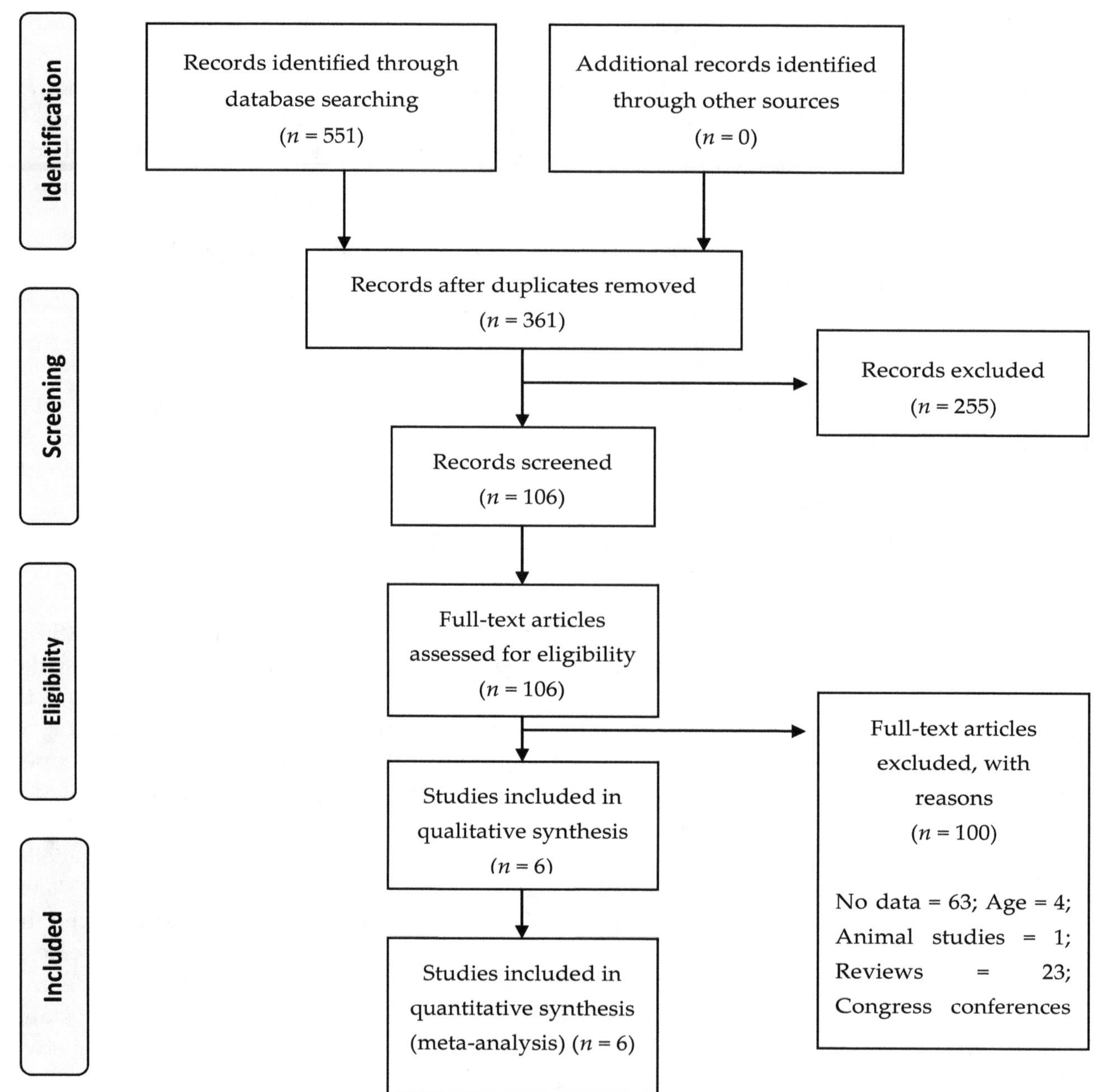

Figure 1. Flow diagram of the process of study selection.

Table 1. Characteristics of the included studies in the meta-analysis.

Extrinsic Variables	Substantive Characteristics											Methodological Characteristics								
															Sleep Well			Sleep Poorly		
Study	Country of the Study	Sex	Alcohol	Tobacco	Level of Physical Activity	Muscle Mass	Sleep Quality	Age	Weight	Height	BMI	Type	Sex	Total	N	Cases	Control	N2	Cases	Control
Buchmann et al.	Berlin	Women	494	46	Moderate	DXA	PSQI	68			25.7	Cross-sectional	M	568	492	79	413	76	27	49
		Women	66	4	Moderate			69			31.2		W	628	508	64	444	120	13	107
		Men	424	59	Moderate			69			26.4		T	1196	1000	143	857	196	40	156
		Men	99	7	Moderate			69			30.2									
Chien et al.	Taiwan	Men			Regular	BIA	PSQI and Self-report	78.7	63.9	162.1	24.3	Cross-sectional	M	224	112	25	87	112	29	83
		Men			Regular			77.8	64.1	163.7	23.9		W	264	76	20	56	188	18	170
		Men			Regular			80	66.8	164.4	24.7		T	488	188	45	143	300	47	253
		Women			Regular			74.4	58.3	151.9	25.3									
		Women			Regular			74.5	57.9	153	24.8									
		Women			Regular			76.2	56.6	152.2	24.3									
Fu et al.	China	48.7% Men	No = 61.1%	No = 37.2%	Moderate	BIA	Self-report	68.24	70.24	163.38	25.9	Cohort study								
		40.5% Men	No = 62.2%	No = 38.9%	Moderate			66.3	67.96	163.91	25.3									
		37.9% Men	No = 59.5%	No = 33.7%	Moderate			67.38	67.16	163.39	25.1		T	920	468	52	416	452	43	409
		54% Men	No = 64.6%	No = 28.8%	Moderate			68.93	68.1	163.37	25.4									
Hu et al.	China	Men	57	62	Moderate	DXA	Self-report	70.8			23.6	Cross-Sectional Study	M	251	63	13	50	188	28	160
		Men	16	19	Moderate			72.6			18.7		W	356	63	14	49	293	57	236
		Women	16	1	Moderate			69.1			23.6		T	607	126	27	99	481	85	396
		Women	5	2	Moderate			72.3			20.3									
Ida et al.	Japan	Men	60%	72.1%		Self-report	PSQI	71.8			24.3	Cross-sectional study	M	189	105	14	91	84	22	62
		Women	17.2%	4,9%				72.8			23.9		W	129	71	11	60	58	24	34
													T	318	176	25	151	142	46	96
Kwon et al.	Korea	Men = 5819; Women = 8118	4.209	3.579	Regular	DXA	Self-report	44				Cross-sectional study	M							
		Men = 1339; Women = 872	635	797	Regular			45.2					W							
													T	16148	4938	819	4119	11210	1486	9724

M, men; W, women; T, total; DXA, densitometry; BIA, bioelectrical impedance analysis and PSQI, pittsburgh sleep quality index.

3.2. Quality of the Studies

The assessment of the methodological quality of the studies included in the quantitative analysis is summarised in Table 2.

Table 2. The score obtained by the studies on the quality scale.

		Q1	Q2	Q3	Q4	Q5	Q6	M.S.	Qi
Buchmann et al. 2016	[19]	1	1	2	3	1	2	10	1
Chien et al. 2015	[36]	1	1	2	3	1	2	9	1
Fu et al. 2019	[37]	1	1	0	3	1	2	7	0.8
Hu et al. 2017	[38]	1	1	2	3	1	2	10	1
Ida et al. 2019	[34]	1	0	0	3	0	2	7	0.6
Kwon et al. 2017	[39]	1	1	2	3	1	2	10	1

TS, Total score; Q1, Were the target population and the observation period well defined?; Q2, Diagnostic criteria; Q3, Method of case ascertainment; Q4, Administration of measurement protocol; Q5, Catchment Area; Q6, Prevalence measure. M.S. mean score; Qi stands for a quality rank.

When estimating a study quality, the mean score was 0.833 (range: 0.7–1). Three studies used bioelectrical impedance analysis (BIA) [33,36], three DXA [19,38,39] and only one study used a self-administered questionnaire [34]. Furthermore, three studies used the Pittsburg Sleep Quality Index (PSQI) [19,34,36], and the other three assessed the sleep duration/quality with self-reports. In addition, two studies [34,37] did not specify the case measurement system. The funnel plots suggest the presence of significant publication bias (Figure 2).

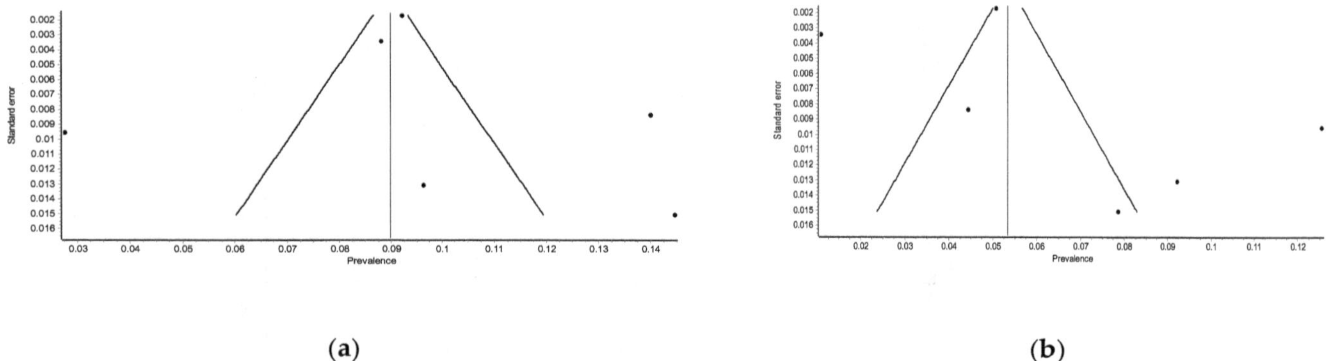

(a) (b)

Figure 2. Funnel plot of the meta-analysis of the published studies. Each plotted point represents the.standard error (SE) and the prevalence. (**a**) Sleep well, (**b**) sleep poorly.

3.3. Meta-Analysis

The overall results of the prevalence of sarcopenia in the studies included in our meta-analysis revealed a high prevalence (Figure 3). When the methodological quality of the studies was considered in the results (Table 2), the prevalence was decreased (Total = 19,677 participants, 2858 cases; 0.144, 95% CI (0.100–0.189); Q = 41.90, $p = 0.0000$) but maintaining a high heterogeneity ($I^2 = 88$).

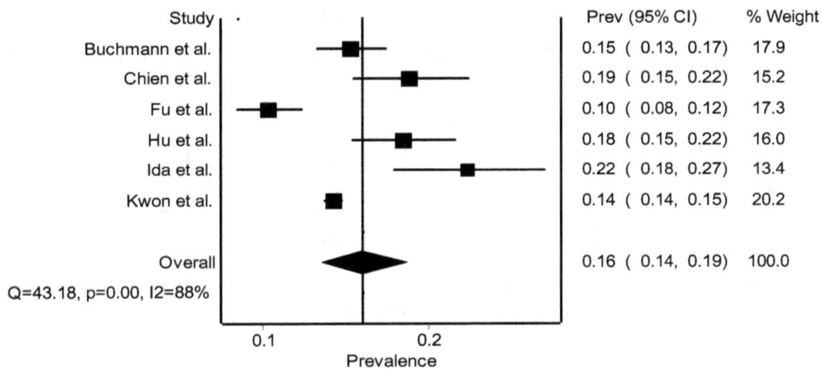

Figure 3. Overall prevalence of studies included in the analysis (method: random effects).

Results by Sleep Categories

The effects of the prevalence of sarcopenia sorted by categories are shown in Table 3. The prevalence values are grouped by sleep quality categories (sleep well and sleep poorly).

Table 3. Prevalence. Pooled results and CIs for three categories by transformation method and model.

Model			Sarcopenia and Self-Report or PSQI							Sarcopenia and Self-Report						
	Transf.	Category	Pooled	LCI	HCI	I^2 (%)	Cochran's Q	x^2 (p)	tau2/ Q-Index	Pooled	LCI	HCI	I^2	Cochran's Q	x^2 (p)	tau2/ Q-Index
Inverse Variance	None	SW	0.056	0.053	0.059	95.786	118.642	0.000		0.052	0.049	0.055	94.549	55.035	0.000	
		SP	0.088	0.084	0.091	95.786	118.642	0.000		0.090	0.086	0.094	94.549	55.035	0.000	
	Logit	SW	0.384	0.052	0.058	95.241	105.072	0.000		0.363	0.049	0.055	90.653	32.094	0.000	
		SP	0.616	0.084	0.092	95.241	105.072	0.000		0.637	0.087	0.095	90.653	32.094	0.000	
	Double arcsine	SW	0.388	0.052	0.059	95.847	120.389	0.000		0.363	0.049	0.055	93.072	43.300	0.000	
		SP	0.612	0.084	0.092	95.847	120.389	0.000		0.637	0.087	0.095	93.072	43.300	0.000	
Random effects	None	SW	0.073	0.044	0.102	95.786	118.642	0.000	0.001	0.060	0.030	0.091	94.549	55.035	0.000	0.001
		SP	0.090	0.061	0.119	95.786	118.642	0.000	0.001	0.093	0.062	0.124	94.549	55.035	0.000	0.001
	Logit	SW	0.460	0.046	0.103	95.241	105.072	0.000	0.264	0.399	0.041	0.083	90.653	32.094	0.000	0.126
		SP	0.540	0.055	0.119	95.241	105.072	0.000	0.264	0.601	0.062	0.122	90.653	32.094	0.000	0.126
	Double arcsine	SW	0.453	0.044	0.102	95.847	120.389	0.000	0.018	0.395	0.036	0.086	93.072	43.300	0.000	0.011
		SP	0.547	0.056	0.120	95.847	120.389	0.000	0.018	0.605	0.061	0.123	93.072	43.300	0.000	0.011
Quality effects	None	SW	0.056	-0.001	0.113	95.786	118.642	0.000	1.698	0.052	0.000	0.104	94.549	55.035	0.000	1.356
		SP	0.088	0.031	0.145	95.786	118.642	0.000	1.698	0.091	0.039	0.143	94.549	55.035	0.000	1.356
	Logit	SW	0.384	0.024	0.118	95.241	105.072	0.000	1.714	0.362	0.028	0.093	90.653	32.094	0.000	0.804
		SP	0.616	0.040	0.182	95.241	105.072	0.000	1.714	0.638	0.051	0.158	90.653	32.094	0.000	0.804
	Double arcsine	SW	0.379	0.011	0.112	95.847	120.389	0.000	1.583	0.353	0.015	0.096	93.072	43.300	0.000	1.013
		SP	0.621	0.030	0.155	95.847	120.389	0.000	1.583	0.647	0.042	0.148	93.072	43.300	0.000	1.013

Transf., transformation; HCI, higher CI; LCI, lower CI; SW, sleep well; SP, sleep poorly.

People who sleep well had lower values than those who sleep poorly and the prevalence in all the sub-analyses was high, suggesting a prevalence of sarcopenia independently of the category. However, the OR value was not significant (OR 0.81; 95% CI (0.41–1.60); Q = 34.04; $p = 0.0000$; test for overall effect, Z = 0.12, $p = 0.91$) when analysing the relationship between sarcopenia and sleep quality. Nonetheless, when the relationship between sleep quality and sarcopenia was analyzed after excluding the Buchmann et al. [19] and Ida et al. [34] studies from the analysis due to high heterogeneity, the sleep quality was associated with sarcopenia (OR 0.76; 95% CI (0.70–0.83); Q = 1.446; $p = 0.695$; test for overall effect, Z = 6.01, $p < 0.00001$). Likewise, the subjects who self-reported fewer sleeping hours showed a higher prevalence of sarcopenia.

Due to the high heterogeneity of the studies included in the meta-analysis, a gender analysis of prevalence was performed (Figure 4). Only four studies provided sex-dependent data. Non-significant associations for men (OR 1.61; 95% CI (0.82–3.16); Q = 11.80; $p = 0.0189$) or women (OR 0.77; 95% CI (0.29–2.03); Q = 21.35; $p = 0.0003$) were observed. However, the heterogeneity still showed high value in all the sub-analyses that were performed (including the quality of the studies and without any transformation), due to the heterogeneity of the methodologies, the types of studies and other parameters that were not taken into consideration for the analysis of the prevalence of sarcopenia.

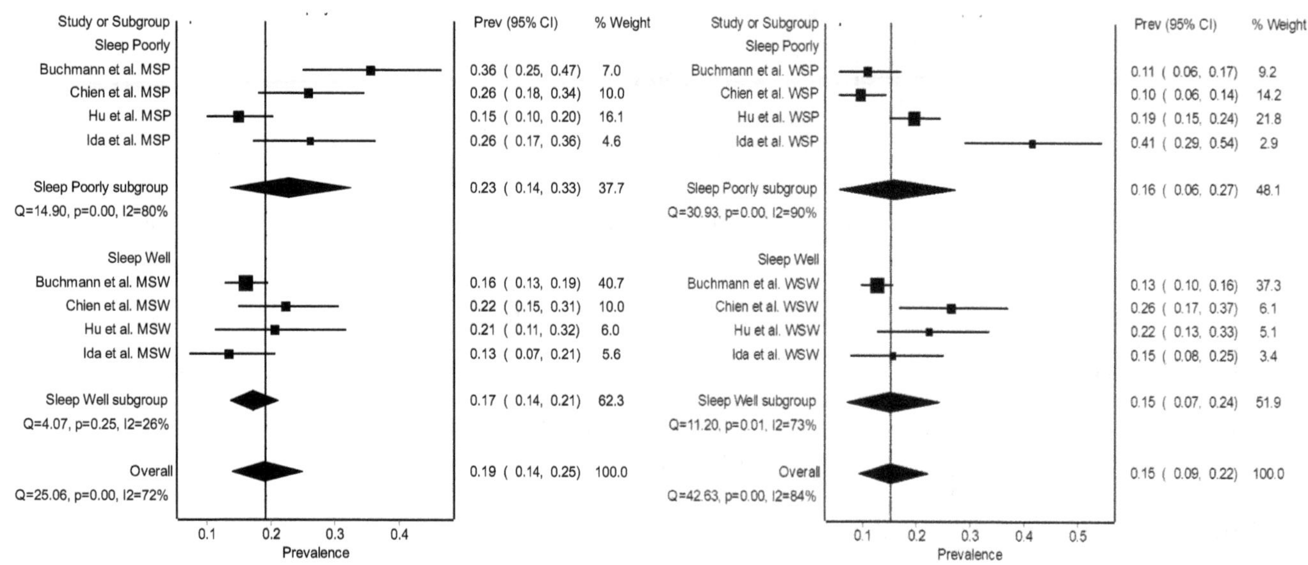

Figure 4. Prevalence of sarcopenia according to the sex of the participants. MSP, men sleep poorly; MSW, men sleep well; SWP, women sleep poorly; and WSW, women sleep well.

4. Discussion

The main finding of this research is that those subjects having inadequate sleep show a higher prevalence of sarcopenia values than those who reported adequate sleep. In addition, our results revealed a high prevalence of sarcopenia in older adults.

The results showed that a higher prevalence of sarcopenia values from those who do not sleep adequately were almost twice the value of the grouped prevalence, according to the model and the transformation that were used in the analysis. In line with our findings, Chien et al. [36], observed a significant association between sleep duration and the prevalence of sarcopenia on a sample of 488 adults (224 men and 264 women) from Taiwan, even though the assessment of sarcopenia was performed by electrical bioimpedance (BIA). Moreover, in the only study carried out in Europe, focused on the German subjects [19], similar results to those described above were observed, with the addition of the association between the sleep length and the quantity of muscle mass and recommending longitudinal studies to better understand the potential association. Similarly, Hu et al. [38] observed a relationship between sleep hours and sarcopenia in a Chinese cohort ($n = 920$, 95 cases). However, in this case, a U-shaped association in the prevalence of sarcopenia was obtained, in which older adults with short or long sleep length obtained higher values compared to those with normal sleep duration.

One plausible explanation to this findings is that the participants with an inefficient sleep may have differences in hormonal regulation (anabolic and catabolic balance), with elevated levels of cortisol (catabolic hormone promoting protein degradation), and low levels of IGF-1 (anabolic hormones promoting protein synthesis), developing a positive balance towards muscle degradation and, therefore, favoring the loss of muscle mass [19,40]. Likewise, Buchmann et al. [19] also observed elevated c-reactive protein (CRP) values. CRP is a pro-inflammatory cytokine and has been proposed as a possible cause of muscular atrophy [41] and also associated with sleep deprivation in high concentrations [42]. The sleep restriction generates hormonal imbalances and pro-inflammatory effects, favoring the loss of muscle mass with age. This could be one reason for the higher prevalence of sarcopenia values of sarcopenia in people with inadequate sleep. We must consider that the losses of muscle strength and muscle mass are associated and, therefore, related to a decrease in the functional capacity and quality of life [43]. Further studies to determine the effects of sleep deprivation in patients diagnosed with sarcopenia are necessary.

Interestingly, our results suggest a higher prevalence of sarcopenia in men compared to women (men = 0.19, 95% CI (0.14–0.25); women = 0.15, 95% CI (0.09–0.22)). These results are in line with previous studies in which the prevalence of sarcopenia can occur at earlier ages, as shown by Kwon et al. [39]. They observed a prevalence of sarcopenia of 14.3% in a group of 16,148 Koreans (44.1 ± 0.2 years), being higher in men (18.7%) than in women (9.7%). This can be explained by the fact that men had a higher muscle mass compared to women, but also a larger magnitude in muscle decrease was observed in men versus women as age increased [14]. On the contrary, in previous studies where the prevalence of sarcopenia was identified at different age intervals, a lower prevalence in men compared to women was observed [44]. Although age is the main causal effect of sarcopenia, the prediction ratio of increased sarcopenia based on age is difficult to verify, due to the multitude of factors that could have an influence in the prevalence values [45]. Nonetheless, it is estimated that the prevalence of clinically significant sarcopenia ranges from 8.8% in elderly women to 17.5% in elderly men, but it should be noted that these values may be higher or lower depending on the environmental factors [46]. In our study, only four articles considered gender as a sarcopenia-modifying variable, with very different methodologies and difficult interpretation. Therefore, the effect of sex on the prevalence of sarcopenia is unclear and more studies are needed to determine this interaction.

In summary, a direct association between sleep duration and prevalence of sarcopenia were confirmed in all the studies included in the quantitative data analysis. However, the interaction of gender and sleep duration/quality is not entirely clear. Hu et al. [38] observed that the prevalence of sarcopenia due to sleep deprivation was more pronounced in women. Similar results were described by Chien et al. [36] and Ida et al. [34]. However, Buchmann et al. [19] reported poor associations between sleep deprivation and the prevalence of sarcopenia in women. This discrepancy could be justified based on the ethnicity of the participants [2] or the age range difference between the studies. This higher and more evident prevalence in women could be associated with the negative effects of menopause. Thus, a decrease in the estrogen levels during menopause could play a potential role in decreasing the muscle mass after the fifth decade of life [13]. In addition, muscle mass seems to play an important role in osteoporosis in women, since muscle contractions involve a mechanical load on the bone that could promote the rate of bone regeneration [47]. Therefore, it could be stated that there is a close link between muscle strength, muscle mass, and bone tissue [48]; and that menopausal women are a sensitive population for the prevalence of sarcopenia, although to determine the gender role of this prevalence more studies would be needed. In addition, physical activity and programmed exercise should be considered, as it could play a relevant role in the prevalence of sarcopenia by improving sleep quality [49].

Finally, the results of this review should be interpreted with caution, since several limitations could be influencing them. For example, the high heterogeneity shown in the analyses could not be corrected by means of the rescaled bias scale. Another point to consider is the origin of the studied population. In five of the analyzed studies, the subjects cohort was from Asia, while only one single study was performed using a European population and the way of measuring the cut-off point and the provenance could be biasing the results [2], resulting in different tendencies between men and women. Other limitations are the way in which the sarcopenia [6] is conceptualized, resulting in prevalence variations due to the different techniques developed to measure sarcopenia, as well as the classification of the pathologic incidence [50] and that sleep quality was only self-reported throughout questionnaires and not objectively monitored; and the low number of articles included for the data for quantitative analysis (low security measure).

5. Conclusions

The main conclusion is the observed association between sleep duration/quality and the prevalence of sarcopenia. In addition, this prevalence seems to be higher in men than in women. These results could have a practical application for the public health since it can help us to consider sleep quality as a risk factor, as well as the need to incorporate therapies in order to improve the sleep quality and to reduce the negative effects of age-associated sarcopenia.

Author Contributions: Conceptualization, J.Á.R.-A., L.A. and R.R.-F.; methodology, R.R.-F.; software, J.Á.R.-A., A.M.-R. and L.M.M.-A.; formal analysis, J.Á.R.-A. and D.J.R.-C.; investigation, J.Á.R.-A., R.R.-F., L.A., L.M.M.-A., A.M.-R. and D.J.R.-C.; writing—original draft preparation, J.Á.R.-A.; writing—review and editing, R.R.-F., L.A., L.M.M.-A., A.M.-R. and D.J.R.-C.; supervision, J.Á.R.-A., R.R.-F., L.A., L.M.M.-A., A.M.-R. and D.J.R.-C.

Acknowledgments: The authors thank to G. Sanz for proofreading in English writing. No sources of funding were used in the preparation of this article.

References

1. Tobergte, D.R.; Curtis, S. Informe Mundial sobre el Envejecimiento y la Salud. *OMS* **2015**.
2. Shafiee, G.; Keshtkar, A.; Soltani, A.; Ahadi, Z.; Larijani, B.; Heshmat, R. Prevalence of sarcopenia in the world: A systematic review and meta-Analysis of general population studies. *J. Diabetes Metab. Disord.* **2017**, *16*, 1–10. [CrossRef] [PubMed]
3. Antunes, A.C.; Araujo, D.A.; Verissimo, M.T.; Amaral, T.F. Sarcopenia and hospitalisation costs in older adults: A cross-Sectional study. *Nutr. Diet.* **2017**, *74*, 46–50. [CrossRef] [PubMed]
4. Beaudart, C.; Zaaria, M.; Pasleau, F.; Reginster, J.Y.; Bruyere, O. Health outcomes of sarcopenia: A systematic review and meta-Analysis. *PLoS ONE* **2017**, *12*, e0169548. [CrossRef] [PubMed]
5. Morley, J.E.; Anker, S.D.; Von Haehling, S. Prevalence, incidence, and clinical impact of sarcopenia: Facts, numbers, and epidemiology—Update 2014. *J. Cachexia Sarcopenia Muscle* **2014**, *5*, 253–259. [CrossRef]
6. Cruz-Jentoft, A.J.; Bahat, G.; Bauer, J.; Boirie, Y.; Bruyere, O.; Cederholm, T.; Cooper, C.; Landi, F.; Rolland, Y.; Sayer, A.A.; et al. Sarcopenia: Revised European consensus on definition and diagnosis. *Age Ageing* **2019**, *48*, 16–31. [CrossRef]
7. Rosenberg, I.H. Sarcopenia: Origins and clinical relevance. *J. Nutr.* **1997**, *127*, 990S–991S. [CrossRef]
8. Lexell, J. Human aging, muscle mass, and fiber type composition. *J. Gerontol. Ser. A Biol. Sci. Med. Sci.* **1995**, *50*, 11–16.
9. Hairi, N.N.; Cumming, R.G.; Naganathan, V.; Handelsman, D.J.; Le Couteur, D.G.; Creasey, H.; Waite, L.M.; Seibel, M.J.; Sambrook, P.N. Loss of muscle strength, mass (sarcopenia), and quality (specific force) and its relationship with functional limitation and physical disability: The concord health and ageing in men project. *J. Am. Geriatr. Soc.* **2010**, *58*, 2055–2062. [CrossRef]
10. Rizzoli, R.; Reginster, J.Y.; Arnal, J.F.; Bautmans, I.; Beaudart, C.; Bischoff-Ferrari, H.; Biver, E.; Boonen, S.; Brandi, M.L.; Chines, A.; et al. Quality of life in sarcopenia and frailty. *Calcif. Tissue Int.* **2013**, *93*, 101–120. [CrossRef]
11. Rantanen, T. Muscle strength, disability and mortality. *Scand. J. Med. Sci. Sports* **2003**, *13*, 3–8. [CrossRef] [PubMed]
12. Arango-Lopera, V.E.; Arroyo, P.; Gutierrez-Robledo, L.M.; Perez-Zepeda, M.U.; Cesari, M. Mortality as an adverse outcome of sarcopenia. *J. Nutr. Health Aging* **2013**, *17*, 259–262. [CrossRef] [PubMed]
13. Messier, V.; Rabasa-Lhoret, R.; Barbat-Artigas, S.; Elisha, B.; Karelis, A.D.; Aubertin-Leheudre, M. Menopause and sarcopenia: A potential role for sex hormones. *Maturitas* **2011**, *68*, 331–336. [CrossRef] [PubMed]
14. Bredella, M.A. *Sex Differences in Body Composition BT-Sex and Gender Factors Affecting Metabolic Homeostasis, Diabetes and Obesity*; Mauvais-Jarvis, F., Ed.; Springer International Publishing: Cham, Germany, 2017; pp. 9–27. ISBN 978-3-319-70178-3.
15. Janssen, I.; Heymsfield, S.B.; Wang, Z.M.; Ross, R. Skeletal muscle mass and distribution in 468 men and women aged 18–88 yr. *J. Appl. Physiol.* **2000**, *89*, 81–88. [CrossRef] [PubMed]
16. Melton, L.J.; Khosla, S.; Riggs, B.L. Epidemiology of sarcopenia. *Mayo Clin. Proc.* **2000**, *48*, 625–630. [CrossRef]
17. Shimokata, H.; Shimada, H.; Satake, S.; Endo, N.; Shibasaki, K.; Ogawa, S.; Arai, H. Chapter 2 Epidemiology of sarcopenia. *Geriatr. Gerontol. Int.* **2018**, *18*, 13–22. [CrossRef]

18. Dodds, R.M.; Roberts, H.C.; Cooper, C.; Sayer, A.A. The Epidemiology of Sarcopenia. *J. Clin. Densitom.* **2015**, *27*, 355–363. [CrossRef]
19. Buchmann, N.; Spira, D.; Norman, K.; Demuth, I.; Eckardt, R.; Steinhagen-Thiessen, E. Sleep, Muscle Mass and Muscle Function in Older People. *Dtsch. Aerzteblatt Int.* **2016**, *113*, 253.
20. Vitale, J.; Bonato, M.; La Torre, A.; Banfi, G. The Role of the Molecular Clock in Promoting Skeletal Muscle Growth and Protecting against Sarcopenia. *Int. J. Mol. Sci.* **2019**, *20*, 4318. [CrossRef]
21. Hirshkowitz, M.; Whiton, K.; Albert, S.M.; Alessi, C.; Bruni, O.; DonCarlos, L.; Hazen, N.; Herman, J.; Katz, E.S.; Kheirandish-Gozal, L.; et al. National Sleep Foundation's sleep time duration recommendations: Methodology and results summary. *Sleep Health* **2015**, *1*, 233–243. [CrossRef]
22. Ancoli-Israel, S.; Cooke, J.R. Prevalence and comorbidity of insomnia and effect on functioning in elderly populations. *J. Am. Geriatr. Soc.* **2005**, *53*, S264–S271. [CrossRef] [PubMed]
23. Zhang, B.; Wing, Y.K. Sex differences in insomnia: A meta-Analysis. *Sleep* **2006**, *29*, 85–93. [CrossRef] [PubMed]
24. Dattilo, M.; Antunes, H.K.M.; Medeiros, A.; Monico Neto, M.; Souza, H.S.; Tufik, S.; De Mello, M.T. Sleep and muscle recovery: Endocrinological and molecular basis for a new and promising hypothesis. *Med. Hypotheses* **2011**, *77*, 220–222. [CrossRef] [PubMed]
25. Cappuccio, F.P.; Cooper, D.; Delia, L.; Strazzullo, P.; Miller, M.A. Sleep duration predicts cardiovascular outcomes: A systematic review and meta-Analysis of prospective studies. *Eur. Heart J.* **2011**, *32*, 1484–1492. [CrossRef]
26. Tuomilehto, H.; Peltonen, M.; Partinen, M.; Lavigne, G.; Eriksson, J.G.; Herder, C.; Aunola, S.; Keinanen-Kiukaanniemi, S.; Ilanne-Parikka, P.; Uusitupa, M.; et al. Sleep duration, lifestyle intervention, and incidence of type 2 diabetes in impaired glucose tolerance: The finnish diabetes prevention study. *Diabetes Care* **2009**, *32*, 1965–1971. [CrossRef]
27. Cappuccio, F.P.; Taggart, F.M.; Kandala, N.B.; Currie, A.; Peile, E.; Stranges, S.; Miller, M.A. Meta-Analysis of short sleep duration and obesity in children and adults. *Sleep* **2008**, *31*, 619–626. [CrossRef]
28. Zhao, H.; Yin, J.Y.; Yang, W.S.; Qin, Q.; Li, T.T.; Shi, Y.; Deng, Q.; Wei, S.; Liu, L.; Wang, X.; et al. Sleep duration and cancer risk: A systematic review and meta-Analysis of prospective studies. *Asian Pac. J. Cancer Prev.* **2013**, *14*, 7509–7515. [CrossRef]
29. Chen, H.C.; Hsu, N.W.; Chou, P. The association between sleep duration and hand grip strength in community-Dwelling older adults: The yilan study, Taiwan. *Sleep* **2017**, *40*, zsx021. [CrossRef]
30. Liberati, A.; Altman, D.G.; Tetzlaff, J.; Mulrow, C.; Gotzsche, P.C.; Ioannidis, J.P.A.; Clarke, M.; Devereaux, P.J.; Kleijnen, J.; Moher, D. The PRISMA statement for reporting systematic reviews and meta-analyses of studies that evaluate health care interventions: Explanation and elaboration. *J. Clin. Epidemiol.* **2009**, *6*, e1000100.
31. Barendregt, J.J.; Doi, S.A. *MetaXL User Guide: Version 5.3*; EpiGear International Pty Ltd.: Queensland, Australia, 2016.
32. Barendregt, J.J.; Doi, S.A.; Lee, Y.Y.; Norman, R.E.; Vos, T. Meta-Analysis of prevalence. *J. Epidemiol. Community Health* **2013**, *67*, 974–978. [CrossRef]
33. Colimon, K.M. *Fundamentos De Epidemiologia*; Diaz de Santos: Madrid, Spain, 1990; ISBN 9788578110796.
34. Ida, S.; Kaneko, R.; Nagata, H.; Noguchi, Y.; Araki, Y.; Nakai, M.; Ito, S.; Ishihara, Y.; Imataka, K.; Murata, K. Association between sarcopenia and sleep disorder in older patients with diabetes. *Geriatr. Gerontol. Int.* **2019**, *19*, 399–403. [CrossRef] [PubMed]
35. Higgins, J.P.T. Measuring inconsistency in meta-Analyses. *BMJ* **2003**, *327*, 557–560. [CrossRef] [PubMed]
36. Chien, M.Y.; Wang, L.Y.; Chen, H.C. The Relationship of Sleep Duration with Obesity and Sarcopenia in Community-Dwelling Older Adults. *Gerontology* **2015**, *61*, 399–406. [CrossRef] [PubMed]
37. Fu, L.; Yu, X.; Zhang, W.; Han, P.; Kang, L.; Ma, Y.; Jia, L.; Yu, H.; Chen, X.; Hou, L.; et al. The Relationship Between Sleep Duration, Falls, and Muscle Mass: A Cohort Study in an Elderly Chinese Population. *Rejuvenation Res.* **2018**. [CrossRef]
38. Hu, X.; Jiang, J.; Wang, H.; Zhang, L.; Dong, B.; Yang, M. Association between sleep duration and sarcopenia among community-Dwelling older adults: A cross-Sectional study. *Medicine* **2017**, *96*, e6268. [CrossRef]
39. Kwon, Y.J.; Jang, S.Y.; Park, E.C.; Cho, A.R.; Shim, J.Y.; Linton, J.A. Long sleep duration is associated with sarcopenia in Korean adults based on data from the 2008–2011 KNHANES. *J. Clin. Sleep Med.* **2017**, *13*, 1097–1104. [CrossRef]

40. Stitt, T.N.; Drujan, D.; Clarke, B.A.; Panaro, F.; Timofeyva, Y.; Kline, W.O.; Gonzalez, M.; Yancopoulos, G.D.; Glass, D.J. The IGF-1/PI3K/Akt pathway prevents expression of muscle atrophy-Induced ubiquitin ligases by inhibiting FOXO transcription factors. *Mol. Cell* **2004**, *14*, 395–403. [CrossRef]
41. Schaap, L.A.; Pluijm, S.M.F.; Deeg, D.J.H.; Visser, M. Inflammatory Markers and Loss of Muscle Mass (Sarcopenia) and Strength. *Am. J. Med.* **2006**, *119*, e9–e526. [CrossRef]
42. Van Leeuwen, W.M.A.; Lehto, M.; Karisola, P.; Lindholm, H.; Luukkonen, R.; Sallinen, M.; Harma, M.; Porkka-Heiskanen, T.; Alenius, H. Sleep restriction increases the risk of developing cardiovascular diseases by augmenting proinflammatory responses through IL-17 and CRP. *PLoS ONE* **2009**, *4*, e4589. [CrossRef]
43. Verlaan, S.; Aspray, T.J.; Bauer, J.M.; Cederholm, T.; Hemsworth, J.; Hill, T.R.; McPhee, J.S.; Piasecki, M.; Seal, C.; Sieber, C.C.; et al. Nutritional status, body composition, and quality of life in community-Dwelling sarcopenic and non-Sarcopenic older adults: A case-Control study. *Clin. Nutr.* **2017**, *36*, 267–274. [CrossRef]
44. Salva, A.; Serra-Rexach, J.A.; Artaza, I.; Formiga, F.; Rojano, I.; Luque, X.; Cuesta, F.; Lopez-Soto, A.; Masanes, F.; Ruiz, D.; et al. La prevalencia de sarcopenia en residencias de Espana: Comparacion de los resultados del estudio multicentrico ELLI con otras poblaciones. *Rev. Esp. Geriatr. Gerontol.* **2016**, *51*, 260–264. [CrossRef] [PubMed]
45. Piovezan, R.D.; Abucham, J.; Dos Santos, R.V.T.; Mello, M.T.; Tufik, S.; Poyares, D. The impact of sleep on age-Related sarcopenia: Possible connections and clinical implications. *Ageing Res. Rev.* **2015**, *23*, 210–220. [CrossRef] [PubMed]
46. Morley, J.E.; Baumgartner, R.; Roubenoff, R.; Mayer, J.; Nair, K.S. Sarcopenia. *J. Lab. Clin. Med.* **2001**, *137*, 231–243. [CrossRef] [PubMed]
47. Schoenau, E. From mechanostat theory to development of the "functional muscle-Bone-Unit". *J. Musculoskelet. Neuronal Interact.* **2005**, *5*, 232.
48. Gregg, E.W.; Kriska, A.M.; Salamone, L.M.; Roberts, M.M.; Anderson, S.J.; Ferrell, R.E.; Kuller, L.H.; Cauley, J.A. The epidemiology of quantitative ultrasound: A review of the relationships with bone mass, osteoporosis and fracture risk. *Osteoporos. Int.* **1997**, *7*, 89–99. [CrossRef]
49. Rubio-Arias, J.; Marin-Cascales, E.; Ramos-Campo, D.J.; Hernandez, A.V.; Perez-Lopez, F.R. Effect of exercise on sleep quality and insomnia in middle-Aged women: A systematic review and meta-Analysis of randomized controlled trials. *Maturitas* **2017**, *100*, 49–56. [CrossRef]
50. Pagotto, V.; Silveira, E.A. Methods, diagnostic criteria, cutoff points, and prevalence of sarcopenia among older people. *Sci. World J.* **2014**, *2014*, 231312. [CrossRef]

9

Preserved Capacity for Adaptations in Strength and Muscle Regulatory Factors in Elderly in Response to Resistance Exercise Training and Deconditioning

Andreas Mæchel Fritzen [1,2,*], Frank D. Thøgersen [1], Khaled Abdul Nasser Qadri [1], Thomas Krag [1], Marie-Louise Sveen [1,3], John Vissing [1] and Tina D. Jeppesen [1]

1 Department of Neurology, Copenhagen Neuromuscular Center, Rigshospitalet, DK-2100 Copenhagen, Denmark; frank.thogersen@gmail.com (F.D.T.); khaled_qadri@hotmail.com (K.A.N.Q.); thomas.krag@regionh.dk (T.K.); mqsv@novonordisk.com (M.-L.S.); john.vissing@regionh.dk (J.V.); tina@dysgaard.dk (T.D.J.)

2 Molecular Physiology Group, Department of Nutrition, Exercise, and Sports, Faculty of Science, University of Copenhagen, DK-2100 Copenhagen, Denmark

3 Novo Nordisk A/S, DK-2860 Søborg, Denmark

* Correspondence: amfritzen@nexs.ku.dk.

Abstract: Aging is related to an inevitable loss of muscle mass and strength. The mechanisms behind age-related loss of muscle tissue are not fully understood but may, among other things, be induced by age-related differences in myogenic regulatory factors. Resistance exercise training and deconditioning offers a model to investigate differences in myogenic regulatory factors that may be important for age-related loss of muscle mass and strength. Nine elderly (82 ± 7 years old) and nine young, healthy persons (22 ± 2 years old) participated in the study. Exercise consisted of six weeks of resistance training of the quadriceps muscle followed by eight weeks of deconditioning. Muscle biopsy samples before and after training and during the deconditioning period were analyzed for MyoD, myogenin, insulin-like growth-factor I receptor, activin receptor IIB, smad2, porin, and citrate synthase. Muscle strength improved with resistance training by 78% (95.0 ± 22.0 kg) in the elderly to a similar extent as in the young participants (83.5%; 178.2 ± 44.2 kg) and returned to baseline in both groups after eight weeks of deconditioning. No difference was seen in expression of muscle regulatory factors between elderly and young in response to exercise training and deconditioning. In conclusion, the capacity to gain muscle strength with resistance exercise training in elderly was not impaired, highlighting this as a potent tool to combat age-related loss of muscle function, possibly due to preserved regulation of myogenic factors in elderly compared with young muscle.

Keywords: resistance exercise training; muscle regulatory factors; sarcopenia; muscle strength; deconditioning; skeletal muscle; elderly; hypertrophy

---

1. Introduction

Sarcopenia means loss of flesh. The term is used to describe the pathological age-related loss of muscle mass, function, and strength that inevitable occurs in humans [1]. From the age of 50 to 85, humans lose 50% of their muscle mass, which is mainly a result of loss of type II muscle fibers [2]. Age-related loss of muscle mass and strength is associated with increasing risk of falling and disability, and thus impairment of basic daily activities.

It is well established that resistance exercise training can counteract the age-related changes in contractile function, strength, hypertrophy, and morphology of aging skeletal muscle [3]. However, whether the potential to adapt to resistance exercise training is completely preserved in skeletal muscles of elderly has been debated. [3]. Although 6–10 weeks of exercise training increased skeletal muscle strength to a similar extent in young and elderly in some studies [4,5], others report greater improvements in young individuals [6,7]. The rate of decline in muscle strength with age is 2–5 times greater than declines in muscle size [8] and strength loss is highly associated with both mortality and physical disability, even when adjusting for sarcopenia, indicating that muscle mass loss may be secondary to the effects of strength loss [9]. It is thus of key interest to elucidate whether increased muscle strength after a period of resistance exercise training occurs to a similar or blunted extent in old compared to young muscle. Moreover, although an aged-associated loss of muscle mass or strength [10,11] appears improved with resistance training in elderly individuals [12–16], several studies find a blunted muscle hypertrophy response [17–19].

Mechanisms responsible for resistance exercise-induced muscle hypertrophy are numerous, but some of the key factors include MyoD, myogenin, and insulin-like growth factor-I (IGF-I) [20–22]. The myogenic regulatory factors (MRF) are transcription factors that promote and regulate the expression of muscle-specific genes, which are essential to the hypertrophic and regenerative response following resistance exercise [23–26]. As MyoD is highly involved in muscle adaptation to resistance exercise, this has been a key factor in studies investigating potential differences in age-related muscle loss [27–29]. Differences in MRFs between young and elderly could be crucial mechanisms behind differences in muscle mass and strength [22,23,30] and in the response to resistance training and deconditioning. Previous studies found elevated levels of MyoD, myogenin, and IGF-I-R mRNA in elderly both at rest [17,31–34] and in response to one bout of resistance exercise [11]. Moreover, 16 weeks of resistance training increased muscle myoD mRNA levels to a similar extent in young and elderly, whereas the training-induced increase in mRNA levels of myogenin was impaired in the elderly [17].

Proteins responsible for negative muscle mass regulation, e.g., actRIIB and smad2, could be upregulated in inactive, aged muscle and be attenuated in response to resistance exercise, resulting in decreased muscle mass. In support, the mRNA level of actRIIB was downregulated after 21 weeks of resistance exercise in elderly [35,36]. The regulation of these molecular pathways involved in negative muscle mass regulation in response to resistance training in young and old muscle is unknown.

Mitochondrial dysfunction is another suggested key contributor loss of muscle mass with age [30]. Resistance exercise training has been found to affect mitochondrial function [37] evidenced by improved mitochondrial respiration and complex protein content after 12 weeks of resistance exercise training in young men [38]. However, whether resistance exercise training induces markers of mitochondrial content in elderly to a similar extent seems not clear.

In the present study, we therefore investigated the effect of resistance exercise training on strength and the protein expression or phosphorylation of factors important for upregulating (MyoD, myogenin, and IGF-I-R) and downregulating (activin receptor IIB (actRIIB) and smad2) skeletal muscle mass and mitochondrial markers in elderly compared to young individuals. In addition, we aimed at elucidating whether subsequent deconditioning affected these parameters in young and elderly similarly.

2. Materials and Methods

2.1. Subjects

Young and elderly volunteers were recruited with the criteria that for the elderly group age should be ≥74 years old and for the younger group age <30 years old. Exclusion criteria were non-sedentary status, illness requiring medical treatment other than treatment for hypertension and antithrombotic treatment, severe back or musculoskeletal pain, rheumatologic or neurological disorders, traumatic musculoskeletal and/or joint injuries, smoking, cardiovascular disease, attendance rate below 80% of total exercise sessions, additional exercise during the exercise phase, or failure to comply with instructions of inactivity during the deconditioning phase. Sedentary was defined as performing a maximum of three kilometers of cycling for transportation a day.

Twenty-two healthy, sedentary participants participated in the study; four were excluded due to noncompliance. Nine elderly, healthy persons—five men and four women (82 ± 7 year old)—fulfilled the inclusion criteria, and completed the resistance exercise training and deconditioning interventions. Data were compared to those found in nine young, healthy persons, also five men and four women (23 ± 3 yrs. of age). All participants completed a detailed medical history and had a normal neurological examination before entering the study. Demographic data of participants are shown in Table 1.

Table 1. General demographic data.

	Young Group		Elderly Group	
Age, years	22.4 ± 2.2		82.3 ± 6.8 ***	
Height, cm	174.8 ± 10.4		167.5 ± 8.6	
Weight, kg	70.9 ± 15.1		64.7 ± 9.7	
BMI, kg/m^2	22.9 ± 2.4		23.5 ± 2.9	
	Pre training	Post training	Pre training	Post training
Body fat (%)	26.2 ± 8.6	26.3 ± 9.5	27.9 ± 4.8	27.1 ± 5.8
LBM (%)	74.5 ± 8.9	74.5 ± 8.8	73.9 ± 6.6	73.7 ± 6.9
LLM (kg)	16.7 ± 4.2	17.0 ± 4.2	14.0 ± 2.9	14.2 ± 2.4

BMI, Body Mass Index; LBM, Lean Body Mass, LLM, lean leg mass. Age, height, weight, and BMI are presented at baseline pre intervention. Body fat, LBM, and LLM was measured before and after six weeks of resistance exercise training in elderly and young men and women. Data are shown as means ± SD. $n = 9$ in both groups. *** Significantly different ($p < 0.001$) from young group.

The study was approved by the Health Research Ethics Committee of the Capital Region of Copenhagen (No. KF-293615) and complied with the guidelines set out in the Declaration of Helsinki. The subjects were all informed about the nature and risks of the study and gave written consent to participate before inclusion.

2.2. Study Design

Nine young and 9 elderly participants completed a six-week resistance exercise training intervention of the lower body (two-legged knee extension) followed by eight weeks of deconditioning (Figure 1). Muscle strength was evaluated by a three-repetition max test before and after resistance exercise training. Skeletal muscle biopsies were taken from the vastus lateralis muscle before and after resistance exercise training and after two, four, six, and eight weeks of deconditioning for measurement of myogenic regulatory factors and mitochondrial markers. DEXA scanning of body composition was performed before and after resistance training.

2.3. DEXA Scanning

A whole-body Dual-Energy X-ray Absorptiometry (DEXA) scan (GE Medical Systems, Lunar, Prodigy, Chicago, IL, USA) was performed prior to the intervention and after the resistance exercise training intervention. The images were analyzed using enCORE™2004 Software (v.8.5) (GE Medical Systems). Reliability of this DEXA scanning was recently described [39].

2.4. Exercise Equipment and Protocol

Testing and exercise training intervention were carried out in a two-legged knee extension resistance exercise model using standard strength exercise equipment machines (Nordic Gym, Technogym, Cesena, Italy). Furthermore, to compensate for muscle imbalances during the selective exercise of the quadriceps, the exercise decline leg press (Nordic Gym) was incorporated into the exercise regimen.

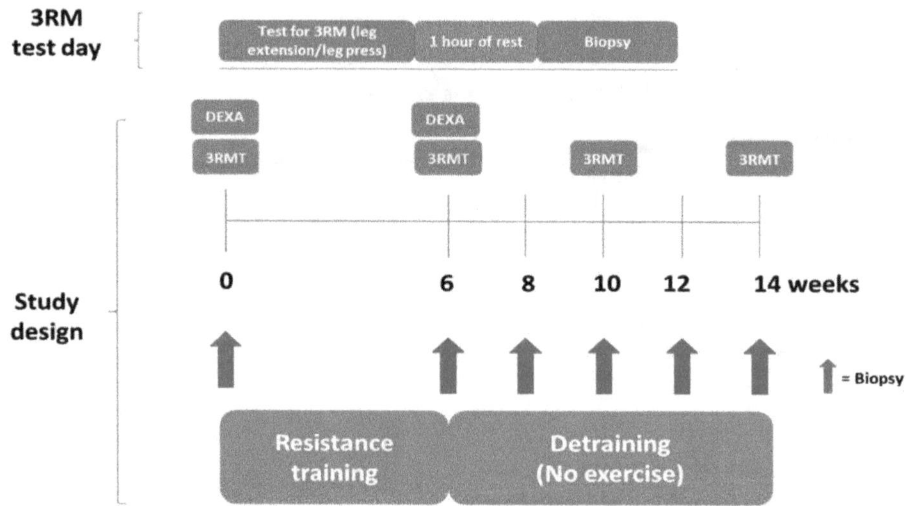

Figure 1. Study design overview. Eighteen participants completed a six-week resistance exercise training intervention followed by eight weeks of deconditioning (detraining—no exercise). Muscle strength was evaluated by a three-repetition max test before and after resistance exercise training. Skeletal muscle biopsies were taken from the vastus lateralis muscle on each test day. Furthermore, a biopsy was taken after two, four, and six weeks of deconditioning.

2.5. *Strength Testing*

Strength testing was performed using a three-repetition maximum (RM) test-protocol. Before initial testing, participants were familiarized with the equipment and test protocol on a separate occasion to reduce the impact that skill learning has on strength performance. The estimated measure of bilateral knee extension muscle strength was recently found to be applicable for monitoring adaptations promoted by physical exercise for older adults with and without sarcopenia [40].

Three repetition maximum test (3RMT): Prior to the 3RMT, participants warmed up using five minutes of low intensity (60–80 watt and 30–50 watt for young and elderly, respectively) cycling ergometer exercise. Afterwards, participants were instructed to execute four repetitions in each attempt. Full range of motion (ROM) for three consecutive repetitions and failure to complete a 4th repetition across a full-ROM was set as a criterion for a successful 3RM estimate. Participants rested 3 min after warm-up, and 1.5 min between all other attempts. After 10 min of rest, the validity of the estimate was evaluated by trying to outperform the current 3RM estimate. 1RM was calculated using Brzycki's formula [41]. 3RMT was measured before and after the resistance training intervention (Figure 1).

2.6. *Resistance Exercise Training and Deconditioning Interventions*

The resistance exercise training intervention lasted for six weeks and consisted of 16 supervised resistance exercise sessions. Resistance exercise followed a progressive protocol in weekly exercise sessions from two to three sessions per week after the first two weeks of exercise. Sessions were divided into three sessions of different load carried on a two-legged knee extension and a decline leg press machine to voluntary failure, and each set was separated by three minutes of rest. The first session encompassed three sets of 10–12 repetitions with 10–12 RM load, followed by three sets of 6–8 repetitions with 6–8 RM load, ending with three sets of 4–6 repetitions with 4–6 RM load. Each session was separated by approximately 48 h of rest.

In addition to and following knee extension resistance exercise, participants exercised in the decline leg press with the same exercise protocol (e.g., three sets of 10–12 reps with 10–12 RM in both exercises in the same session). After six weeks of resistance exercise training, participants stopped the exercise program and returned to their habitual sedentary lifestyle and were instructed not to initiate any new form of exercise the following eight weeks. This was ensured by participants wearing accelerometers and weekly interviews of the participants.

2.7. Skeletal Muscle Biopsy

A skeletal muscle biopsy was performed in vastus lateralis right leg muscle before and after the six weeks resistance exercise training intervention, and after two, four, six, and eight weeks of deconditioning (post2w, post4w, post6w, and post8w) approximately one hour post the acute 3RMT on the experimental days. The biopsy was performed as previously described using a 5 mm percutaneous Bergström needle [42]. Needle entry was at least three centimeters away from the previous insertion to avoid scar tissue and interference with data due to post-biopsy edema, regeneration, and cellular infiltration. Muscle samples were immediately frozen in isopentane cooled by liquid nitrogen before storage at −80 °C for later analysis.

2.8. Western Blotting Analysis

Western blot analysis was performed as previously described [43]. Biopsies were sectioned on a cryostat at −20 °C and homogenized in ice-cold lysis buffer with protease and phosphatase inhibitors (10 mM Tris, pH 7.4, 0.1% Triton-X 100, 0.5% sodium deoxycholate, 0.07 U/mL aprotinin, 20 M leupeptin, 20 M pepstatin, 1 mM phenylmethanesulfonyl fluoride (PMSF), 1 mM EDTA, 1 mM EGTA, 1 mM DTT, 5 mM β-glycerophosphate, 1 mM sodium fluoride, 1.15 mM sodium molybdate, 2 mM sodium pyrophosphate decahydrate, 1 mM sodium orthovanadate, 4 mM sodium tartrate, 2 mM imidazole, 10 nM calyculin, and 5 mM cantharidin; Sigma-Aldrich, St. Louis, MO, USA) using a Bullet Blender bead-mill at 4 °C (Next Advance, Averill, NY, USA). The homogenate was directly centrifuged at 15,000× *g* for 5 min at 4 °C. The supernatant was immediately transferred to new Eppendorf tubes and added 4× sample buffer including beta mercapto-ethanol. Equal amounts of extracted muscle proteins (10 μL) were separated on 4–15% polyacrylamide gels (Bio-Rad, Hercules, CA, USA) at 200 V for 40–50 min along with molecular weight markers (Bio-Rad). Proteins were transferred to PVDF membranes at 2.5 A for 5 min using a Trans-Blot Turbo (Bio-Rad) and blocked in Bailey's Irish cream (R. J. Bailey & Co, Dublin, Ireland) for 30 min and washed in TBS-T to remove excess Bailey's (3 × 10 min). The study investigated the expression and/or phosphorylation of proteins involved in muscle development/regeneration (IGF-I-R, MyoD, myogenin) and negative regulators of muscle mass (actRIIB and smad2) as well as porin [44], a mitochondrial membrane protein, to assess any changes in mitochondrial content. Thus, to investigate MRFs, antibodies against MyoD (45 kDa; diluted 1:1000; host: mouse; Thermo Fisher Scientific, Waltham, MA, USA) and myogenin (F5D) (40/25 kDa; diluted 1:1000; host: mouse; Developmental Studies Hybridoma Bank (DSHB), University of Iowa, IA, USA) were used. Antibodies against phosphorylated insulin-like growth factor 1 receptor (p-IGF-IR beta Y1135/1136; 95 kDa; diluted 1:500; host: rabbit; Cell Signaling Technology, Danvers, MA, USA), activin IIB receptor (58 kDa; diluted 1:1000; host: rabbit; ab180185, Abcam, Cambridge, UK), and phospho-smad2/3 (pSer250; 58 kDa; diluted 1:1000; host rabbit; Cell Signaling Technology) were used to investigate if muscle growth regulation had changed. Antibodies against porin (30–33 kDa; diluted 1:50,000; host: mouse; Thermo Fisher Scientific) were used to investigate a marker of mitochondrial content.

Antibodies against glyceraldehyde-3-phosphate dehydrogenase (GAPDH) were used at 1:5000 (ab22555; Abcam, Cambridge, UK) as loading control. Secondary goat anti-rabbit and goat anti-mouse antibodies coupled with horseradish peroxidase at concentration 1:10,000 were used to detect primary antibodies (DAKO, Glostrup, Denmark). Immunoreactive bands were detected by chemiluminescence using Clarity Max, (BioRad), quantified using a GBox XT16 darkroom, and GeneTools software was used to measure the intensities of immunoreactive bands (Syngene, Cambridge, UK). Immunoreactive band intensities were normalized to the intensity of the GAPDH bands for each subject to correct for differences in total muscle protein loaded on the gel.

2.9. *Muscle Histology and Immunohistochemistry*

Cryosections (10 µm) were cut from biopsies mounted in Tissue-Tek (Sakura Finetek Europe B.V., AJ Alphen aan den Rijn Netherlands), mounted on glass slides, and stored at −20 °C until stained. To assess myosin heavy chain (MHC) muscle fiber type distribution, sections were stained with MHC antibody clone BA-D5 (DSHB) for MHC type I, and a secondary goat anti-mouse antibody was used (GAM IgG2b Alexa Fluor 594, Thermo Fisher Scientific). For MHC type II assessment, sections were stained with MHC antibody clone A4.74 (DSHB), and a secondary goat anti-mouse antibody (GAM IgG1 Alexa Fluor 488) was used. All sections were observed at room temperature using a Nikon 20× Plan Apo VC N/A 0.75 mounted on a Nikon Ti-E epifluorescence microscope (Nikon Instruments, Melville, NY, USA). Images of the entire sections were acquired at 20× with a 5-Mpixel Andor Neo camera for fluorescence imaging (Andor, Belfast, Northern Ireland), using NIS-Elements Advanced Research (AR) software (Nikon Instruments) and merged in software.

2.10. *Mitochondrial Citrate Synthase Enzyme Activity*

Citrate synthase enzyme activity was investigated in muscle biopsies pre-exercise, post-exercise, and after 8 weeks of deconditioning. In short, skeletal muscle tissue (~200 mg) was sectioned on a cryostat (Microm HM550, Thermo Fisher, by, stat) at −20 °C and homogenized in ice-cold CelLytic MT (Mammalian tissue lysis/extraction reagent) containing protease inhibitor cocktail. The tissue was homogenized using a Bullet Blender bead-mill at 4 °C (Next Advance, Averill, NY, USA). The homogenate was directly centrifuged at 15,000× *g* for 5 min at 4 °C. The supernatant was transferred to new Eppendorf tubes and used for subsequent analysis. The assay was carried out according to the manufacturer's instructions (#CS0720, Sigma-Aldrich). Briefly, the assay solutions were heated at 25 °C. A master mix consisting of 1× assay buffer, 30 mM Acetyl-CoA solution, and 10 mM DTNB solution were mixed and added in the lysate to perform triple measurements per sample. Citrate synthase was measured by reading absorbance at 412 nm every 10th second for 1.5 min, and thereafter adding 10 mM OAA solution and then remeasured again every 10 s for 1.5 min at 412 nm.

2.11. *Statistical Analysis*

All statistical analyses were carried out using Excel 2010 (Microsoft®, Redmond, WA, USA) and GraphPad PRISM 8 (GraphPad, San Diego, CA, USA). A Shapiro–Wilkinson test was performed to test for normal distribution of data. Baseline subject characteristics were evaluated with unpaired *t*-tests between young and elderly groups and by a repeated measures two-way ANOVA for DEXA data before and after training (Table 1).The differences among groups were analyzed by a three-way repeated measures ANOVA in Figure 2A and a two-way repeated measures ANOVA in Figure 2B, Figure 3, and Table 2, followed by Tukey's multiple comparison tests when ANOVA revealed significant interactions. Prior to this, an additional two-way ANOVA was performed to ensure no gender differences prior to pooling data for male and females.). Correlation analyses were performed with the Pearson's product-moment correlation coefficient. All data are presented as means ± standard deviation (SD). Differences were considered to be statistically significant when $p < 0.05$.

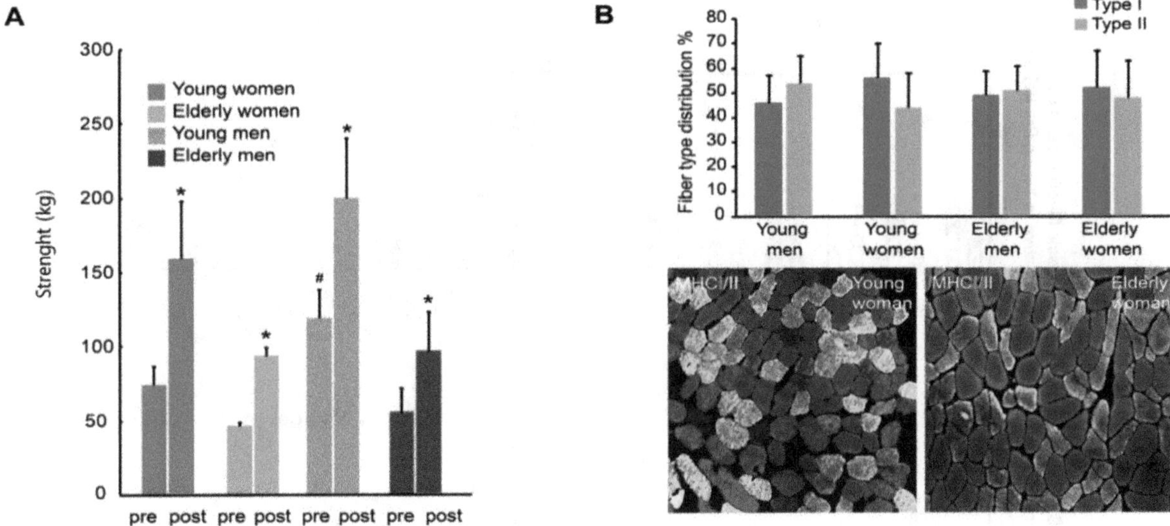

Figure 2. Muscle strength and muscle fiber type composition. (**A**) Quadriceps muscle strength measured in a three repetition maximum test before and after six weeks of resistance exercise training in elderly and young men and women. (**B**) Pre-intervention muscle fiber type distribution shown as bar graph and by representative cross-sectional images of m. vastus lateralis in a younger and older woman showing fiber type distribution of myosin heavy chain (MHC) type I (red) and type II (green). * $p < 0.05$, post-exercise vs. pre-exercise within the same group. # $p < 0.05$, pre-exercise, young men vs. young women. $n = 5$ elderly men, $n = 4$ elderly women, $n = 5$ young men, and $n = 4$ young women. All data are presented as means ± SD.

Table 2. Mitochondrial markers.

	Young Group			Elderly Group		
	Pre Training	Post Training	Post Deconditioning	Pre Training	Post Training	Post Deconditioning
Porin protein content relative to young pre training (AU)	1.00 ± 0.4	0.98 ± 1.1	1.60 ± 1.3	1.19 ± 1.2	1.53 ± 1.3	2.40 ± 1.9
CS activity, µmol/min/mg w.w.	1.7 ± 1.0	2.2 ± 1.3	2.0 ± 0.6	1.0 ± 0.6	1.7 ± 1.9	1.4 ± 0.9

Porin protein content and maximal muscle citrate synthase (CS) activity measured pre-training, following six weeks of resistance exercise training (post training), and after eight weeks of subsequent deconditioning (post decondition). Porin protein content is expressed relative to young pre training. Data are shown as means ± SD. $n = 9$ in both groups.

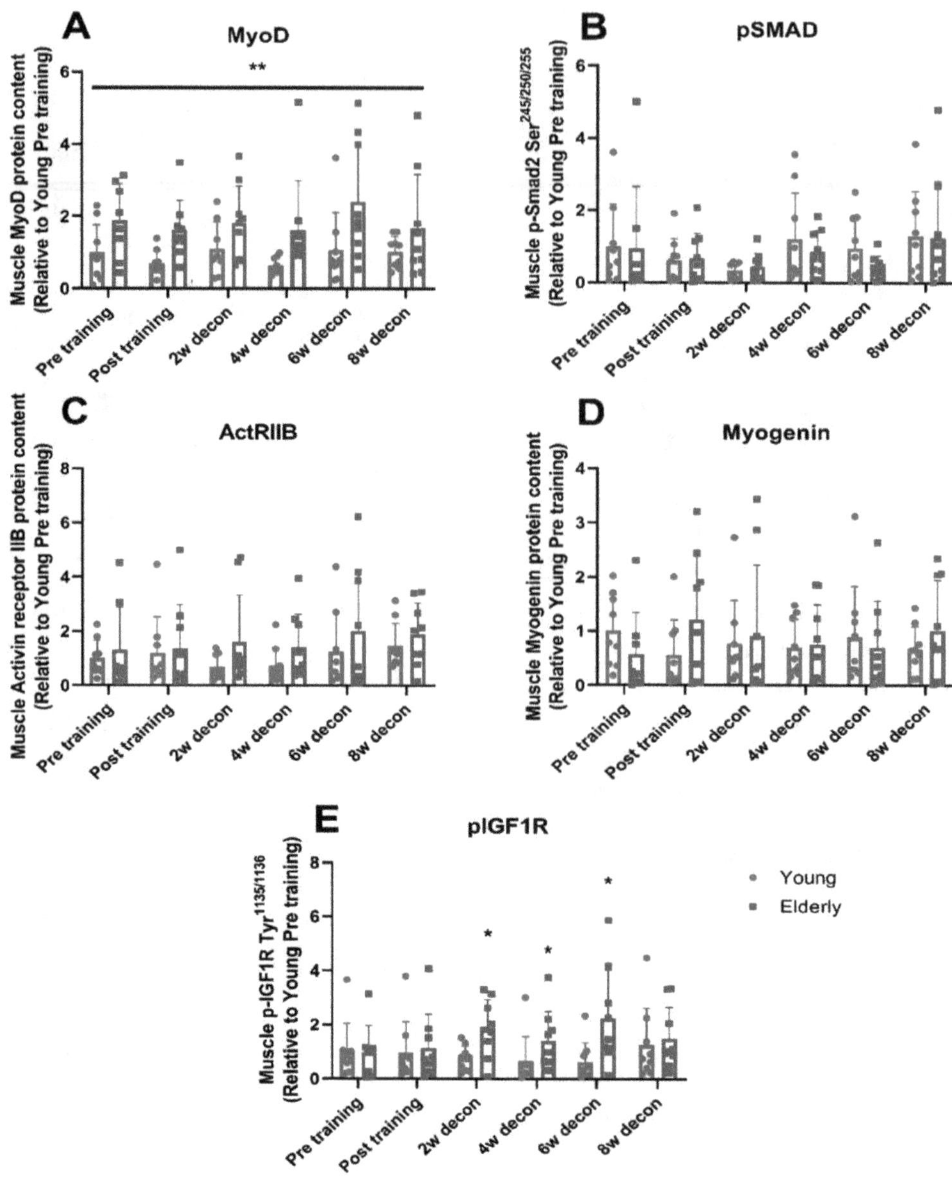

Figure 3. Muscle regulatory factors. Muscle regulatory factors measured in skeletal muscle pre and post six weeks of resistance exercise training and during 2, 4, 6, and 8 weeks into a subsequent deconditioning period in young (red bars) and elderly (blue bars) individuals. (**A**) Protein expression of activin receptor IIB, (**B**). Phosphorylation level of smad2 at Ser245/250/255. (**C**) Protein expression of MyoD. (**D**) Protein expression of myogenin. (**E**) Phosphorylation level of IGF-I-R at Tyr1135 /1136. Measurements have been performed as single determinations by Western blotting. Representative Western blots are shown in Supplementary Figure S1. $n = 9$ in young group and $n = 9$ in the elderly group. Values are arbitrary units (means ± SD) and expressed relative to young group pre training. * $p < 0.05$, young vs. elderly group, ** $p < 0.01$, main effect of age independently of training and deconditioning. ANOVA F-values ($F_{time}/F_{age}/F_{time \times age}$): (**A**) 1.08/11.62/0.32; (**B**) 0.76/0.58/0.49; (**C**) 0.77/2.97/0.23; (**D**) 0.09/0.15/1.20; (**E**) 0.54/8.62/1.41.

3. Results

3.1. Anthropometry

Total body weight, body mass index (BMI), body fat %, and lean body mass % were similar between the young and the elderly group (Table 1). Six weeks of resistance exercise training did not lead to changes in whole body fat %, lean body mass %, or lean leg mass, as a read out for muscle mass, in the trained legs in neither the young nor the elderly individuals.

3.2. *Muscle Strength*

Six weeks of resistance exercise training increased quadriceps muscle strength in the elderly group by 78% (53.4 ± 14.3 kg (pre-exercise) vs. 95.0 ± 22.0 kg (post-exercise); $p < 0.05$), which was similar to that found in the young healthy persons (83.5%; 97.1 ± 27.5 kg (pre-exercise) vs. 178.2 ± 44.2 kg (post-exercise); $p < 0.05$) (Figure 2A). Pre-exercise, the elderly men did not have a significantly greater muscle strength compared to elderly women (56.2 ± 16.1 kg vs. 46.5 ± 2.5 kg), whereas a gender difference in muscle strength was observed in the younger group, in which the younger men had a 59% greater muscle strength at pre-training compared to younger women (119.2 ± 19.5 kg vs. 75 ± 12.6 kg; $p < 0.05$) (Figure 2A). No significant differences in strength between genders were observed post-exercise within the elderly or young group (Figure 2A).

3.3. *Muscle Fiber Type Composition*

No pre-exercise fiber type differences were seen between gender, young, and elderly participants (Figure 2B).

3.4. *Myogenic Regulatory Factors*

Six weeks of resistance exercise training and 8 weeks of deconditioning did not change the protein expression of MyoD, actRIIB, and myogenin and phosphorylation of Smad2 and IGF-I- receptor in the elderly and the young group (Figure 3A–E).

MyoD protein expression were overall higher ($p < 0.01$) in muscles of elderly compared with young individuals (Figure 3A).

No differences in total protein expression of actRIIB and myogenin and phosphorylation of Smad2 and IGF-I-R were observed pre-training or after six weeks following resistance training in young versus elderly participants (Figure 3B–E). IGF-I receptor phosphorylation at Tyr1135 /1136 was lower in the younger group of healthy persons compared to the elderly group two weeks post-exercise (post2w) (0.7 ± 0.5 vs. 1.9 ± 1.1, $p < 0.05$), four weeks post-exercise (post4w) (0.6 ± 0.9 vs. 1.4 ± 1.1, $p < 0.05$) and six weeks post-exercise (post6w) (0.6 ± 0.7 vs. 2.6 ± 2.7, $p < 0.05$) (Figure 3E). There was no difference between genders at all time points in both groups in all protein and phosphorylation levels investigated, why these data were pooled in the data shown.

3.5. *Mitochondrial Markers: Porin and Citrate Synthase*

The protein expression of porin did not change with six weeks of resistance exercise training and remained unchanged after deconditioning in both the young and the elderly and was not significantly different between the groups (Table 2).

The maximal muscle enzyme activity of citrate synthase in the elderly was not significantly different from that found in the young participants (Table 2). Maximal muscle enzyme activity of citrate synthase in the elderly group remained unchanged with resistance exercise training and subsequent deconditioning, which was similar to that found in the young group (Table 2). There was no difference in the citrate synthase activity among genders in the elderly and young groups, which is why these data were pooled (Table 2).

3.6. *Correlation between Myogenic and Mitochondrial Factors and Muscle Strength*

There was no association between any of the studied MRFs (MyoD, myogenin, actRIIB protein expression, and IGF-I-R and smad2 phosphorylation) or mitochondrial factors (citrate synthase activity and porin protein expression) and absolute or relative change in muscle strength after six weeks of resistance exercise training in the elderly or the young group.

4. Discussion

Resistance exercise training and deconditioning offer a unique opportunity to investigate differences in myogenic regulatory factors that may be crucial in the age-related loss of muscle mass and strength. The aim of this study was to investigate regulation of myogenic factors prior and in response to resistance exercise training and deconditioning in elderly (74–92 years of age) versus young, healthy, gender-matched individuals. The primary findings were (1) six weeks of intensive resistance exercise training induced the same increase in muscle strength in young and older individuals, (2) the key myogenic regulating factors (MyoD, myogenin, and IGF-I-R) were similar in muscles of young and elderly individuals and not differently regulated by six weeks of resistance exercise training or subsequent eight weeks of deconditioning, and (3) no change was found in markers of oxidative capacity and mitochondrial content after six weeks of resistance exercise training in either elderly or young healthy persons.

Age-related loss of muscle strength is inevitable and cannot be explained by age-related decreased physical activity level alone [45]. It has been suggested that elderly persons have a blunted muscle hypertrophy response to resistance exercise training [17–19]. Thus, it could be that differences in muscle mass and function between young and elderly are driven by age-related changes in the ability to gain and/or maintain muscle strength with age. However, the present study showed that six weeks of intensive resistance exercise training resulted in the same increase in quadriceps muscle strength in elderly compared to that found in young, gender-matched, sedentary individuals. Therefore, skeletal muscle of elderly has the same capacity to increase strength in response to resistance training as in young healthy individuals. This finding is important in a translational perspective, emphasizing that resistance exercise training benefits elderly as much as in young persons and therefore seems to be a valid tool to combat loss of muscle function and strength in aging.

Myogenic regulatory factors promote and regulate the expression of muscle-specific genes after muscle injury or strenuous resistance exercise leading to muscle hypertrophy [46]. It has been hypothesized that the inevitably age-related muscle strength loss may relate to downregulation of MRFs, and thus skeletal muscle atrophy, which we were unable to corroborate. With the same levels of MRFs in elderly compared to young persons in the present study, our findings contrast the majority of previous studies measuring on mRNA levels. Previous studies found elevated levels of MyoD, myogenin, and IGF-I-R mRNA in elderly both at rest [17,31–34] and in response to exercise training compared to younger individuals [17,47–50]. This suggests that the increase in MRF mRNA levels represented a continuous compensatory mechanism to preserve muscle protein and mass with aging [17]. The present study is the first to investigate protein levels of MRFs, obviating the issues with changes in mRNA levels that may not translate into similar changes in protein expression due to post-translational regulation [51]. The present study suggests that the myogenic program is intact in the elderly, as the levels of MyoD, myogenin, and IGF-I-R are activated to the same extent as in younger skeletal muscle. An overall higher level of MyoD protein expression in the elderly compared with the young muscle, and a higher IGF-I-R phosphorylation 2, 4, and 6 weeks into the deconditioning period in the elderly compared with young individuals support that compensatory mechanisms in MRF regulation contribute to preserve muscle protein and mass in aging. Importantly, our study underscores that protein and phosphorylation levels should be measured in favor of mRNA. Our finding further suggests that an intact anabolic muscle response seems able to compensate in part for the loss of muscle.

As the expression of MRFs are time-dependent in relation to external and internal stimuli, it could be hypothesized that lack of differences in MRFs in the present versus other studies (measuring mRNA levels though) investigating this could be related to the timing of the muscle biopsy sampling. In the present study, the muscle biopsy intervention was taken one hour post-exercise. As the expression of the proteins that was investigated in the present study is expected to be stable and not affected by an acute bout of exercise, timing of muscle sample seems not have an impact on the data presented in the present study. This is supported by findings in post-exercise muscle biopsy intervention (3 h post-exercise), in which no increase was found in key myogenic factors (MyoD, myf-6), except for myogenin [52], underscoring that timing of muscle biopsy sampling likely did not impact the protein levels of MRFs in the present study.

Muscle growth is tightly regulated through the myostatin, actRIIB, and smad2 pathway [53]. In response to muscle disuse, this and other pathways mediate a decrease in muscle mass [54]. In line with this, studies have shown that inhibition of myostatin-actRIIB-smad pathway leads to skeletal muscle hypertrophy in mice [55]. Studies by Hulmi et al. [35,36] have indicated that factors downregulating muscle mass in aged muscle could be attenuated in response to resistance exercise, as the mRNA level of actRIIB was downregulated after 21 weeks of resistance exercise in elderly (62.3 ± 6.3 years of age). The findings from that study indicate that proteins responsible for negative muscle mass regulation, e.g., actRIIB and smad2, could be upregulated in inactive aged muscle, resulting in decreased muscle mass and thus strength. However, our results did not support that finding. Instead, our data demonstrate that skeletal muscles of elderly have the same dynamics of MRF-mediated hypo- and hypertrophy, indicating that resistance exercise and deconditioning regulatory effects on skeletal muscle anabolism is the same irrespective of age.

Citrate synthase is a key mitochondrial matrix enzyme and a strong indicator of oxidative capacity in skeletal muscle [56–59] and maximal citrate synthase activity was also found to strongly correlate with mitochondrial volume measured by electron microscopy in skeletal muscles of healthy, young men [58]. Porin (also known as voltage dependent anion channel, VDAC1) is a pore-forming protein localized in the outer membrane of mitochondria, and is used as a marker of mitochondrial content [60,61]. Alterations in mitochondrial function and content has been proposed to be a factor underlying sarcopenia and muscle atrophy [62,63]. In order to investigate whether age-related decline in muscle strength was accompanied by muscle mitochondrial impairments in response to resistance training, muscle citrate synthase activity, and porin protein expression were measured before and after six weeks of resistance exercise training and eight weeks of deconditioning. Data showed that there was no change in oxidative capacity and indices of mitochondrial content after six weeks of resistance exercise training in either elderly or young healthy individuals, indicating that the gain in muscle strength was not associated with any changes in mitochondrial content.

It has been hypothesized that change in age-related muscle mass is driven by loss of muscle fiber type II number with age. However, findings regarding age-related changes in muscle fiber type II number have been ambiguous [64–67]. In the present study, the elderly individuals were older than those previously studied (+74 years old), and despite an age difference of 60 years between the young and elderly participants, there was no difference in number of type I and II fibers between elderly and younger persons. In the present study, we did not measure fiber type composition after training and deconditioning. Fiber type composition is in most studies not changed with exercise training [68] especially not within 6 weeks of resistance training. However, we cannot exclude that fiber type composition was mildly affected by exercise training in the present study. Furthermore, it was not within the scope of the present investigation to evaluate fiber size changes with resistance exercise training and deconditioning and it remains to be established, whether muscle fiber sizes are affected by 6 weeks of resistance training and subsequent 8 weeks of deconditioning in skeletal muscle of young and elderly.

5. Conclusions

Despite the fact that aging is associated with substantial loss of muscle mass resulting in a net loss of muscle strength and function, our study showed that elderly (aged 74+ years old) are remarkably capable of gaining muscle strength compared to younger participants in response to resistance exercise training. This underlines the applicability of resistance exercise training as an important instrument to diminish age-related loss of muscle function. Interestingly, the preserved ability to gain muscle strength with resistance exercise training was associated with a similar interaction between myogenic factors for up- and downregulation of skeletal muscle in elderly and young individuals. Thus, our data suggests that the entire myogenic regulatory program is not impaired in aged relative to younger skeletal muscle.

Supplementary Materials: The following are available online at Figure S1: Representative Western blots.

Author Contributions: Conceptualization, F.D.T and T.D.J.; methodology, T.K., K.A.N.Q.; formal analysis, K.A.N.Q., A.M.F.; investigation, A.M.F., F.D.T., K.A.N.Q., T.K., M.-L.S., T.D.J.; resources, J.V.; data curation, A.M.F., F.D.T., K.A.N.Q.; writing—original draft preparation, A.M.F., K.A.N.Q., T.D.J.; writing—review and editing A.M.F., F.D.T., K.A.N.Q., T.K., M.-L.S., J.V., T.D.J.; visualization, A.M.F., K.A.N.Q., T.D.J.; supervision, T..K., J.V., T.D.J.; project administration, F.D.T., T.D.J.; funding acquisition, J.V. All authors have read and agree to the published version of the manuscript.

Acknowledgments: We thank Tessa Munkeboe Hornsyld and Danuta Goralska-Olsen for excellent technical assistance.

References

1. Fuggle, N.; Shaw, S.; Dennison, E.; Cooper, C. Sarcopenia. *Best Pract. Res. Clin. Rheumatol.* **2017**, *31*, 218–242. [CrossRef] [PubMed]
2. Drey, M. Sarcopenia—Pathophysiology and clinical relevance. *Wien Med. Wochenschr.* **2011**, *161*, 402–408. [CrossRef] [PubMed]
3. Fragala, M.S.; Cadore, E.L.; Dorgo, S.; Izquierdo, M.; Kraemer, W.J.; Peterson, M.D.; Ryan, E.D. Resistance Training for Older Adults: Position Statement from the National Strength and Conditioning Association. *J. Strength Cond. Res.* **2019**, *33*, 2019–2052. [CrossRef]
4. Newton, R.U.; Hakkinen, K.; Hakkinen, A.; McCormick, M.; Volek, J.; Kraemer, W.J. Mixed-methods resistance training increases power and strength of young and older men. *Med. Sci. Sports Exerc.* **2002**, *34*, 1367–1375. [CrossRef]
5. HÃkkinen, K.; Newton, R.U.; Gordon, S.E.; McCormick, M.; Volek, J.S.; Nindl, B.C.; Gotshalk, L.A.; Campbell, W.W.; Evans, W.J.; HÃ¤kkinen, A.; et al. Changes in muscle morphology, electromyographic activity, and force production characteristics during progressive strength training in young and older men. *J. Gerontol. A Biol. Sci. Med. Sci.* **1998**, *53*, B415–B423. [CrossRef] [PubMed]
6. Lemmer, J.T.; Hurlbut, D.E.; Martel, G.F.; Tracy, B.L.; Ivey, F.M.; Metter, E.J.; Fozard, J.L.; Fleg, J.L.; Hurley, B.F. Age and gender responses to strength training and detraining. *Med. Sci. Sports Exerc.* **2000**, *32*, 1505–1512. [CrossRef] [PubMed]
7. Macaluso, A.; De Vito, G.; Felici, F.; Nimmo, M.A. Electromyogram changes during sustained contraction after resistance training in women in their 3rd and 8th decades. *Eur. J. Appl. Physiol.* **2000**, *82*, 418–424. [CrossRef] [PubMed]
8. Delmonico, M.J.; Harris, T.B.; Visser, M.; Park, S.W.; Conroy, M.B.; Velasquez-Mieyer, P.; Boudreau, R.; Manini, T.M.; Nevitt, M.; Newman, A.B.; et al. Longitudinal study of muscle strength, quality, and adipose tissue infiltration. *Am. J. Clin. Nutr.* **2009**, *90*, 1579–1585. [CrossRef]
9. Clark, B.C.; Manini, T.M. Functional consequences of sarcopenia and dynapenia in the elderly. *Curr. Opin. Clin. Nutr. Metab. Care* **2010**, *13*, 271–276. [CrossRef]
10. Karlsen, A.; Bechshoft, R.L.; Malmgaard-Clausen, N.M.; Andersen, J.L.; Schjerling, P.; Kjaer, M.; Mackey, A.L. Lack of muscle fibre hypertrophy, myonuclear addition, and satellite cell pool expansion with resistance training in 83-94-year-old men and women. *Acta Physiol.* **2019**, *227*, e13271. [CrossRef]
11. Snijders, T.; Verdijk, L.B.; Smeets, J.S.; McKay, B.R.; Senden, J.M.; Hartgens, F.; Parise, G.; Greenhaff, P.; van Loon, L.J. The skeletal muscle satellite cell response to a single bout of resistance-type exercise is delayed with aging in men. *Age* **2014**, *36*, 9699. [CrossRef]
12. Verdijk, L.B.; Gleeson, B.G.; Jonkers, R.A.; Meijer, K.; Savelberg, H.H.; Dendale, P.; van Loon, L.J. Skeletal muscle hypertrophy following resistance training is accompanied by a fiber type-specific increase in satellite cell content in elderly men. *J. Gerontol. A Biol. Sci. Med. Sci.* **2009**, *64*, 332–339. [CrossRef] [PubMed]

13. Leenders, M.; Verdijk, L.B.; van der Hoeven, L.; van Kranenburg, J.; Nilwik, R.; van Loon, L.J. Elderly men and women benefit equally from prolonged resistance-type exercise training. *J. Gerontol. A Biol. Sci. Med. Sci.* **2013**, *68*, 769–779. [CrossRef] [PubMed]
14. Snijders, T.; Nederveen, J.P.; Joanisse, S.; Leenders, M.; Verdijk, L.B.; van Loon, L.J.; Parise, G. Muscle fibre capillarization is a critical factor in muscle fibre hypertrophy during resistance exercise training in older men. *J. Cachexia Sarcopenia Muscle* **2017**, *8*, 267–276. [CrossRef] [PubMed]
15. Karlsen, A.; Soendenbroe, C.; Malmgaard-Clausen, N.M.; Wagener, F.; Moeller, C.E.; Senhaji, Z.; Damberg, K.; Andersen, J.L.; Schjerling, P.; Kjaer, M.; et al. Preserved capacity for satellite cell proliferation, regeneration, and hypertrophy in the skeletal muscle of healthy elderly men. *FASEB J.* **2020**, *34*, 6418–6436. [CrossRef] [PubMed]
16. Blocquiaux, S.; Gorski, T.; Van Roie, E.; Ramaekers, M.; Van Thienen, R.; Nielens, H.; Delecluse, C.; De Bock, K.; Thomis, M. The effect of resistance training, detraining and retraining on muscle strength and power, myofibre size, satellite cells and myonuclei in older men. *Exp. Gerontol.* **2020**, *133*, 110860. [CrossRef] [PubMed]
17. Kosek, D.J.; Kim, J.S.; Petrella, J.K.; Cross, J.M.; Bamman, M.M. Efficacy of 3 days/wk resistance training on myofiber hypertrophy and myogenic mechanisms in young vs. older adults. *J. Appl. Physiol.* **2006**, *101*, 531–544. [CrossRef] [PubMed]
18. Mero, A.A.; Hulmi, J.J.; Salmijarvi, H.; Katajavuori, M.; Haverinen, M.; Holviala, J.; Ridanpaa, T.; Hakkinen, K.; Kovanen, V.; Ahtiainen, J.P.; et al. Resistance training induced increase in muscle fiber size in young and older men. *Eur. J. Appl. Physiol.* **2013**, *113*, 641–650. [CrossRef]
19. Brook, M.S.; Wilkinson, D.J.; Mitchell, W.K.; Lund, J.N.; Phillips, B.E.; Szewczyk, N.J.; Greenhaff, P.L.; Smith, K.; Atherton, P.J. Synchronous deficits in cumulative muscle protein synthesis and ribosomal biogenesis underlie age-related anabolic resistance to exercise in humans. *J. Physiol.* **2016**, *594*, 7399–7417. [CrossRef]
20. Hwa, V.; Fang, P.; Derr, M.A.; Fiegerlova, E.; Rosenfeld, R.G. IGF-I in human growth: Lessons from defects in the GH-IGF-I axis. *Nestle Nutr. Inst. Workshop Ser.* **2013**, *71*, 43–55. [CrossRef]
21. Stilling, F.; Wallenius, S.; Michaelsson, K.; Dalgard, C.; Brismar, K.; Wolk, A. High insulin-like growth factor-binding protein-1 (IGFBP-1) is associated with low relative muscle mass in older women. *Metabolism* **2017**, *73*, 36–42. [CrossRef] [PubMed]
22. Zanou, N.; Gailly, P. Skeletal muscle hypertrophy and regeneration: Interplay between the myogenic regulatory factors (MRFs) and insulin-like growth factors (IGFs) pathways. *Cell. Mol. Life Sci.* **2013**, *70*, 4117–4130. [CrossRef] [PubMed]
23. Hernandez-Hernandez, J.M.; Garcia-Gonzalez, E.G.; Brun, C.E.; Rudnicki, M.A. The myogenic regulatory factors, determinants of muscle development, cell identity and regeneration. *Semin. Cell Dev. Biol.* **2017**, *72*, 10–18. [CrossRef]
24. Seward, D.J.; Haney, J.C.; Rudnicki, M.A.; Swoap, S.J. bHLH transcription factor MyoD affects myosin heavy chain expression pattern in a muscle-specific fashion. *Am. J. Physiol. Cell Physiol.* **2001**, *280*, C408–C413. [CrossRef] [PubMed]
25. Mozdziak, P.E.; Greaser, M.L.; Schultz, E. Myogenin, MyoD, and myosin heavy chain isoform expression following hindlimb suspension. *Aviat. Space Environ. Med.* **1999**, *70*, 511–516. [PubMed]
26. Mozdziak, P.E.; Greaser, M.L.; Schultz, E. Myogenin, MyoD, and myosin expression after pharmacologically and surgically induced hypertrophy. *J. Appl. Physiol.* **1998**, *84*, 1359–1364. [CrossRef] [PubMed]
27. Steffl, M.; Bohannon, R.W.; Sontakova, L.; Tufano, J.J.; Shiells, K.; Holmerova, I. Relationship between sarcopenia and physical activity in older people: A systematic review and meta-analysis. *Clin. Interv. Aging* **2017**, *12*, 835–845. [CrossRef]
28. Schoene, D.; Kiesswetter, E.; Sieber, C.C.; Freiberger, E. Musculoskeletal factors, sarcopenia and falls in old age. *Z. Gerontol. Geriatr.* **2019**, *52*, 37–44. [CrossRef]
29. Distefano, G.; Goodpaster, B.H. Effects of Exercise and Aging on Skeletal Muscle. *Cold Spring Harb. Perspect. Med.* **2018**, *8*, a029785. [CrossRef]
30. Tieland, M.; Trouwborst, I.; Clark, B.C. Skeletal muscle performance and ageing. *J. Cachexia Sarcopenia Muscle* **2018**, *9*, 3–19. [CrossRef] [PubMed]
31. Haddad, F.; Adams, G.R. Aging-sensitive cellular and molecular mechanisms associated with skeletal muscle hypertrophy. *J. Appl. Physiol.* **2006**, *100*, 1188–1203. [CrossRef] [PubMed]

32. Hameed, M.; Orrell, R.W.; Cobbold, M.; Goldspink, G.; Harridge, S.D. Expression of IGF-I splice variants in young and old human skeletal muscle after high resistance exercise. *J. Physiol.* **2003**, *547*, 247–254. [CrossRef] [PubMed]
33. Kim, J.S.; Kosek, D.J.; Petrella, J.K.; Cross, J.M.; Bamman, M.M. Resting and load-induced levels of myogenic gene transcripts differ between older adults with demonstrable sarcopenia and young men and women. *J. Appl. Physiol.* **2005**, *99*, 2149–2158. [CrossRef]
34. Raue, U.; Slivka, D.; Jemiolo, B.; Hollon, C.; Trappe, S. Myogenic gene expression at rest and after a bout of resistance exercise in young (18–30 yr) and old (80–89 yr) women. *J. Appl. Physiol.* **2006**, *101*, 53–59. [CrossRef] [PubMed]
35. Hulmi, J.J.; Ahtiainen, J.P.; Kaasalainen, T.; Pollanen, E.; Hakkinen, K.; Alen, M.; Selanne, H.; Kovanen, V.; Mero, A.A. Postexercise myostatin and activin IIb mRNA levels: Effects of strength training. *Med. Sci. Sports Exerc.* **2007**, *39*, 289–297. [CrossRef] [PubMed]
36. Hulmi, J.J.; Kovanen, V.; Selanne, H.; Kraemer, W.J.; Hakkinen, K.; Mero, A.A. Acute and long-term effects of resistance exercise with or without protein ingestion on muscle hypertrophy and gene expression. *Amino Acids* **2009**, *37*, 297–308. [CrossRef]
37. Groennebaek, T.; Vissing, K. Impact of Resistance Training on Skeletal Muscle Mitochondrial Biogenesis, Content, and Function. *Front. Physiol.* **2017**, *8*, 713. [CrossRef]
38. Porter, C.; Reidy, P.T.; Bhattarai, N.; Sidossis, L.S.; Rasmussen, B.B. Resistance Exercise Training Alters Mitochondrial Function in Human Skeletal Muscle. *Med. Sci. Sports Exerc.* **2015**, *47*, 1922–1931. [CrossRef]
39. Dordevic, A.L.; Bonham, M.; Ghasem-Zadeh, A.; Evans, A.; Barber, E.; Day, K.; Kwok, A.; Truby, H. Reliability of Compartmental Body Composition Measures in Weight-Stable Adults Using GE iDXA: Implications for Research and Practice. *Nutrients* **2018**, *10*, 1484. [CrossRef]
40. Abdalla, P.P.; Carvalho, A.D.S.; Dos Santos, A.P.; Venturini, A.C.R.; Alves, T.C.; Mota, J.; Machado, D.R.L. One-repetition submaximal protocol to measure knee extensor muscle strength among older adults with and without sarcopenia: A validation study. *BMC Sports Sci. Med. Rehabil.* **2020**, *12*, 29. [CrossRef]
41. Abdul-Hameed, U.; Rangra, P.; Shareef, M.Y.; Hussain, M.E. Reliability of 1-repetition maximum estimation for upper and lower body muscular strength measurement in untrained middle aged type 2 diabetic patients. *Asian J. Sports Med.* **2012**, *3*, 267–273. [CrossRef] [PubMed]
42. Bergstrom, J. Percutaneous needle biopsy of skeletal muscle in physiological and clinical research. *Scand. J. Clin. Lab. Invest.* **1975**, *35*, 609–616. [CrossRef] [PubMed]
43. Fritzen, A.M.; Thogersen, F.B.; Thybo, K.; Vissing, C.R.; Krag, T.O.; Ruiz-Ruiz, C.; Risom, L.; Wibrand, F.; Hoeg, L.D.; Kiens, B.; et al. Adaptations in Mitochondrial Enzymatic Activity Occurs Independent of Genomic Dosage in Response to Aerobic Exercise Training and Deconditioning in Human Skeletal Muscle. *Cells* **2019**, *8*, 237. [CrossRef]
44. Ben-Hail, D.; Shoshan-Barmatz, V. VDAC1-interacting anion transport inhibitors inhibit VDAC1 oligomerization and apoptosis. *Biochim. Biophys. Acta* **2016**, *1863*, 1612–1623. [CrossRef] [PubMed]
45. Brioche, T.; Pagano, A.F.; Py, G.; Chopard, A. Muscle wasting and aging: Experimental models, fatty infiltrations, and prevention. *Mol. Aspects Med.* **2016**, *50*, 56–87. [CrossRef]
46. Kopantseva, E.E.; Belyavsky, A.V. Key regulators of skeletal myogenesis. *Mol. Biol. (Mosk.)* **2016**, *50*, 195–222. [CrossRef] [PubMed]
47. Agergaard, J.; Reitelseder, S.; Pedersen, T.G.; Doessing, S.; Schjerling, P.; Langberg, H.; Miller, B.F.; Aagaard, P.; Kjaer, M.; Holm, L. Myogenic, matrix, and growth factor mRNA expression in human skeletal muscle: Effect of contraction intensity and feeding. *Muscle Nerve* **2013**, *47*, 748–759. [CrossRef]
48. Heinemeier, K.M.; Olesen, J.L.; Schjerling, P.; Haddad, F.; Langberg, H.; Baldwin, K.M.; Kjaer, M. Short-term strength training and the expression of myostatin and IGF-I isoforms in rat muscle and tendon: Differential effects of specific contraction types. *J. Appl. Physiol.* **2007**, *102*, 573–581. [CrossRef] [PubMed]
49. Luo, L.; Lu, A.M.; Wang, Y.; Hong, A.; Chen, Y.; Hu, J.; Li, X.; Qin, Z.H. Chronic resistance training activates autophagy and reduces apoptosis of muscle cells by modulating IGF-1 and its receptors, Akt/mTOR and Akt/FOXO3a signaling in aged rats. *Exp. Gerontol.* **2013**, *48*, 427–436. [CrossRef]
50. Mathers, J.L.; Farnfield, M.M.; Garnham, A.P.; Caldow, M.K.; Cameron-Smith, D.; Peake, J.M. Early inflammatory and myogenic responses to resistance exercise in the elderly. *Muscle Nerve* **2012**, *46*, 407–412. [CrossRef]

51. Myers, J.; Prakash, M.; Froelicher, V.; Do, D.; Partington, S.; Atwood, J.E. Exercise capacity and mortality among men referred for exercise testing. *N. Engl. J. Med.* **2002**, *346*, 793–801. [CrossRef] [PubMed]
52. Bamman, M.M.; Ragan, R.C.; Kim, J.S.; Cross, J.M.; Hill, V.J.; Tuggle, S.C.; Allman, R.M. Myogenic protein expression before and after resistance loading in 26- and 64-yr-old men and women. *J. Appl. Physiol.* **2004**, *97*, 1329–1337. [CrossRef] [PubMed]
53. Marcotte, G.R.; West, D.W.; Baar, K. The molecular basis for load-induced skeletal muscle hypertrophy. *Calcif. Tissue Int.* **2015**, *96*, 196–210. [CrossRef] [PubMed]
54. Schiaffino, S.; Dyar, K.A.; Ciciliot, S.; Blaauw, B.; Sandri, M. Mechanisms regulating skeletal muscle growth and atrophy. *FEBS J.* **2013**, *280*, 4294–4314. [CrossRef]
55. Bogdanovich, S.; Krag, T.O.; Barton, E.R.; Morris, L.D.; Whittemore, L.A.; Ahima, R.S.; Khurana, T.S. Functional improvement of dystrophic muscle by myostatin blockade. *Nature* **2002**, *420*, 418–421. [CrossRef]
56. Cai, Q.; Zhao, M.; Liu, X.; Wang, X.; Nie, Y.; Li, P.; Liu, T.; Ge, R.; Han, F. Reduced expression of citrate synthase leads to excessive superoxide formation and cell apoptosis. *Biochem. Biophys. Res. Commun.* **2017**, *485*, 388–394. [CrossRef]
57. Kadenbach, B. Introduction to mitochondrial oxidative phosphorylation. *Adv. Exp. Med. Biol.* **2012**, *748*, 1–11. [CrossRef]
58. Larsen, S.; Nielsen, J.; Hansen, C.N.; Nielsen, L.B.; Wibrand, F.; Stride, N.; Schroder, H.D.; Boushel, R.; Helge, J.W.; Dela, F.; et al. Biomarkers of mitochondrial content in skeletal muscle of healthy young human subjects. *J. Physiol.* **2012**, *590*, 3349–3360. [CrossRef]
59. Proctor, D.N.; Joyner, M.J. Skeletal muscle mass and the reduction of VO2max in trained older subjects. *J. Appl. Physiol.* **1997**, *82*, 1411–1415. [CrossRef]
60. Meierhofer, D.; Mayr, J.A.; Foetschl, U.; Berger, A.; Fink, K.; Schmeller, N.; Hacker, G.W.; Hauser-Kronberger, C.; Kofler, B.; Sperl, W. Decrease of mitochondrial DNA content and energy metabolism in renal cell carcinoma. *Carcinogenesis* **2004**, *25*, 1005–1010. [CrossRef]
61. Van Moorsel, D.; Hansen, J.; Havekes, B.; Scheer, F.A.; Jorgensen, J.A.; Hoeks, J.; Schrauwen-Hinderling, V.B.; Duez, H.; Lefebvre, P.; Schaper, N.C.; et al. Demonstration of a day-night rhythm in human skeletal muscle oxidative capacity. *Mol. Metab.* **2016**, *5*, 635–645. [CrossRef]
62. Calvani, R.; Joseph, A.M.; Adhihetty, P.J.; Miccheli, A.; Bossola, M.; Leeuwenburgh, C.; Bernabei, R.; Marzetti, E. Mitochondrial pathways in sarcopenia of aging and disuse muscle atrophy. *Biol. Chem.* **2013**, *394*, 393–414. [CrossRef] [PubMed]
63. Romanello, V.; Sandri, M. Mitochondrial Quality Control and Muscle Mass Maintenance. *Front. Physiol.* **2016**, *6*, 422. [CrossRef] [PubMed]
64. Green, H.; Goreham, C.; Ouyang, J.; Ball-Burnett, M.; Ranney, D. Regulation of fiber size, oxidative potential, and capillarization in human muscle by resistance exercise. *Am. J. Physiol.* **1999**, *276*, R591–R596. [CrossRef]
65. Hiatt, W.R.; Regensteiner, J.G.; Wolfel, E.E.; Carry, M.R.; Brass, E.P. Effect of exercise training on skeletal muscle histology and metabolism in peripheral arterial disease. *J. Appl. Physiol.* **1996**, *81*, 780–788. [CrossRef]
66. Kirkendall, D.T.; Garrett, W.E., Jr. The effects of aging and training on skeletal muscle. *Am. J. Sports Med.* **1998**, *26*, 598–602. [CrossRef]
67. Miljkovic, N.; Lim, J.Y.; Miljkovic, I.; Frontera, W.R. Aging of skeletal muscle fibers. *Ann. Rehabil. Med.* **2015**, *39*, 155–162. [CrossRef]
68. Wilson, J.M.; Loenneke, J.P.; Jo, E.; Wilson, G.J.; Zourdos, M.C.; Kim, J.S. The effects of endurance, strength, and power training on muscle fiber type shifting. *J. Strength Cond. Res.* **2012**, *26*, 1724–1729. [CrossRef]

10

Resistance Exercise, Electrical Muscle Stimulation and Whole-Body Vibration in Older Adults

Nejc Šarabon [1,2,3,*], Žiga Kozinc [1,4], Stefan Löfler [5,6] and Christian Hofer [7]

1 Faculty of Health Sciences, University of Primorska, Polje 42, SI-6310 Izola, Slovenia; ziga.kozinc@fvz.upr.si
2 InnoRenew CoE, Human Health Department, Livade 6, SI6310 Izola, Slovenia
3 S2P, Science to practice, Ltd., Laboratory for Motor Control and Motor Behavior, Tehnološki Park 19, SI-1000 Ljubljana, Slovenia
4 Andrej Marušič Institute, University of Primorska, Muzejski Trg 2, SI-6000 Koper, Slovenia
5 Physiko- & Rheumatherapie, Institute for Physical Medicine and Rehabilitation, 3100 St. Pölten, Austria; stefan.loefler@rehabilitationresearch.eu
6 Centre of Active Ageing—Competence Centre for Health, Prevention and Active Ageing, 3100 St. Pölten, Austria
7 Ludwig Boltzmann Institute for Rehabilitation Research, 3100 St. Pölten, Austria; christian.hofer@rehabilitationresearch.eu
* Correspondence: nejc.sarabon@fvz.upr.si.

Abstract: It has been shown that resistance exercise (RT) is one of the most effective approaches to counteract the physical and functional changes associated with aging. This systematic review with meta-analysis compared the effects of RT, whole-body vibration (WBV), and electrical muscle stimulation (EMS) on muscle strength, body composition, and functional performance in older adults. A thorough literature review was conducted, and the analyses were limited to randomized controlled trials. In total, 63 studies were included in the meta-analysis (48 RT, 11 WBV, and 4 EMS). The results showed that RT and WBV are comparably effective for improving muscle strength, while the effects of EMS remains debated. RT interventions also improved some outcome measures related to functional performance, as well as the cross-sectional area of the quadriceps. Muscle mass was not significantly affected by RT. A limitation of the review is the smaller number of WBV and particularly EMS studies. For this reason, the effects of WBV and EMS could not be comprehensively compared to the effect of RT for all outcome measures. For the moment, RT or combinations of RT and WBV or EMS, is probably the most reliable way to improve muscle strength and functional performance, while the best approach to increase muscle mass in older adults remains open to further studies.

Keywords: sarcopenia; falls; elderly; resistance exercise; vibration; electrical stimulation

1. Introduction

With rising life expectancy and the increasing proportion of older adults in the population [1,2], effective interventions that promote lifelong well-being and health are more needed than ever before. There is no doubt that performing physical exercise is one of the most effective ways for older adults to maintain functional independence, maintain physical abilities, and reduce the risk of various diseases and injuries [3–7]. One of the most notable changes associated with aging is sarcopenia, which is characterized by a loss of muscle mass and other subsequent changes, such as reduced muscle strength and impaired functional ability [8]. Together with nutritional interventions, resistance exercise training

(RT) seems to be the most effective approach to prevent and treat sarcopenia [9–11]. Falls are also one of the major problems in the older adult population [12] and are thus given considerable attention in terms of prevention. It has been shown that the best way to prevent falls is by performing RT alone or in combination with other exercise types or other interventions [13,14]. Despite extensive research regarding the effects of resistance exercise on sarcopenia, fall risk, and general health of older adults, the recommendations for prescribing exercises in this population are still relatively vague and generic [3,11,15]. In contrast, previous studies have investigated several factors that are worth considering in order to maximize the effects of RT for older adults, such as intensity [16], speed of movement [17], and supervision of the training sessions [18]. Certain types of RT, such as speed-power training [19], are also increasingly being investigated as potentially superior to traditional resistance exercise.

Recent literature reviews have found numerous barriers, such as decreased physical ability, walking disability, lack of companionship, and lack of motivation, that are decreasing the participation of older adults in exercise programs [20,21]. For this reason, different methods to combat sarcopenia, prevent falls, and increase well-being in older adults should be considered as an alternative to RT. Recently, whole-body vibration (WBV) has been shown to improve postural balance [22] and muscle strength [23] and to reduce the likelihood of falls in older adults [24]. WBV is therefore a possible alternative to RT; however, direct comparisons between the effects of RT and WBV are lacking. Roelants et al., reported similar improvements in knee extension strength, jumping performance, and speed of movement after 12 and 24 weeks of RT and WBV interventions in older women [25]. Similarly, Bogaerts et al., showed comparable effects of WBV and RT on muscle mass and muscle strength in older men [26]. Another promising alternative to RT is electrical muscle stimulation (EMS) [27–31]. EMS has been shown to improve functional performance of aging muscles [27,31] and to counteract muscle decline in old age [30]. Moreover, EMS has been appreciated as a convenient intervention for older adults with lower physical abilities or low motivation to exercise [32].

Although many positive effects of RT, WBV, and EMS in older adults have been consistently demonstrated, it is not entirely clear which interventions should be prioritized for the best health benefits. Moreover, studies often follow only a limited set of outcome measures, making comparisons between interventions difficult. Therefore, the objective of this work was to provide a comprehensive systematic review with meta-analysis of high-quality studies that assessed the effects of RT, WBV, or ES in older adults. To obtain a broad overview of these effects, we included studies that assessed various outcome measures, including muscle strength, body composition, and muscle morphology, and the outcomes of functional performance tests. In addition, the aim of this review was to examine the effects of several independent variables, pertaining to the intervention programs, such as (but not limited to) intervention duration, weekly frequency, volume, intensity, supervision, and compliance. We hypothesized that RT, WBV, and EMS will have similar effects on body composition, muscle strength, and functional performance.

2. Materials and Methods

2.1. Inclusion Criteria

Study inclusion criteria were structured according to PICOS tool [33]:

- Population (P): Male or female older adults. The criterion for inclusion was mean sample age ≥ 65.0 years. Patients with sarcopenia were included if they met this criterion (age ≥ 65.0 years); however, sarcopenia was not an inclusion criterion.
- Intervention (I): RT, EMS, or WBW interventional programs of any duration. Studies exploring multimodal interventional programs (e.g., RT programs combined with stretching exercise) were excluded.

- Comparisons (C): Control groups, receiving no intervention or placebo intervention. Groups that received cognitive training or other non-physical interventions were also accepted as control groups. Studies in which control groups received any type of exercise, vibration intervention, electrical stimulation, or nutritional supplementation were excluded.
- Outcomes (O): (a) Muscular strength or power, not limited to type of testing or body part; (b) body composition and muscle architecture (including body fat, fat free mass, muscle mass, regional muscle mass, skeletal muscle mass, cross-sectional muscle area, circumference measures, and sarcopenia index) and (c) functional mobility outcomes (timed up-and-go test, stepping tests, sit-stand tests, functional reach tests, etc.).
- Study design (S): Only randomized controlled trials (RCT) that included at least one intervention group (RT, EMS, or WBV) and control group.

2.2. Search Strategy

Multiple databases of scientific literature (PubMed, Cochrane Central Register of Controlled Trials, PEDro, and ScienceDirect) were searched in May 2020 without regard to the date of publication. For the databases that enable using Boolean search operators, we used the following combination of search key words: (sarcopenia OR muscle atrophy OR muscle wasting) and (training OR exercise OR vibration OR electrical stimulation OR electrostimulation OR magnetic stimulation OR vibration training OR physical therapy) and (strength OR power OR muscle mass OR muscle diameter) and (elderly OR older OR older adults OR ageing OR age-related). Otherwise, we used several reduced combinations of key words, including, but not limited to resistance exercise older adults, vibration training elderly, electrical stimulation elderly and older adults sarcopenia intervention. Additionally, reference lists of several review articles describing interventions for older adults were carefully scrutinized. Finally, we carefully reviewed reference lists of all articles that were already retrieved through the database search and were published within the last 4 years. The database search was performed independently by two authors (N.Š. and Ž.K.). Two reviewers (N.Š. and S.L.) also screened the titles and the abstracts independently. Potentially relevant articles were screened in full text, followed by additional screening for their eligibility by the additional reviewers.

2.3. Data Extraction

The data extraction was carried out independently by two authors (Ž.K. and C.H.) and disagreements were resolved through consultation with other authors. The extracted data included: (a) baseline and post-intervention means and standard deviations for all eligible outcome measures for interventional and control groups; (b) baseline demographics of participants (gender, age, body height, body mass, body mass index); (c) intervention characteristics (target body area (upper, lower or whole-body), duration of the intervention, number of sessions per week, volume (number of exercises, sets, and repetitions), breaks between exercises and sets, supervision, and progression of exercise difficulty). For studies examining RT, we also extracted the type of load used (bodyweight, machine, elastics, weights, etc.) and intensity as a percentage of 1-maximum repetition (1RM) or subjective measures, such as the Borg scale. For EMS studies, we further extracted the stimulation frequency and amplitude, the stimulated body parts, pulse shapes, and breaks between repetitions or sets. For WBV studies, we additionally extracted the amplitude and the frequency that was used during training. Data were carefully entered into Microsoft Excel 2016 (Microsoft, Redmond, WA, USA). If the data were presented in a graphical rather than tabular form, we used Adobe Illustrator Software (version CS5, Adobe Inc., San Jose, CA, USA) to accurately determine the means and standard deviations. In case of missing data, the corresponding author of the respective articles was contacted by e-mail. If no response was received after 21 days, the author was contacted again. If the author did not reply to the second inquiry, the data was considered irretrievable.

2.4. Assessment of Study Quality

Two authors (Ž.K. and N.Š.) evaluated the quality of the studies using the PEDro tool [34], which assesses study quality based on a ten-level scale. Potential disagreements between ratings were resolved by consulting the other authors. Studies scoring from 9–10 were considered as "excellent," 6–8 as "good," 4–5 as "fair," and less than 4 as "poor" quality. The PEDro scale was chosen because it was developed specifically to assess the quality of randomized controlled trial studies evaluating physical therapist interventions [34].

2.5. Data Analysis and Synthesis

The main data analyses were carried out in Review Manager (Version 5.3, Copenhagen: The Nordic Cochrane Centre, The Cochrane Collaboration, 2014, London, UK). Before the results were entered into the meta-analytical model, the pre-post differences and pooled standard deviations were calculated according to the following formula $SD = \sqrt{[(SD_{pre}^2 + SD_{post}^2) - (2 \times r \times SD_{pre} \times SD_{post})}$. The correction value (r), which represents the pre-test–post-test correlation of outcome measures, was conservatively set at 0.75. It should be noted that a change in the correction value in the range between 0.5 and 0.9 had little effect on the pooled SD and would not change the outcomes of the meta-analyses. For the meta-analyses, the inverse variance method for continuous outcomes with a random-effects model was used. The pooled effect sizes were expressed as mean difference (MD) where possible, which allows the effect size to be expressed in units of measurement. Where this was not possible due to the heterogeneity of the outcome variables (e.g., muscle strength reported in kg, N, Nm, N/kg, and Nm/kg), the effect sizes were expressed as standardized mean difference (SMD). For MD and SMD, the respective 95% confidence intervals were also calculated and reported.

Basic analysis compared the effects of the RT, EMS, and WBV interventions. Further subgroup analyses were conducted where possible (depending on the number of studies reporting a given outcome) based on several independent variables, related to the characteristics of the interventions (e.g., weekly number of sessions). Some outcomes did not appear in EMS and WBV studies and were thereby only analyzed in view of RT studies. Statistical heterogeneity among studies was determined by calculating the I2 statistics. According to Cochrane guidelines, the I2 statistics of 0% to 40% might not be important, 30% to 60% may represent moderate heterogeneity, 50% to 90% may represent substantial heterogeneity, and 75% to 100% indicates considerable heterogeneity [35]. The threshold for statistical significance was set at $p \leq 0.05$ for the main effect size and the subgroup difference tests.

Sensitivity analysis was performed when deemed necessary i.e., by examining the effect of exclusion of certain studies from the analyses (e.g., studies that could have included subsets of previous studies, studies with very low compliance, studies that did not report intensity, studies with and without elderly with sarcopenia, etc.). The sensitivity analyses showed no or very little effect on the main results (SMD changes = 0.01–0.10), except where noted and reported in the results.

3. Results

3.1. Summary of Search Results

The results of the search steps are summarized in Figure 1. The search resulted in 64 studies in total, 48 of which included RT interventions (55 intervention groups in total), 12 included WBV interventions (14 intervention groups in total) and 4 included EMS interventions (4 intervention groups in total). A table encompassing all the details regarding the participants, interventions and outcomes of individual studies is included in Supplementary data 1.

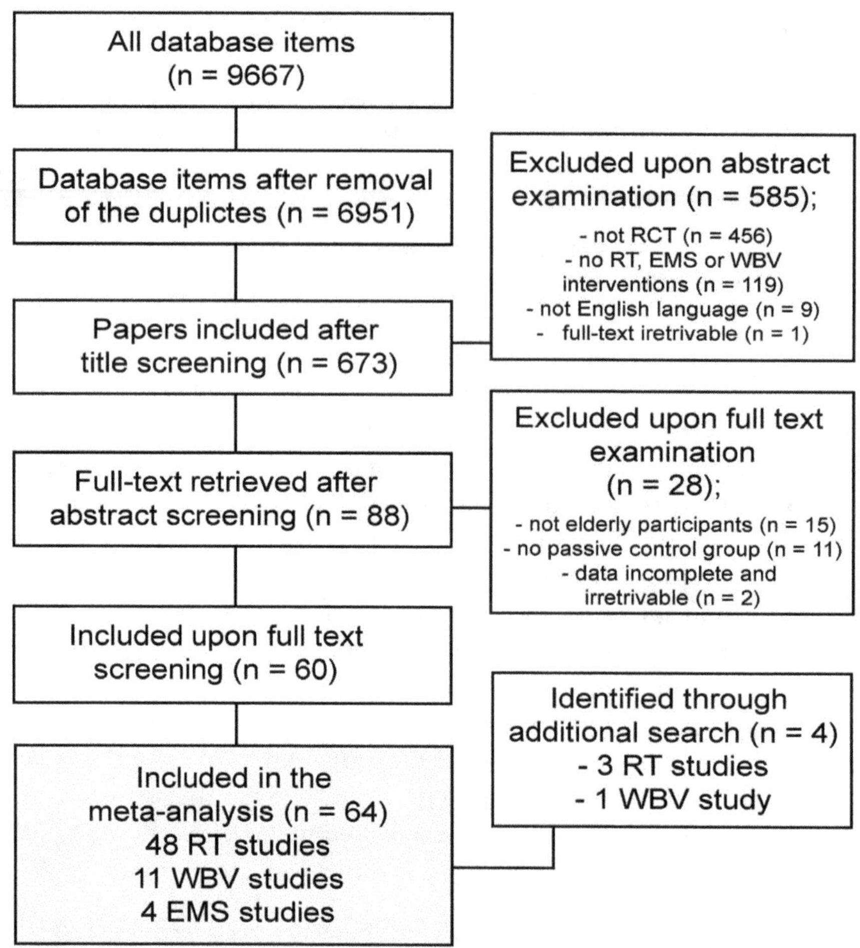

Figure 1. Summary of search results. RT—resistance training; WBV—whole-body vibration; EMS—electrical muscle stimulation.

3.2. Study Quality Assessment

The PEDro scale scores indicated overall fair to good quality of the RT studies (mean = 5.25 ± 1.26; median = 5.0; range = 2–8) and WBV studies (mean = 5.41 ± 1.24; median = 5.5; range = 4–7). Studies exploring EMS were all rated as good (mean = 6.52 ± 1.03; median = 6.0; range = 6–8). The most common items that almost all studies failed to satisfy were blinding of the subjects, therapists and assessors.

3.3. Participant Data and Intervention Characteristics

In total, there were 2017 participants (1158 in intervention groups and 1026 in control groups) in the RT studies, 606 in WBV studies (325 in intervention groups and 284 in control groups), and 192 in the EMS studies (99 in intervention groups and 93 in control groups). Across all studies, the pooled participant age was 73.5 ± 4.8 years (range of means: 65–92 years), the pooled participant body mass was 65.8 ± 10.33 kg (range of means: 40.5–101.8 kg), and the pooled body mass index was 26.39 ± 3.77 kg/m^2 (range of means: 18.8–36.7 kg/m^2). In total, 36 included participants of both genders, 24 studies included only females, and 4 studies included only males. In 16 RT studies, sarcopenia was listed as an inclusion criterion. In 47 studies, the interventions were supervised, while the interventions in the remaining studies were not supervised (n = 9) or the information regarding the supervision was missing (n = 7). The most typical duration of the interventions was 12 weeks (n = 28), while 12 interventions were shorter (4 interventions lasted 5–6 weeks, and 8 interventions lasted 8–11 weeks) and 23 interventions were longer (12 interventions lasted 13–24 weeks, and 11 interventions lasted 25 weeks or more). Most interventions included either 2 (n = 23) or 3 (n = 32) sessions per week, while 5 interventions were performed once per week and 3 interventions were performed 4–5 times per week. Only 4 WBV and 19 RT studies reported adherence to the intervention program, with mean values of 90 ± 3% and 84 ± 9%, respectively.

Across the RT studies, 14 intervention programs used machines, 6 used free weights, 5 used elastic resistance, 4 implemented bodyweight exercises, 1 used weighted tai-chi exercises, and 1 used isoinertial exercises on a flywheel device. The remaining 17 studies used mixed approaches (5 combined bodyweight and elastic exercise, 2 combined free weights and bodyweight exercises, 3 combined free weights and machines, and 7 used more three or four types of load). RT interventions included either full body workout (n = 32) or focused on the lower limb muscles (n = 16), while no interventions focused only on the trunk or the upper limbs. Most often (n = 29), the intervention included a combination of single-joint and multi-joint exercises; however, some interventions included predominantly single-joint (n = 12) or multi-joint (n = 7) exercises. The volume of exercise varied substantially between studies, with the number of exercises ranging from 1 to 12 (mean: 5.9 ± 2.9), the number of sets ranging from 1 to 5 (mean: 2.7 ± 0.8), and number of repetitions within sets ranging from 7 to 25 (mean: 11.0 ± 3.5). Intensity was set as percentage of 1-repetition-maximum in 27 studies (mean: 66.2 ± 15.3%; range: 20–80%) or using the 6–20 Borg scale for assessment of the rate of perceived exertion in 10 studies (all studies used 13 as the target value). One study determined the intensity as percentage of maximal heart rate (set between 60 and 80%). The remaining 12 studies did not report the intensity of the exercise. Breaks between sets were reported in 11 studies and ranged from 30 s to 150 s (mean: 100 ± 45 s). Breaks between exercises were only reported in 5 studies (range: 90–180 s).

In WBV studies, the number of exercises ranged from 1 to 9 (mean: 3.8 ± 3.1) and the number of sets ranged from 1 to 10 (mean: 3.5 ± 2.7). With the exception of 1 study, which used highly varying vibration frequency (27–114 Hz), the frequencies used ranged from 20 to 60 Hz (mean: 35.7 ± 10.1 Hz). The amplitude of the vibration ranged from 2 to 6 mm (mean: 3.8 ± 1.4 mm). Breaks between sets ranged from 30 to 180 s (mean: 75 ± 53.8 s).

Finally, 3 EMS studies targeted full body (all used stimulation frequency of 85 Hz, impulse width at 350 μs, moderate intensity (subjectively determined) and lasted 20 min per session), while 1 study stimulated only the lower limbs (frequency: 100 Hz; amplitude: 40–120 mA; impulse width: 400 μs).

3.4. *Effects of RT and WBV on Muscle Strength*

Knee extension strength was by far the most common outcome across studies and was reported in 2 EMS studies with 2 intervention groups [36,37], 6 WBW studies with 8 intervention groups [25,26,38–42], and 26 RT studies with 29 intervention groups [25,43–67]. In total, 5 studies measured isokinetic strength (1 study at 30°/s, 3 studies at 60°/s and 1 study sat 90°/s), and the rest measured isometric strength. Figure 2 displays the main analysis, comparing the effect of WBV, RT, and EMS on knee strength. Due to substantial discrepancy between the studies in terms of units of reporting, only the SMD could be computed.

There was a statistically significant increase in knee extension strength in the intervention groups across all studies compared to control groups (SMD = 1.12 (0.86–1.37); $p < 0.001$; $I^2 = 83\%$). Both WBV interventions (SMD = 0.97 (0.34–1.59); $p = 0.00$; $I^2 = 90\%$) and RT interventions (SMD = 1.24 (0.96–1.52); $p < 0.001$; $I^2 =79\%$) improved knee extension strength, while EMS did not (SMD = −0.08 (−1.08–0.91); $p = 0.88$; $I^2 = 81\%$). RT appeared superior to WBV; however, the difference between intervention types was not statistically significant ($p = 0.32$). For WBV, the subgroup analysis was performed for intervention duration and indicated that interventions longer than 24 weeks have a higher effect (SMD = 1.61 (0.35–2.87) than interventions lasting up to 12 weeks (SMD = 0.55 (0.21–0.88) or interventions lasting 13–24 weeks (SMD = 0.55 (−0.29–1.40)), although the subgroup test showed that this difference was not statistically significant ($p = 0.28$). Within the RT studies, most interventions lasted 12 weeks (17/26 studies). Subgroup analyses showed no effect of intervention duration on knee strength increases (SMD = 0.94–1.26 across subgroups). The effect of RT was the highest in studies with participants aged > 80 years (SMD = 1.76 (1.01–2.52), lower in the < 70-year-old subgroup (SMD =

1.17 (0.73–1.61) and the lowest in the 70–80-year-old subgroup (SMD = 0.95 (0.65–1.25)) ($p = 0.14$ for subgroup differences). The effect was comparable in studies using predominantly single-joint (SMD = 1.38 (0.70–2.07), predominantly multi-joint (SMD = 1.12 (0.33–1.90)), or a combination of single- and multi-joint exercises (SMD = 1.27 (0.91–1.62)) ($p = 0.88$ for subgroup differences). No differences between studies were found ($p = 0.68$) based on the type of resistance, though there was a trend for higher effect of interventions based on machine training (SMD = 1.36 (0.97–1.75)) and free weights (SMD = 1.33 (0.37–2.29)) compared to elastic resistance (SMD = 0.91 (0.20–1.63)) and approaches that combined multiple types of resistance (SMD = 0.98 (0.49–1.47)). Finally, studies were grouped according to number of sessions per week and no differences were found between interventions performed ≤2 times per week (SMD = 1.30 (0.92–1.68)) and ≥3 times per week (SMD = 1.15 (0.75–1.55)) ($p = 0.59$ for subgroup differences).

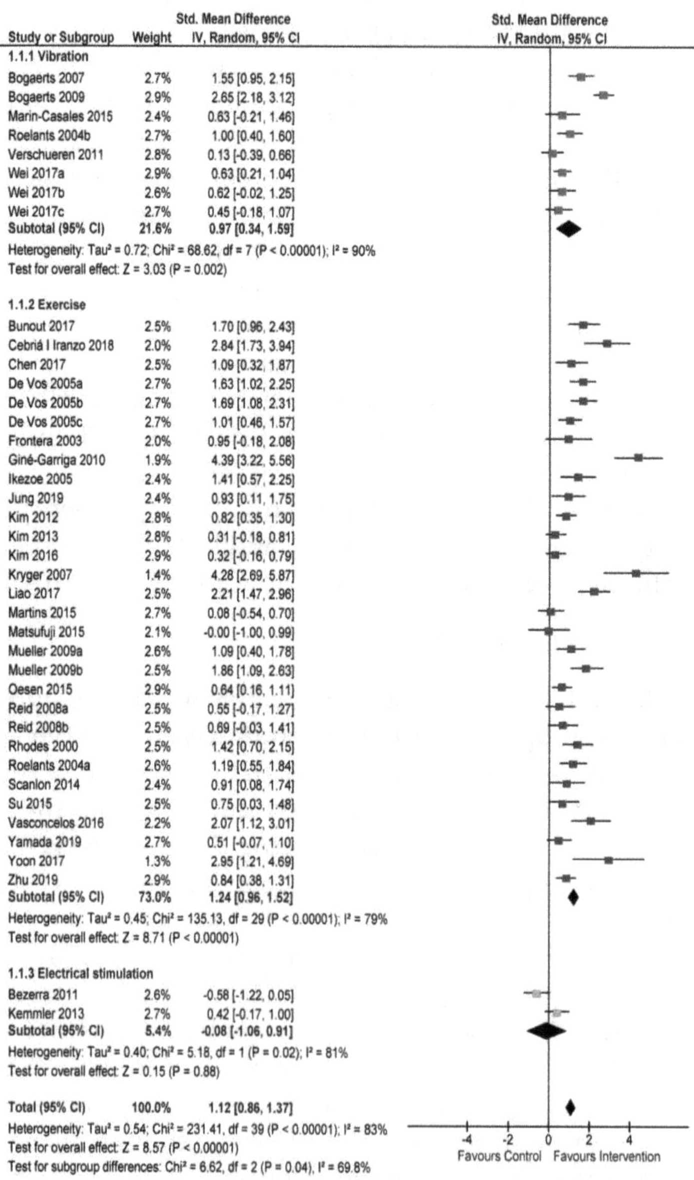

Figure 2. Effects of whole-body vibration, resistance exercise, and electrical muscle stimulation interventions on knee extension strength.

Sensitivity analysis was performed to examine the effect of certain concerns regarding the studies. Since it was not entirely clear if Bogaerts et al. (2007 and 2009, see Figure 2, top section) reported the data for entirely different sample in the two studies, we excluded the study with smaller sample size. The pooled effect of WBV was decreased from 0.97 to 0.88; however, it was still statistically significant

($p = 0.01$). Furthermore, 4 WBV studies included in this analysis involved some component (lunges, squats) of RT. Therefore, it is unclear if this RT component contributed to the overall improvements. Removing these studies from the analysis yields a lower overall effect (SMD = 0.59 (0.30–0.87), which is statistically still significant ($p = 0.03$); however, with this reduction in studies, the subgroup analyses indicate statistically significant difference ($p = 0.001$) between RT and WBV, indicating the superiority of RT compared to WBV without any RT components. Additionally, we repeated the analysis with exclusion of RT studies on sarcopenia patients (SMD increased from 1.24 to 1.34) and vice versa (SMD dropped to 1.01). Therefore, a slight tendency for larger effect in healthy older adults was indicated. A final sensitivity analysis was performed for type of measurement. Removing the studies that measured isokinetic strength increased the main effect slightly (from 1.24 to 1.33). However, the studies with isokinetic measurements also had large and statistically significant pooled effect (SMD = 0.88; $p < 0.001$), which suggest isokinetic and isometric strength both substantially increased with RT.

Leg press strength was reported in 5 RT studies (8 interventional groups) [46,60,61,68,69]. There was a statistically significant increase in intervention groups across studies (SMD = 1.45 (0.85–2.06); $p < 0.001$; $I^2 = 83\%$) (Figure 3). Interventions performed 3 times per week tended to have a larger effect (SMD = 1.98 (0.50–3.45)) than interventions performed 2 times per week (SMD = 1.12 (0.78–1.47)), but the subgroup difference was not statistically significant ($p = 0.27$ for subgroup differences). Two RT studies reported back extensor strength [45,70] and showed a statistically significant increase (MD = 7.97 kg (3.07–12.88 kg); $p < 0.001$; $I^2 = 0.0\%$) (Figure 3). Three RT studies [71–73] reported a composite score for strength (i.e., sum of several strength tasks). There was a statistically significant improvement in intervention groups (SMD = 3.55 (2.28–4.83); $p < 0.001$; $I^2 = 90\%$) (Figure 3). Grip strength was reported in 19 RT studies [44,45,49,52,53,55,56,59,61,65,67,69,70,74–79]. There was a mean increase of 1.48 kg (0.26–2–23 kg; $p < 0.001$) across studies with pre-post mean differences ranging from −1.00 to 5.70 kg.

3.5. Effects of RT on Body Composition

Muscle mass was reported in 7 RT studies (8 intervention groups) [45,52,70,71,74,78,80]. Compared to control groups, there was not a statistically significant increase in muscles mass in intervention groups across studies (MD = 0.60 kg (−0.18–1.37 kg); $p = 0.13$; $I^2 = 83\%$) (Figure 4). There were no differences between interventions performed 2 times a week (MD = 0.60 kg (−1.01–2.22 kg)) and 3 times a week (MD = 0.68 kg (0.23–1.14 kg)) ($p = 0.93$ for subgroup differences). Appendicular muscle mass was reported in 7 RT studies [51–53,65,70,80–82]. The pooled effect showed no change after RT interventions compared to control groups (MD = 0.01 kg (−0.26–0.28 kg); $p = 0.92$; $I^2 = 8\%$) (Figure 4). Lower-limb muscle mass was reported in 8 RT studies [51–53,55,56,67,80,82], with an overall small and statistically non-significant increase (MD = 0.18 kg (−0.11—0.47 kg); $p = 0.22$; $I^2 = 45\%$) (Figure 4). No statistically significant differences were shown between interventions performed 3 times per week (MD = 0.55 kg (−0.44–1.55 kg)) compared to interventions performed 2 times per week (MD = 0.10 kg (−0.10–0.31 kg)) ($p = 0.39$ for subgroup differences). Upper limb muscle mass was reported in 5 RT studies [53,56,67,80,82], and the pooled effect was negligible (MD = 0.01 kg (−0.11–0.13 kg); $p = 0.84$; $I^2 = 0\%$) (Figure 4).

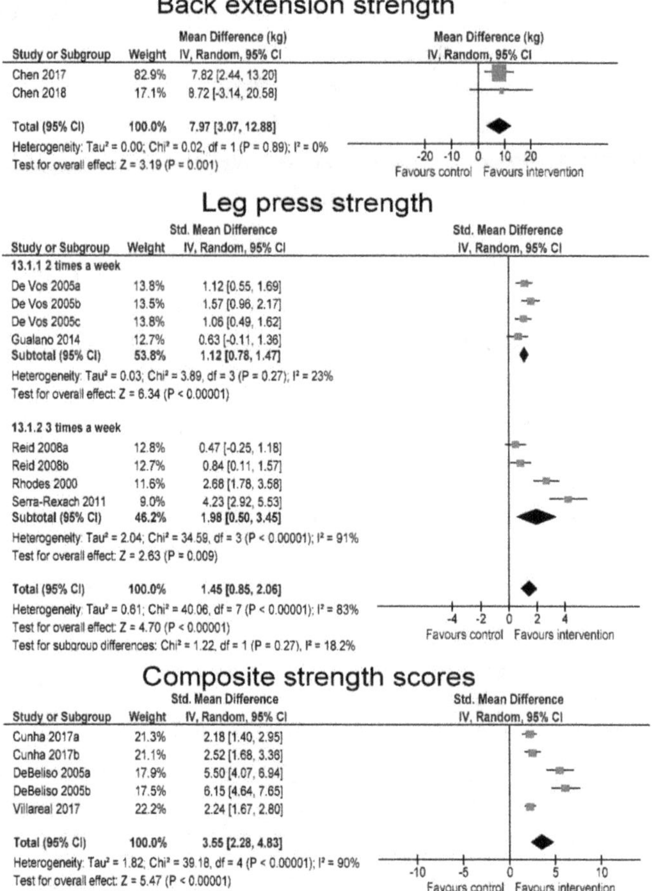

Figure 3. Effect of resistance exercise interventions on back extension, leg press, and composite strength scores.

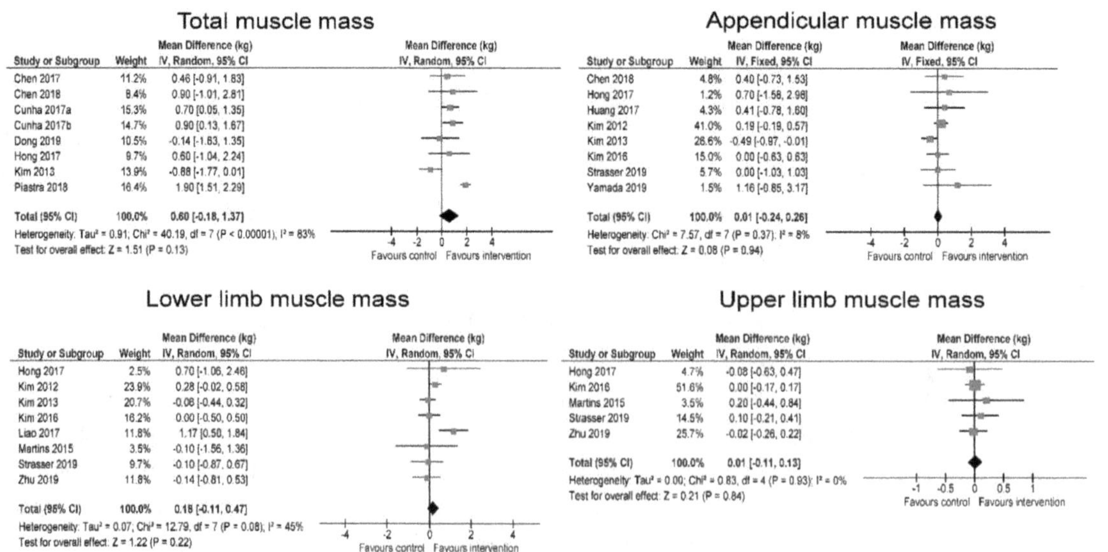

Figure 4. Effect of resistance exercise interventions on muscle mass.

Fat-free mass was recorded in 2 WBV [39,83], 7 RT [55,62,73–76,81], and 1 EMS studies [84], with a very small and statistically non-significant reduction across studies (MD = −0.27 kg (−0.84–0.31 kg); $p = 0.46$; $I^2 = 0\%$). The pooled effect of the two WBV studies showed a slight increase (MD = 0.53 kg (−1.75–2.81 kg); $p = 0.15$), as did one EMS study (MD = 0.61 kg (−0.81–2.03 kg); $p = 0.40$), while there was a small and statistically non-significant decrease across RT interventions (MD = −0.60 kg

(−1.28–0.09 kg); $p = 0.09$). The differences between WBV, RT, and EMS were not statistically significant ($p = 0.25$).

Body fat mass was reported in 2 WBV [39,41] and 14 RT (16 intervention groups) studies [45,50,53,55,58,62,70,71,73,74,76,80,81,85], with a statistically significant decrease overall (SMD = −0.65 (−1.09–−0.21); $p < 0.001$; $I^2 = 86\%$). For the purposes of MD calculation, three studies (4 intervention groups) [45,58,74] that reported body mass in kg instead of the percentage of body weight were removed and the analysis was repeated. SMD slightly increased (SMD = −0.74) and MD calculation showed a mean reduction of body fat mass percentage of −1.99% (−3.75–−0.22%).

Nine RT studies [44,50,67,70,74,77,78,82] and one EMS study [86] also reported the sarcopenia index (sometimes termed skeletal muscle index) (Figure 5). Mainly (7 studies), the index was computed as the ratio of appendicular skeletal muscle mass and the square body height. However, since two studies did not report the exact calculation of the index, we opted for SMD in order analyses to be conservative. There was a moderate, but statistically non-significant improvement across all studies (SMD = 0.65 (−0.02–1.32); $p = 0.06$; $I^2 = 90\%$). Subgroup analyses favored RT interventions, performed 2 times weekly ($p = 0.008$); this is being heavily influenced by one RT study that showed substantial improvement (SMD = 3.44). Most of the studies showed very small negative or very small positive effects, while the pooled effect was heavily influenced by the aforementioned study. Furthermore, 3 WBV studies [42,87,88] (5 intervention groups) and 3 RT studies [47,62,66] reported the quadriceps muscle (or individual heads of quadriceps muscle) cross-sectional area. In order to obtain a sufficient number of studies for meaningful comparison, these results were compared together and expressed as SMD. Overall, there was a statistically significant effect of interventions (SMD = 0.29 (0.03–0.55); $p = 0.03$; $I^2 = 0\%$) (Figure 5). Subgroup differences showed no differences between RT (SMD = 0.61 (0.04–1.18)) and WBV (SMD = 0.20 (−0.09–0.49) ($p = 0.21$ for subgroup differences). For the RT studies (all reported the cross-sectional area for the full quadriceps muscle), the MD was 1.80 (0.51–3.09) cm^2. One RT study [57] reported thigh circumference, with no effect of the intervention (MD = −0.10 cm (−2.55–2.35 cm); $p = 0.94$; I^2 not applicable).

Two RT studies [58,89] reported the percentage of type I fibers, with small and statistically non-significant pooled effect (MD = 0.14% (−1.38–1.66%); $p = 0.86$; $I^2 = 0\%$). The same two studies reported the percentage of type IIa fibers, showing slight but statistical non-significant increase (MD = 1.03% (−0.43–2.48%); $p = 0.17$; $I^2 = 11\%$). Finally, one RT study [58] reported a statistically significant increase in the percentage of type IIx fibers (MD = 2.42% (1.96–2.88); $p < 0.001$; I^2 not applicable).

3.6. *Effects of RT and WBV on Body Functional Performance*

The results on functional performance are summarized in Figure 6. The timed up-and-go test was performed in 2 WBV [87,88] and 6 RT studies [52,55,69,75,90]. Overall, there were no differences between intervention and control groups across all studies (MD = −0.12 s (−1.36–1.12 s); $p = 0.85$; $I^2 = 93\%$). There were also no differences between the WBV and RT (MD = 0.20 and −0.08 s, respectively; $p = 0.89$ for subgroup differences). The 30-s sit-stand test was performed in 6 RT studies [55,59,68,76,80,85], with an overall improvement of 2.68 repetitions (1.90–3.47 repetitions, $p < 0.001$; $I^2 = 0.50\%$). There was no difference between interventions performed 2 times per week (MD = 2.85 (1.16–4.54 repetitions)) and 3 times per week (MD = 2.73 (2.07–3.39 repetitions)) ($p = 0.90$ for subgroup differences). The 5-repetition sit-stand test was recorded in 4 RT studies [65,67,75,76], and there was a significant improvement (i.e., decreased time to complete the test) across all studies (MD = −2.36 s (−3.9–−0.82 s); $p = 0.003$; $I^2 = 83\%$).

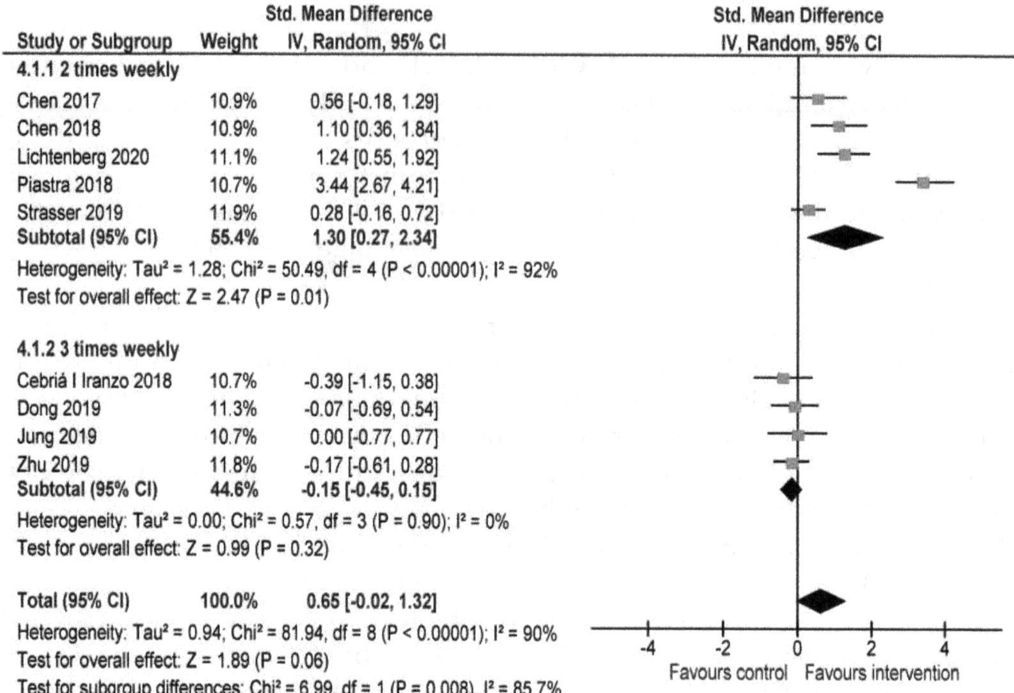

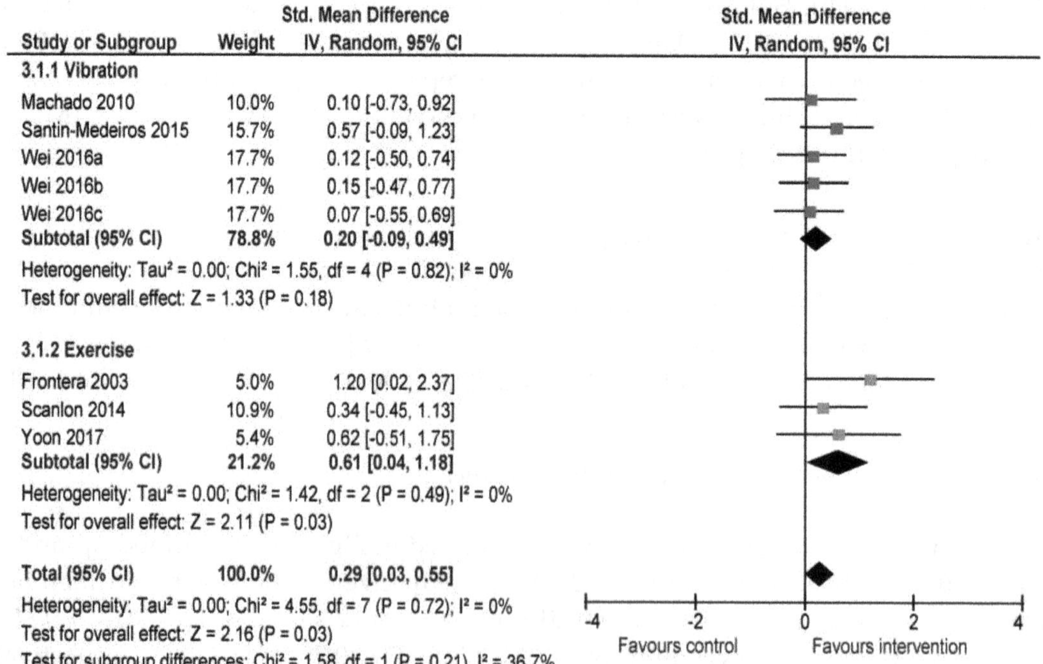

Figure 5. Effects of whole-body vibration and resistance exercise on sarcopenia index and quadriceps cross-sectional area.

Timed-up-and-go test

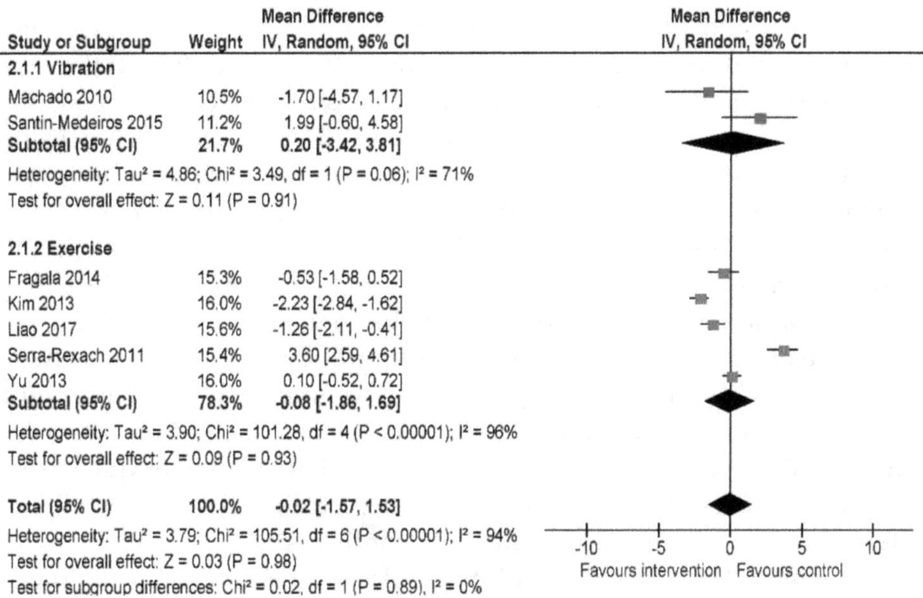

30-second sit-stand test

Study or Subgroup	Weight	Mean Difference IV, Random, 95% CI
15.2.1 12 weeks		
Hong 2017	7.4%	2.10 [-0.46, 4.66]
Krause 2019	26.7%	2.90 [2.14, 3.66]
Liao 2017	14.5%	2.24 [0.66, 3.82]
Subtotal (95% CI)	**48.7%**	**2.73 [2.07, 3.39]**
Heterogeneity: Tau² = 0.00; Chi² = 0.79, df = 2 (P = 0.67); I² = 0%		
Test for overall effect: Z = 8.07 (P < 0.00001)		
15.2.2 24-32 weeks		
Gualano 2014	19.6%	1.30 [0.11, 2.49]
Oesen 2015	15.7%	4.00 [2.52, 5.48]
Sousa 2013	16.1%	3.40 [1.95, 4.85]
Subtotal (95% CI)	**51.3%**	**2.85 [1.16, 4.54]**
Heterogeneity: Tau² = 1.74; Chi² = 9.14, df = 2 (P = 0.01); I² = 78%		
Test for overall effect: Z = 3.31 (P = 0.0009)		
Total (95% CI)	**100.0%**	**2.68 [1.90, 3.47]**
Heterogeneity: Tau² = 0.45; Chi² = 9.94, df = 5 (P = 0.08); I² = 50%		
Test for overall effect: Z = 6.71 (P < 0.00001)		
Test for subgroup differences: Chi² = 0.02, df = 1 (P = 0.90), I² = 0%		

-10 -5 0 5 10
Favours control Favours experimental

5-repetition sit-stand test

Study or Subgroup	Weight	Mean Difference IV, Random, 95% CI
Fragala 2014	25.9%	-1.84 [-3.17, -0.51]
Krause 2019	31.4%	-1.30 [-1.70, -0.90]
Yamada 2019	19.7%	-1.59 [-3.75, 0.57]
Zhu 2019	23.0%	-5.06 [-6.77, -3.35]
Total (95% CI)	**100.0%**	**-2.36 [-3.90, -0.82]**
Heterogeneity: Tau² = 1.93; Chi² = 17.90, df = 3 (P = 0.0005); I² = 83%		
Test for overall effect: Z = 3.00 (P = 0.003)		

-10 -5 0 5 10
Favours intervention Favours control

Figure 6. Effects of whole-body vibration and resistance exercise on functional mobility tests.

4. Discussion

The purpose of this systematic review with meta-analysis was to investigate the effects of RT, WBV, and EMS interventions on muscle strength, body composition, and functional performance in older adults. It included randomized controlled trials involving at least one intervention group (RT, EMS, or WBV) and a control group were included. In total, 64 studies were included in the meta-analysis (48 RT studies, 12 WBV studies, and 4 EMS studies). The main findings of the present systematic reviews are: (1) knee extension strength was improved by RT and WBV, but not ES; (2) the remaining strength outcomes were only assessed in RT studies and significant positive effects were observed; (3) the effects of RT on body composition were small, while the effects of WBV and EMS are unclear due to the small number of studies; (4) there were small effects on sarcopenia index, while quadriceps cross-sectional area was improved in RT studies, but not WBV studies; (5) functional performance was improved by RT interventions, though not in all tests. Overall, the RT interventions proved to be effective for improving muscle strength, muscle cross-sectional area and functional performance, while the effects on body composition were small or non-existent. WBV seems to be comparably effective for improving muscle strength, but not muscle cross-sectional area. A major limitation of the review is the smaller number of WBV and particularly EMS studies. Comparisons between the different intervention types were therefore limited and were not possible for several outcome measures. Subgroup analyses revealed that some of the independent variables (duration of intervention, weekly frequency, type of resistance in RT studies, and age of participants) might have influenced the results; however, these findings were not statistically significant and cannot be conclusively confirmed.

The positive effects of RT, WBV, and EMS in older adults have been reported numerous times [9–11,13,14,19,22,23,25,26,30,31,91–93]. In this review, we included only randomized controlled trials that included at least one group that did not receive any interventions (control group). While the positive effects of RT were clearly demonstrated, the effects of WBV, and in particular EMS, were smaller or absent. Individual studies that directly compared RT and WBV have shown similar effects of the two interventions related to muscle strength and power outcomes [25,26]. In a non-controlled single-group study, improvements in muscle strength and power and functional performance were also observed after 9 weeks of WBV [94]. While the present review showed improvements in muscle strength after WBV interventions, only 2 WBV studies that assessed functional performance were included. Therefore, the effects of WBV on functional performance remain unclear. Since improvements in functional performance are often observed in parallel with increases in muscle strength [92,95,96] and muscle power [97], it can be expected that WBV will also increase functional performance. In addition to increases on muscle strength and possible improvements in functional performance after WBV, previous research also showed positive effects of WBV on postural balance [22], cardiovascular outcomes [98] and possibly muscle activation [99] in older adults. Overall, we can recommend the prescription of WBV to older adults, but it cannot be guaranteed that WBV will produce comparable effects to RT in view of all outcomes relevant to health and well-being.

EMS has been used extensively in people who cannot engage in normal physical activity and has been shown to produce somewhat similar responses to exercise at the muscular level [100]. In this review, a very limited amount of randomized controlled trials has been identified to investigate the effects of EMS in older adults. Our analyses could not confirm or indicate any effects of EMS interventions. EMS has previously been shown to be effective in counteracting muscle weakness in advanced disease [101] and sarcopenia in older adults [30,32], and even to provide additive effects in terms of morphological outcomes when combined with RT in healthy adults [102]. However, the effect of EMS on functional performance of the older adults are less consistent [103]. Nevertheless, the above-mentioned promising results should be re-evaluated in randomized controlled trials to strengthen the findings and enable better comparison to RT and WBV. Based on the results of this and previous research [92], the use of EMS should be encouraged when performing physical activities is not possible or older adults are not motivated to perform it.

Across all interventions, the improvements in muscle strength were much more evident than improvements in muscle mass. It is known that improvements in strength due to neural adaptations occur much earlier before a meaningful increase in muscle mass is seen [104]. While most of the interventions in the present review lasted 12 weeks or longer, improvements in muscle mass could nonetheless be expected. It is possible that muscle mass measurements are not reliable enough to detect the effect of the interventions. Alternatively, the cross-sectional area of the quadriceps was statistically significantly increased across RT studies in this review. Moreover, a previous review also reported notable increases in the cross-sectional area of thigh muscles (+2.31 cm^2) in older adults aged >75 years [105]. Interestingly, the latter review reported such effects for WBV, while the pooled effects of the WBV studies in our review were small.

The results on functional performance were different across outcome measures. Neither WBV, RT nor EMS improved the performance of the timed up-and-go test. Conversely, the sit-stand performance was significantly improved by RT interventions (an increase of 2.68 repetitions in 30-s sit-stand task and a decrease of 2.36 s in the 5-repetition sit-stand task time). It should be noted that the results regarding functional performance were significantly influenced by the heterogeneity of the studies. In particular, the timed up-and-go test performance was substantially improved (−1.77 s) in one study and reduced even more in the second study (+1.99 s). Similarly, most RT studies showed improvements in this test, but one study [69] showed a large reduction (+3.6 s), which led to a negligible pooled effect. This particular study was conducted on very old participants (> 90 years) and included a short-term resistance exercise program, based on light to moderate loads. If this study is excluded from the analysis, the pooled effect size would show statistically significant positive improvements (MD = −0.93 s; $p < 0.001$).

The secondary aim of this paper was to determine the independent variables, related to the interventions, that can influence the magnitude of the outcomes. Most of the subgroup analyses that could be conducted as the number of studies was sufficient, showed no such statistically significant effects. There were statistically non-significant trends for lower limb muscle mass and leg press strength to be improved more with a higher (≥3) weekly session frequency. The literature in the field of sports science [106,107] suggests that weekly frequency is not an independent factor for improvements in muscle strength and muscle mass. A recent meta-analysis suggested that similar is true for older adults [108], although a minimum of 2 sessions per week is typically recommended. Our results also indicated a potentially higher effect of interventions based on machine training and free weights, compared to elastic resistance and approaches combining several types of resistance. In the general population, the effect of elastic resistance appears to be essentially the same as machine-based resistance and free weights [109]. Note that our observation on lesser effects of elastic resistance compared to machines and free weights is limited to knee extension strength and that the difference between the effect of elastic resistance (SMD = 0.91) and machine-based resistance (SMD = 1.36) and free weights (SMD = 1.33) was not statistically significant ($p = 0.68$). Therefore, it is probably appropriate to include elastic resistance in RT programs for older adults.

The first limitation of this systematic review with meta-analysis is the inclusion of only randomized controlled trials. While this was done to compile only high-quality evidence, important findings from studies with different designs were omitted. In particular, the number of EMS studies was very small. It should be emphasized that the lack of reported effects of EMS in the review is partly due to the lack of randomized controlled trials and not necessarily because the EMS is not effective. Furthermore, a major limitation of the review is the high heterogeneity of the studies, which precluded more subgroup analyses and is potentially a major confounding factor. Partially, we investigated this issue with several sensitivity analyses which showed that the results were not heavily influenced by certain factors, such as type of measurements (for knee strength), presence of sarcopenia (though somewhat smaller effects were observed in elderly sarcopenia patients), and adherence to studies. Because there are several factors that can influence response to resistance exercise (in particular, the characteristics of the intervention in addition to those mentioned above), we did our best to perform subgroup analyses to exclude or confirm several factors, such as exercise frequency, intervention duration, and resistance exercise type. Nevertheless, some of the variability between the interventions could not be accounted for. Therefore, we strongly emphasize that these results should be viewed with high caution. Future studies and practitioners should not use the numbers we obtained as a standalone guideline, but rather view our analyses as an exploration of general trends in the field of interventions for older adults.

5. Conclusions

This paper reviewed RCT studies that examined the effects of RT, WBV, and EMS on muscle strength, body composition, and functional performance of older adults. It was found that RT and WBV are effective for increasing muscle strength, while the data was very limited for EMS. RT interventions also improve functional performance and increase muscle-cross sectional area but have no effect on muscle mass. Further studies exploring the effect of WBV and in particular of EMS are needed for better comparison with RT. For the time being, EMS can be recommended for people that are unable to perform RT or WBV. Otherwise, RT or a combination of RT and WBV or EMS is probably the most efficient way to improve muscle strength and functional performance, while the best approach to increase muscle mass in older adults still needs to be determined by further studies. Due to the several limitations of this review, we urge the readers to view the results with caution.

Supplementary Materials: The following are available online at Supplementary data 1: Detailed data regarding study outcomes, interventions and participants.

Author Contributions: Conceptualization, N.S. and Ž.K.; methodology, N.Š., Ž.K., S.L., C.H.; software, Ž.K.; formal analysis, N.Š., Ž.K., S.L., C.H.; investigation, N.Š., Ž.K., S.L., C.H.; resources, N.S., S.L.; data curation, N.Š., Ž.K., S.L., C.H.; writing—original draft preparation, N.Š., Ž.K.; writing—review and editing, S.L., C.H.; visualization, N.Š, Ž.K.; supervision, N.S.; project administration, N.Š. funding acquisition, S.L. All authors have read and agreed to the published version of the manuscript.

Acknowledgments: We want to acknowledge the support of the European Regional Development Fund and Physiko- and Rheumatherapie institute through the Centre of Active Ageing project in the Interreg Slovakia-Austria cross-border cooperation program (partners: Faculty for Physical Education and Sports, Comenius University in Bratislava: Institute for Physical Medicine and Rehabilitation, Physiko- & Rheumatherapie GmbH). Authors NS and ZK acknowledge the European Commission for funding the InnoRenew CoE project (Grant Agreement 739574) under the Horizon2020 Widespread-Teaming program.

References

1. Cheng, X.; Yang, Y.; Schwebel, D.C.; Liu, Z.; Li, L.; Cheng, P.; Ning, P.; Hu, G. Population ageing and mortality during 1990-2017: A global decomposition analysis. *PLoS Med.* **2020**, *17*, e1003138. [CrossRef] [PubMed]
2. Lutz, W.; Sanderson, W.; Scherbov, S. The coming acceleration of global population ageing. *Nature* **2008**, *451*, 716–719. [CrossRef] [PubMed]
3. Galloza, J.; Castillo, B.; Micheo, W. Benefits of Exercise in the Older Population. *Phys. Med. Rehabil. Clin. N. Am.* **2017**, *28*, 659–669. [CrossRef] [PubMed]
4. De Labra, C.; Guimaraes-Pinheiro, C.; Maseda, A.; Lorenzo, T.; Millán-Calenti, J.C. Effects of physical exercise interventions in frail older adults: A systematic review of randomized controlled trials. *BMC Geriatr.* **2015**, *15*, 154. [CrossRef] [PubMed]
5. Lopez, P.; Pinto, R.S.; Radaelli, R.; Rech, A.; Grazioli, R.; Izquierdo, M.; Cadore, E.L. Benefits of resistance training in physically frail elderly: A systematic review. *Aging Clin. Exp. Res.* **2018**, *30*, 889–899. [CrossRef] [PubMed]
6. Barreto, P.D.S.; Rolland, Y.; Vellas, B.; Maltais, M. Association of Long-term Exercise Training with Risk of Falls, Fractures, Hospitalizations, and Mortality in Older Adults: A Systematic Review and Meta-analysis. *JAMA Intern. Med.* **2019**, *179*, 394–405. [CrossRef]
7. Cvecka, J.; Tirpakova, V.; Sedliak, M.; Kern, H.; Mayr, W.; Hamar, D. Physical activity in elderly. *Eur. J. Transl. Myol.* **2015**, *25*, 249–252. [CrossRef]

8. Cruz-Jentoft, A.J.; Bahat, G.; Bauer, J.; Boirie, Y.; Bruyère, O.; Cederholm, T.; Cooper, C.; Landi, F.; Rolland, Y.; Sayer, A.A.; et al. Sarcopenia: Revised European consensus on definition and diagnosis. *Age Ageing* **2019**, *48*, 16–31. [CrossRef]
9. Phu, S.; Boersma, D.; Duque, G. Exercise and Sarcopenia. *J. Clin. Densitom.* **2015**, *18*, 488–492. [CrossRef]
10. Landi, F.; Marzetti, E.; Martone, A.M.; Bernabei, R.; Onder, G. Exercise as a remedy for sarcopenia. *Curr. Opin. Clin. Nutr. Metab. Care* **2014**, *17*, 25–31. [CrossRef]
11. Marzetti, E.; Calvani, R.; Tosato, M.; Cesari, M.; Di Bari, M.; Cherubini, A.; Broccatelli, M.; Savera, G.; D'Elia, M.; Pahor, M.; et al. Physical activity and exercise as countermeasures to physical frailty and sarcopenia. *Aging Clin. Exp. Res.* **2017**, *29*, 35–42. [CrossRef] [PubMed]
12. Cuevas-Trisan, R. Balance Problems and Fall Risks in the Elderly. *Phys. Med. Rehabil. Clin. N. Am.* **2017**, *28*, 727–737. [CrossRef] [PubMed]
13. Tricco, A.C.; Thomas, S.M.; Veroniki, A.A.; Hamid, J.S.; Cogo, E.; Strifler, L.; Khan, P.A.; Robson, R.; Sibley, K.M.; MacDonald, H.; et al. Comparisons of interventions for preventing falls in older adults: A systematic review and meta-analysis. *JAMA J. Am. Med. Assoc.* **2017**, *318*, 1687–1699. [CrossRef] [PubMed]
14. Sherrington, C.; Michaleff, Z.A.; Fairhall, N.; Paul, S.S.; Tiedemann, A.; Whitney, J.; Cumming, R.G.; Herbert, R.D.; Close, J.C.T.; Lord, S.R. Exercise to prevent falls in older adults: An updated systematic review and meta-analysis. *Br. J. Sports Med.* **2017**, *51*, 1749–1757. [CrossRef]
15. Aguirre, L.E.; Villareal, D.T. Physical Exercise as Therapy for Frailty. *Nestle Nutr. Inst. Workshop Ser.* **2015**, *83*, 83–92. [CrossRef]
16. Csapo, R.; Alegre, L.M. Effects of resistance training with moderate vs heavy loads on muscle mass and strength in the elderly: A meta-analysis. *Scand. J. Med. Sci. Sports* **2016**, *26*, 995–1006. [CrossRef]
17. Watanabe, Y.; Tanimoto, M.; Oba, N.; Sanada, K.; Miyachi, M.; Ishii, N. Effect of resistance training using bodyweight in the elderly: Comparison of resistance exercise movement between slow and normal speed movement. *Geriatr. Gerontol. Int.* **2015**, *15*, 1270–1277. [CrossRef]
18. Lacroix, A.; Hortobágyi, T.; Beurskens, R.; Granacher, U. Effects of Supervised vs. Unsupervised Training Programs on Balance and Muscle Strength in Older Adults: A Systematic Review and Meta-Analysis. *Sports Med.* **2017**, *47*, 2341–2361. [CrossRef]
19. Šarabon, N.; Smajla, D.; Kozinc, Ž.; Kern, H. Speed-power based training in the elderly and its potential for daily movement function enhancement. *Eur. J. Transl. Myol.* **2020**, *30*, 8898. [CrossRef]
20. Yarmohammadi, S.; Saadati, H.M.; Ghaffari, M.; Ramezankhani, A. A systematic review of barriers and motivators to physical activity in elderly adults in Iran and worldwide. *Epidemiol. Health* **2019**, *41*, e2019049. [CrossRef]
21. Freiberger, E.; Kemmler, W.; Siegrist, M.; Sieber, C. Frailty und Trainingsinterventionen: Evidenz und Barrieren für Bewegungsprogramme. *Z. Gerontol. Geriatr.* **2016**, *49*, 606–611. [CrossRef] [PubMed]
22. Rogan, S.; Taeymans, J.; Radlinger, L.; Naepflin, S.; Ruppen, S.; Bruelhart, Y.; Hilfiker, R. Effects of whole-body vibration on postural control in elderly: An update of a systematic review and meta-analysis. *Arch. Gerontol. Geriatr.* **2017**, *73*, 95–112. [CrossRef] [PubMed]
23. Rogan, S.; de Bruin, E.D.; Radlinger, L.; Joehr, C.; Wyss, C.; Stuck, N.J.; Bruelhart, Y.; de Bie, R.A.; Hilfiker, R. Effects of whole-body vibration on proxies of muscle strength in old adults: A systematic review and meta-analysis on the role of physical capacity level. *Eur. Rev. Aging Phys. Act.* **2015**, *12*, 12. [CrossRef] [PubMed]
24. Jepsen, D.B.; Thomsen, K.; Hansen, S.; Jørgensen, N.R.; Masud, T.; Ryg, J. Effect of whole-body vibration exercise in preventing falls and fractures: A systematic review and meta-analysis. *BMJ Open* **2017**, *7*, e018342. [CrossRef]
25. Roelants, M.; Delecluse, C.; Verschueren, S.M. Whole-body-vibration training increases knee-extension strength and speed of movement in older women. *J. Am. Geriatr. Soc.* **2004**, *52*, 901–908. [CrossRef]
26. Bogaerts, A.; Delecluse, C.; Claessens, A.; Coudyzer, W.; Boonen, S.; Verschueren, S. Impact of Whole-Body Vibration Training Versus Fitness Training on Muscle Strength and Muscle Mass in Older Men: A 1-Year Randomized Controlled Trial. *J. Gerontol. Ser. A* **2007**, *62*, 630–635. [CrossRef]
27. Mayr, W. Neuromuscular electrical stimulation for mobility support of elderly. *Eur. J. Transl. Myol.* **2015**, *25*, 263–268. [CrossRef]
28. Pette, D.; Vrbová, G. The contribution of neuromuscular stimulation in elucidating muscle plasticity revisited. *Eur. J. Transl. Myol.* **2017**, *27*, 33–39. [CrossRef]

29. Taylor, M.J.; Schils, S.; Ruys, A.J. Home FES: An exploratory review. *Eur. J. Transl. Myol.* **2019**, *29*, 283–292. [CrossRef]
30. Kern, H.; Barberi, L.; Löfler, S.; Sbardella, S.; Burggraf, S.; Fruhmann, H.; Carraro, U.; Mosole, S.; Sarabon, N.; Vogelauer, M.; et al. Electrical stimulation (ES) counteracts muscle decline in seniors. *Front. Aging Neurosci.* **2014**, *6*. [CrossRef]
31. Zampieri, S.; Mosole, S.; Löfler, S.; Fruhmann, H.; Burggraf, S.; Cvečka, J.; Hamar, D.; Sedliak, M.; Tirptakova, V.; Šarabon, N.; et al. Physical exercise in Aging: Nine weeks of leg press or electrical stimulation training in 70 years old sedentary elderly people. *Eur. J. Transl. Myol.* **2015**, *25*, 237–242. [CrossRef] [PubMed]
32. O'Connor, D.; Brennan, L.; Caulfield, B. The use of neuromuscular electrical stimulation (NMES) for managing the complications of ageing related to reduced exercise participation. *Maturitas* **2018**, *113*, 13–20. [CrossRef] [PubMed]
33. Methley, A.M.; Campbell, S.; Chew-Graham, C.; McNally, R.; Cheraghi-Sohi, S. PICO, PICOS and SPIDER: A comparison study of specificity and sensitivity in three search tools for qualitative systematic reviews. *BMC Health Serv. Res.* **2014**, *14*, 579. [CrossRef] [PubMed]
34. Maher, C.G.; Sherrington, C.; Herbert, R.D.; Moseley, A.M.; Elkins, M. Reliability of the PEDro Scale for Rating Quality of Randomized Controlled Trials. *Phys. Ther.* **2003**, *83*, 713–721. [CrossRef]
35. Higgins, J.P.T.; Green, S. Cochrane Handbook for Systematic Reviews of Interventions|Cochrane Training. Available online: https://training.cochrane.org/handbook/current (accessed on 15 May 2020).
36. Kemmler, W.; von Stengel, S. Whole-body electromyostimulation as a means to impact muscle mass and abdominal body fat in lean, sedentary, older female adults: Subanalysis of the TEST-III trial. *Clin. Interv. Aging* **2013**, *8*, 1353–1364. [CrossRef]
37. Bezerra, P.; Zhou, S.; Crowley, Z.; Davie, A.; Baglin, R. Effects of electromyostimulation on knee extensors and flexors strength and steadiness in older adults. *J. Mot. Behav.* **2011**, *43*, 413–421. [CrossRef]
38. Bogaerts, A.C.; Delecluse, C.; Claessens, A.L.; Troosters, T.; Boonen, S.; Verschueren, S.M. Effects of whole body vibration training on cardiorespiratory fitness and muscle strength in older individuals (a 1-year randomised controlled trial). *Age Ageing* **2009**, *38*. [CrossRef]
39. Marín-Cascales, E.; Rubio-Arias, J.A.; Romero-Arenas, S.; Alcaraz, P.E. Effect of 12 weeks of whole-body vibration versus multi-component training in post-menopausal women. *Rejuvenation Res.* **2015**, *18*, 508–516. [CrossRef]
40. Verschueren, S.M.; Bogaerts, A.; Delecluse, C.; Claessens, A.L.; Haentjens, P.; Vanderschueren, D.; Boonen, S. The effects of whole-body vibration training and vitamin D supplementation on muscle strength, muscle mass, and bone density in institutionalized elderly women: A 6-month randomized, controlled trial. *J. Bone Miner. Res.* **2011**, *26*, 42–49. [CrossRef]
41. Zheng, A.; Sakari, R.; Cheng, S.M.; Hietikko, A.; Moilanen, P.; Timonen, J.; Fagerlund, K.M.; Kärkkäinen, M.; Alèn, M.; Cheng, S. Effects of a low-frequency sound wave therapy programme on functional capacity, blood circulation and bone metabolism in frail old men and women. *Clin. Rehabil.* **2009**, *23*, 897–908. [CrossRef]
42. Wei, N.; Pang, M.Y.C.; Ng, S.S.M.; Ng, G.Y.F. Optimal frequency/time combination of whole-body vibration training for improving muscle size and strength of people with age-related muscle loss (sarcopenia): A randomized controlled trial. *Geriatr. Gerontol. Int.* **2017**, *17*, 1412–1420. [CrossRef] [PubMed]
43. Bunout, D.; Barrera, G.; de la Maza, P.; Avendaño, M.; Gattas, V.; Petermann, M.; Hirsch, S. The impact of nutritional supplementation and resistance training on the health functioning of free-living Chilean elders: Results of 18 months of follow-up. *J. Nutr.* **2001**, *131*, 2441S–2446S. [CrossRef] [PubMed]
44. Iranzo, M.A.C.; Balasch-Bernat, M.; Tortosa-Chuliá, M.; Balasch-Parisi, S. Effects of resistance training of peripheral muscles versus respiratory muscles in older adults with sarcopenia who are institutionalized: A randomized controlled trial. *J. Aging Phys. Act.* **2018**, *26*, 637–646. [CrossRef] [PubMed]
45. Chen, H.T.; Chung, Y.C.; Chen, Y.J.; Ho, S.Y.; Wu, H.J. Effects of Different Types of Exercise on Body Composition, Muscle Strength, and IGF-1 in the Elderly with Sarcopenic Obesity. *J. Am. Geriatr. Soc.* **2017**, *65*, 827–832. [CrossRef] [PubMed]
46. De Vos, N.J.; Singh, N.A.; Ross, D.A.; Stavrinos, T.M.; Orr, R.; Singh, M.A.F. Optimal load for increasing muscle power during explosive resistance training in older adults. *J. Gerontol. Ser. A* **2005**, *60*, 638–647. [CrossRef] [PubMed]
47. Frontera, W.R.; Hughes, V.A.; Krivickas, L.S.; Kim, S.K.; Foldvari, M.; Roubenoff, R. Strength training in older women: Early and late changes in whole muscle and single cells. *Muscle Nerve* **2003**, *28*, 601–608. [CrossRef]

48. Giné-Garriga, M.; Guerra, M.; Pagès, E.; Manini, T.M.; Jiménez, R.; Unnithan, V.B. The effect of functional circuit training on physical frailty in frail older adults: A randomized controlled trial. *J. Aging Phys. Act.* **2010**, *18*, 401–424. [CrossRef]
49. Ikezoe, T.; Tsutou, A.; Asakawa, Y.; Tsuboyama, T. Low Intensity Training for Frail Elderly Women: Long-term Effects on Motor Function and Mobility. *J. Phys. Ther. Sci.* **2005**, *17*, 43–49. [CrossRef]
50. Jung, W.S.; Kim, Y.Y.; Park, H.Y. Circuit Training Improvements in Korean Women with Sarcopenia. *Percept. Mot. Skills* **2019**, *126*, 828–842. [CrossRef]
51. Kim, H.K.; Suzuki, T.; Saito, K.; Yoshida, H.; Kobayashi, H.; Kato, H.; Katayama, M. Effects of exercise and amino acid supplementation on body composition and physical function in community-dwelling elderly Japanese sarcopenic women: A randomized controlled trial. *J. Am. Geriatr. Soc.* **2012**, *60*, 16–23. [CrossRef]
52. Kim, H.; Suzuki, T.; Saito, K.; Yoshida, H.; Kojima, N.; Kim, M.; Sudo, M.; Yamashiro, Y.; Tokimitsu, I. Effects of exercise and tea catechins on muscle mass, strength and walking ability in community-dwelling elderly Japanese sarcopenic women: A randomized controlled trial. *Geriatr. Gerontol. Int.* **2013**, *13*, 458–465. [CrossRef]
53. Kim, H.; Kim, M.; Kojima, N.; Fujino, K.; Hosoi, E.; Kobayashi, H.; Somekawa, S.; Niki, Y.; Yamashiro, Y.; Yoshida, H. Exercise and Nutritional Supplementation on Community-Dwelling Elderly Japanese Women With Sarcopenic Obesity: A Randomized Controlled Trial. *J. Am. Med. Dir. Assoc.* **2016**, *17*, 1011–1019. [CrossRef] [PubMed]
54. Kryger, A.I.; Andersen, J.L. Resistance training in the oldest old: Consequences for muscle strength, fiber types, fiber size, and MHC isoforms. *Scand. J. Med. Sci. Sports* **2007**, *17*, 422–430. [CrossRef] [PubMed]
55. De Liao, C.; Tsauo, J.Y.; Lin, L.F.; Huang, S.W.; Ku, J.W.; Chou, L.C.; Liou, T.H. Effects of elastic resistance exercise on body composition and physical capacity in older women with sarcopenic obesity. *Medicine* **2017**, *96*, e7115. [CrossRef]
56. Martins, W.R.; Safons, M.P.; Bottaro, M.; Blasczyk, J.C.; Diniz, L.R.; Fonseca, R.M.C.; Bonini-Rocha, A.C.; De Oliveira, R.J. Effects of short term elastic resistance training on muscle mass and strength in untrained older adults: A randomized clinical trial. *BMC Geriatr.* **2015**, *15*, 99. [CrossRef]
57. Matsufuji, S.; Shoji, T.; Yano, Y.; Tsujimoto, Y.; Kishimoto, H.; Tabata, T.; Emoto, M.; Inaba, M. Effect of Chair Stand Exercise on Activity of Daily Living: A Randomized Controlled Trial in Hemodialysis Patients. *J. Ren. Nutr.* **2015**, *25*, 17–24. [CrossRef] [PubMed]
58. Mueller, M.; Breil, F.A.; Vogt, M.; Steiner, R.; Klossner, S.; Hoppeler, H.; Däpp, C.; Lippuner, K.; Popp, A. Different response to eccentric and concentric training in older men and women. *Eur. J. Appl. Physiol.* **2009**, *107*, 145–153. [CrossRef]
59. Oesen, S.; Halper, B.; Hofmann, M.; Jandrasits, W.; Franzke, B.; Strasser, E.M.; Graf, A.; Tschan, H.; Bachl, N.; Quittan, M.; et al. Effects of elastic band resistance training and nutritional supplementation on physical performance of institutionalised elderly—A randomized controlled trial. *Exp. Gerontol.* **2015**, *72*, 99–108. [CrossRef]
60. Reid, K.F.; Callahan, D.M.; Carabello, R.J.; Phillips, E.M.; Frontera, W.R.; Fielding, R.A. Lower extremity power training in elderly subjects with mobility limitations: A randomized controlled trial. *Aging Clin. Exp. Res.* **2008**, *20*, 337–343. [CrossRef]
61. Rhodes, E.C.; Martin, A.D.; Taunton, J.E.; Donnelly, M.; Warren, J.; Elliot, J. Effects of one year of resistance training on the relation between muscular strength and bone density in elderly women. *Br. J. Sports Med.* **2000**, *34*, 18–22. [CrossRef]
62. Scanlon, T.C.; Fragala, M.S.; Stout, J.R.; Emerson, N.S.; Beyer, K.S.; Oliveira, L.P.; Hoffman, J.R. Muscle architecture and strength: Adaptations to short-term resistance training in older adults. *Muscle Nerve* **2014**, *49*, 584–592. [CrossRef]
63. Su, Z.; Zhao, J.; Wang, N.; Chen, Y.; Guo, Y.; Tian, Y. Effects of weighted tai chi on leg strength of older adults. *J. Am. Geriatr. Soc.* **2015**, *63*, 2208–2210. [CrossRef] [PubMed]
64. Vasconcelos, K.S.S.; Dias, J.M.D.; Araújo, M.C.; Pinheiro, A.C.; Moreira, B.S.; Dias, R.C. Effects of a progressive resistance exercise program with high-speed component on the physical function of older women with sarcopenic obesity: A randomized controlled trial. *Brazilian J. Phys. Ther.* **2016**, *20*, 432–440. [CrossRef]
65. Yamada, M.; Kimura, Y.; Ishiyama, D.; Nishio, N.; Otobe, Y.; Tanaka, T.; Ohji, S.; Koyama, S.; Sato, A.; Suzuki, M.; et al. Synergistic effect of bodyweight resistance exercise and protein supplementation on

skeletal muscle in sarcopenic or dynapenic older adults. *Geriatr. Gerontol. Int.* **2019**, *19*, 429–437. [CrossRef] [PubMed]

66. Yoon, S.J.; Lee, M.J.; Lee, H.M.; Lee, J.S. Effect of low-intensity resistance training with heat stress on the HSP72, anabolic hormones, muscle size, and strength in elderly women. *Aging Clin. Exp. Res.* **2017**, *29*, 977–984. [CrossRef] [PubMed]
67. Zhu, L.Y.; Chan, R.; Kwok, T.; Cheng, K.C.C.; Ha, A.; Woo, J. Effects of exercise and nutrition supplementation in community-dwelling older Chinese people with sarcopenia: A randomized controlled trial. *Age Ageing* **2019**, *48*, 220–228. [CrossRef] [PubMed]
68. Gualano, B.; Macedo, A.R.; Alves, C.R.R.; Roschel, H.; Benatti, F.B.; Takayama, L.; de Sá Pinto, A.L.; Lima, F.R.; Pereira, R.M.R. Creatine supplementation and resistance training in vulnerable older women: A randomized double-blind placebo-controlled clinical trial. *Exp. Gerontol.* **2014**, *53*, 7–15. [CrossRef]
69. Serra-Rexach, J.A.; Bustamante-Ara, N.; Hierro Villarán, M.; González Gil, P.; Sanz Ibáñez, M.J.; Blanco Sanz, N.; Ortega Santamaría, V.; Gutiérrez Sanz, N.; Marín Prada, A.B.; Gallardo, C.; et al. Short-term, light- to moderate-intensity exercise training improves leg muscle strength in the oldest old: A randomized controlled trial. *J. Am. Geriatr. Soc.* **2011**, *59*, 594–602. [CrossRef]
70. Chen, H.T.; Wu, H.J.; Chen, Y.J.; Ho, S.Y.; Chung, Y.C. Effects of 8-week kettlebell training on body composition, muscle strength, pulmonary function, and chronic low-grade inflammation in elderly women with sarcopenia. *Exp. Gerontol.* **2018**, *112*, 112–118. [CrossRef]
71. Cunha, P.M.; Ribeiro, A.S.; Tomeleri, C.M.; Schoenfeld, B.J.; Silva, A.M.; Souza, M.F.; Nascimento, M.A.; Sardinha, L.B.; Cyrino, E.S. The effects of resistance training volume on osteosarcopenic obesity in older women. *J. Sports Sci.* **2018**, *36*, 1564–1571. [CrossRef]
72. DeBeliso, M.; Harris, C.; Spitzer-Gibson, T.; Adams, K.J. A comparison of periodised and fixed repetition training protocol on strength in older adults. *J. Sci. Med. Sport* **2005**, *8*, 190–199. [CrossRef]
73. Villareal, D.T.; Aguirre, L.; Gurney, A.B.; Waters, D.L.; Sinacore, D.R.; Colombo, E.; Armamento-Villareal, R.; Qualls, C. Aerobic or Resistance Exercise, or Both, in Dieting Obese Older Adults. *N. Engl. J. Med.* **2017**, *376*, 1943–1955. [CrossRef] [PubMed]
74. Dong, Z.J.; Zhang, H.L.; Yin, L.X. Effects of intradialytic resistance exercise on systemic inflammation in maintenance hemodialysis patients with sarcopenia: A randomized controlled trial. *Int. Urol. Nephrol.* **2019**, *51*, 1415–1424. [CrossRef] [PubMed]
75. Fragala, M.S.; Fukuda, D.H.; Stout, J.R.; Townsend, J.R.; Emerson, N.S.; Boone, C.H.; Beyer, K.S.; Oliveira, L.P.; Hoffman, J.R. Muscle quality index improves with resistance exercise training in older adults. *Exp. Gerontol.* **2014**, *53*, 1–6. [CrossRef] [PubMed]
76. Krause, M.; Crognale, D.; Cogan, K.; Contarelli, S.; Egan, B.; Newsholme, P.; De Vito, G. The effects of a combined bodyweight-based and elastic bands resistance training, with or without protein supplementation, on muscle mass, signaling and heat shock response in healthy older people. *Exp. Gerontol.* **2019**, *115*, 104–113. [CrossRef] [PubMed]
77. Lichtenberg, T.; Von Stengel, S.; Sieber, C.; Kemmler, W. The favorable effects of a high-intensity resistance training on sarcopenia in older community-dwelling men with osteosarcopenia: The randomized controlled frost study. *Clin. Interv. Aging* **2019**, *14*, 2173–2186. [CrossRef]
78. Piastra, G.; Perasso, L.; Lucarini, S.; Monacelli, F.; Bisio, A.; Ferrando, V.; Gallamini, M.; Faelli, E.; Ruggeri, P. Effects of Two Types of 9-Month Adapted Physical Activity Program on Muscle Mass, Muscle Strength, and Balance in Moderate Sarcopenic Older Women. *BioMed Res. Int.* **2018**, *2018*, 5095673. [CrossRef]
79. Tsuzuku, S.; Kajioka, T.; Sakakibara, H.; Shimaoka, K. Slow movement resistance training using body weight improves muscle mass in the elderly: A randomized controlled trial. *Scand. J. Med. Sci. Sports* **2018**, *28*, 1339–1344. [CrossRef]
80. Hong, J.; Kim, J.; Kim, S.W.; Kong, H.J. Effects of home-based tele-exercise on sarcopenia among community-dwelling elderly adults: Body composition and functional fitness. *Exp. Gerontol.* **2017**, *87*, 33–39. [CrossRef]
81. Huang, S.W.; Ku, J.W.; Lin, L.F.; Liao, C.D.; Chou, L.C.; Liou, T.H. Body composition influenced by progressive elastic band resistance exercise of sarcopenic obesity elderly women: A pilot randomized controlled trial. *Eur. J. Phys. Rehabil. Med.* **2017**, *53*, 556–563. [CrossRef]
82. Strasser, E.M.; Hofmann, M.; Franzke, B.; Schober-Halper, B.; Oesen, S.; Jandrasits, W.; Graf, A.; Praschak, M.; Horvath-Mechtler, B.; Krammer, C.; et al. Strength training increases skeletal muscle quality but not muscle

mass in old institutionalized adults: A randomized, multi-arm parallel and controlled intervention study. *Eur. J. Phys. Rehabil. Med.* **2018**, *54*, 921–933. [CrossRef] [PubMed]

83. Gómez-Cabello, A.; González-Agüero, A.; Ara, I.; Casajús, J.A.; Vicente-Rodríguez, G. Efectos de una intervención de vibración corporal total sobre la masa magra en personas ancianas. *Nutr. Hosp.* **2013**, *28*, 1255–1258. [CrossRef] [PubMed]
84. Kemmler, W.; Bebenek, M.; Engelke, K.; Von Stengel, S. Impact of whole-body electromyostimulation on body composition in elderly women at risk for sarcopenia: The Training and ElectroStimulation Trial (TEST-III). *Age (Omaha)* **2014**, *36*, 395–406. [CrossRef] [PubMed]
85. Sousa, N.; Mendes, R.; Abrantes, C.; Sampaio, J.; Oliveira, J. Is once-weekly resistance training enough to prevent sarcopenia? *J. Am. Geriatr. Soc.* **2013**, *61*, 1423–1424. [CrossRef]
86. Kemmler, W.; Teschler, M.; Weissenfels, A.; Bebenek, M.; von Stengel, S.; Kohl, M.; Freiberger, E.; Goisser, S.; Jakob, F.; Sieber, C.; et al. Whole-body electromyostimulation to fight sarcopenic obesity in community-dwelling older women at risk. Resultsof the randomized controlled FORMOsA-sarcopenic obesity study. *Osteoporos. Int.* **2016**, *27*, 3261–3270. [CrossRef] [PubMed]
87. Machado, A.; García-López, D.; González-Gallego, J.; Garatachea, N. Whole-body vibration training increases muscle strength and mass in older women: A randomized-controlled trial. *Scand. J. Med. Sci. Sports* **2010**, *20*, 200–207. [CrossRef]
88. Santin-Medeiros, F.; Rey-López, J.P.; Santos-Lozano, A.; Cristi-Montero, C.S.; Vallejo, N.G. Effects of Eight Months of Whole-Body Vibration Training on the Muscle Mass and Functional Capacity of Elderly Women. *J. Strength Cond. Res.* **2015**, *29*, 1863–1869. [CrossRef]
89. Strandberg, E.; Ponsot, E.; Piehl-Aulin, K.; Falk, G.; Kadi, F. Resistance training alone or combined with N-3 PUFA-rich diet in older women: Effects on muscle Fiber hypertrophy. *J. Gerontol. Ser. A* **2019**, *74*, 489–494. [CrossRef]
90. Yu, W.; An, C.; Kang, H. Effects of resistance exercise using Thera-band on balance of elderly adults: A randomized controlled trial. *J. Phys. Ther. Sci.* **2013**, *25*, 1471–1473. [CrossRef]
91. Carraro, U.; Gava, K.; Baba, A.; Marcante, A.; Piccione, F. To contrast and reverse skeletal muscle atrophy by full-body in-bed gym, a mandatory lifestyle for older olds and borderline mobility-impaired persons. In *Advances in Experimental Medicine and Biology*; Springer: New York, NY, USA, 2018; Volume 1088, pp. 549–560.
92. Sajer, S.; Guardiero, G.S.; Scicchitano, B.M. Myokines in home-based functional electrical stimulation-induced recovery of skeletal muscle in elderly and permanent denervation. *Eur. J. Transl. Myol.* **2018**, *28*, 337–345. [CrossRef]
93. Oreská, L'.; Slobodová, L.; Vajda, M.; Kaplánová, A.; Tirpáková, V.; Cvečka, J.; Buzgó, G.; Ukropec, J.; Ukropcová, B.; Sedliak, M. The effectiveness of two different multimodal training modes on physical performance in elderly. *Eur. J. Transl. Myol.* **2020**, *30*, 8920. [CrossRef]
94. Cristi, C.; Collado, P.S.; Márquez, S.; Garatachea, N.; Cuevas, M.J. Whole-body vibration training increases physical fitness measures without alteration of inflammatory markers in older adults. *Eur. J. Sport Sci.* **2014**, *14*, 611–619. [CrossRef] [PubMed]
95. Mazini Filho, M.L.; Aidar, F.J.; Gama De Matos, D.; Costa Moreira, O.; Patrocínio De Oliveira, C.E.; Rezende De Oliveira Venturini, G.; Magalhäes Curty, V.; Menezes Touguinha, H.; Caputo Ferreira, M.E. Circuit strength training improves muscle strength, functional performance and anthropometric indicators in sedentary elderly women. *J. Sports Med. Phys. Fitness* **2018**, *58*, 1029–1036. [CrossRef] [PubMed]
96. Lima, A.B.; de Souza Bezerra, E.; da Rosa Orssatto, L.B.; de Paiva Vieira, E.; Picanço, L.A.A.; dos Santos, J.O.L. Functional resistance training can increase strength, knee torque ratio, and functional performance in elderly women. *J. Exerc. Rehabil.* **2018**, *14*, 654–659. [CrossRef]
97. Bean, J.F.; Kiely, D.K.; Larose, S.; Goldstein, R.; Frontera, W.R.; Leveille, S.G. Are changes in leg power responsible for clinically meaningful improvements in mobility in older adults? *J. Am. Geriatr. Soc.* **2010**, *58*, 2363–2368. [CrossRef] [PubMed]
98. Licurci, M.D.; de Almeida Fagundes, A.; Arisawa, E.A. Acute effects of whole body vibration on heart rate variability in elderly people. *J. Bodyw. Mov. Ther.* **2018**, *22*, 618–621. [CrossRef]
99. Wei, N.; Ng, G.Y.F. The effect of whole body vibration training on quadriceps voluntary activation level of people with age-related muscle loss (sarcopenia): A randomized pilot study. *BMC Geriatr.* **2018**, *18*, 240. [CrossRef]

100. Barberi, L.; Scicchitano, B.M.; Musarò, A. Molecular and cellular mechanisms of muscle aging and sarcopenia and effects of electrical stimulation in seniors. *Eur. J. Transl. Myol.* **2015**, *25*, 231. [CrossRef]
101. Jones, S.; Man, W.D.C.; Gao, W.; Higginson, I.J.; Wilcock, A.; Maddocks, M. Neuromuscular electrical stimulation for muscle weakness in adults with advanced disease. *Cochrane Database Syst. Rev.* **2016**, *2016*, CD009419. [CrossRef]
102. Evangelista, A.; Teixeira, C.; Barros, B.M.; de Azevedo, J.; Paunksnis, M.; Souza, C.; Wadhi, T.; Rica, R.; Braz, T.V.; Bocalini, D. Does Whole-Body Electrical Muscle Stimulation Combined With Strength Training Promote Morphofunctional Alterations? *Clinics* **2019**, *74*, e1334. [CrossRef]
103. Langeard, A.; Bigot, L.; Chastan, N.; Gauthier, A. Does neuromuscular electrical stimulation training of the lower limb have functional effects on the elderly?: A systematic review. *Exp. Gerontol.* **2017**, *91*, 88–98. [CrossRef] [PubMed]
104. Hughes, D.C.; Ellefsen, S.; Baar, K. Adaptations to endurance and strength training. *Cold Spring Harb. Perspect. Med.* **2018**, *8*, a029769. [CrossRef] [PubMed]
105. Stewart, V.H.; Saunders, D.H.; Greig, C.A. Responsiveness of muscle size and strength to physical training in very elderly people: A systematic review. *Scand. J. Med. Sci. Sports* **2014**, *24*, e1–e10. [CrossRef] [PubMed]
106. Schoenfeld, B.J.; Ogborn, D.; Krieger, J.W. Effects of Resistance Training Frequency on Measures of Muscle Hypertrophy: A Systematic Review and Meta-Analysis. *Sports Med.* **2016**, *46*, 1689–1697. [CrossRef]
107. Ralston, G.W.; Kilgore, L.; Wyatt, F.B.; Buchan, D.; Baker, J.S. Weekly Training Frequency Effects on Strength Gain: A Meta-Analysis. *Sports Med. Open* **2018**, *4*, 36. [CrossRef]
108. Grgic, J.; Schoenfeld, B.J.; Davies, T.B.; Lazinica, B.; Krieger, J.W.; Pedisic, Z. Effect of Resistance Training Frequency on Gains in Muscular Strength: A Systematic Review and Meta-Analysis. *Sports Med.* **2018**, *48*, 1207–1220. [CrossRef]
109. Lopes, J.S.S.; Machado, A.F.; Micheletti, J.K.; de Almeida, A.C.; Cavina, A.P.; Pastre, C.M. Effects of training with elastic resistance versus conventional resistance on muscular strength: A systematic review and meta-analysis. *SAGE Open Med.* **2019**, *7*, 205031211983111. [CrossRef]

Impact of Psychological Distress and Sleep Quality on Balance Confidence, Muscle Strength and Functional Balance in Community-Dwelling Middle-Aged and Older People

Raquel Fábrega-Cuadros, Agustín Aibar-Almazán *, Antonio Martínez-Amat and Fidel Hita-Contreras

Department of Health Sciences, Faculty of Health Sciences, University of Jaén, 23071 Jaén, Spain; rfabrega@ujaen.es (R.F.-C.); amamat@ujaen.es (A.M.-A.); fhita@ujaen.es (F.H.-C.)

* Correspondence: aaibar@ujaen.es.

Abstract: The objective was to evaluate the associations of psychological distress and sleep quality with balance confidence, muscle strength, and functional balance among community-dwelling middle-aged and older people. An analytical cross-sectional study was conducted (n = 304). Balance confidence (Activities-specific Balance Confidence scale, ABC), muscle strength (hand grip dynamometer), and functional balance (Timed Up-and-Go test) were assessed. Psychological distress and sleep quality were evaluated by the Hospital Anxiety and Depression Scale and the Pittsburgh Sleep Quality Index, respectively. Age, sex, physical activity level, nutritional status, and fatigue were included as possible confounders. Multivariate linear and logistic regressions were performed. Higher values of anxiety (OR = 1.10), fatigue (OR = 1.04), and older age (OR = 1.08) were associated with an increased risk of falling (ABC < 67%). Greater muscle strength was associated with male sex and improved nutritional status (adjusted R^2 = 0.39). On the other hand, being older and using sleeping medication were linked to poorer functional balance (adjusted R^2 = 0.115). In conclusion, greater anxiety levels and the use of sleep medication were linked to a high risk of falling and poorer functional balance, respectively. No associations were found between muscle strength and sleep quality, anxiety, or depression.

Keywords: fall risk; balance; muscle strength; anxiety; depression; sleep quality

---

1. Introduction

Aging brings with it a series of changes that can affect the mobility and independence of people [1]. These changes affect the mood and attitude towards their environment, and this depends largely on the degree of acceptance of aging since it contributes to the feeling of happiness and satisfaction with life, whose lack can cause feelings of loneliness and sadness [2].

Certain disorders associated with this process, such as anxiety and/or depression, are psychological indicators of a decrease in quality of life [3]. Specifically, the prevalence of depression in the geriatric population worldwide is 7%, and its incidence increases with age [4]. Conversely, the prevalence of anxiety in people over 60 years old ranges between 0.7% and 18.6%, values far below those of younger adults [5].

Sleep quality is a key contributor to good health, and its importance among the older population cannot be overstated, given that sleep disorders and the difficulty to fall asleep become more common with age [6]. It has been shown that although the need to sleep remains the same throughout an individual's life, the ability to get enough sleep does in fact decrease with age. This brings about several adverse health outcomes such as reduced physical function, depression, increased risk of falls, and mortality [7].

Falls represent a major health care problem among older people and are linked to increased morbidity, mortality, and health costs [8]. Around 30% of older people living in the community experience a fall each year [9]. Fall risk factors have been studied in detail and include demographic, environmental, and health-related factors [10]. Balance confidence is one of the most important psychological factors linked to falls and the deterioration of balance, and its decrease can lead to diminished independence and participation in activities of daily living, thus creating a vicious circle that affects the quality of life and creates more isolated and dependent people [11]. On the other hand, the impaired functional balance has been shown to be one of the most important predictors of falls [12].

Muscle strength also declines with age more sharply than muscle mass [13]. It has been reported that muscle loss in older women decreases 3.7% per decade, however, strength decreases 15% per decade until age 70 when the loss accelerates considerably [14]. Moreover, in 2018 the European Working Group on Sarcopenia (EWGSOP2) listed low strength as a primary indicator of probable sarcopenia [15]. A decrease in muscle strength contributes to an elevated prevalence of falls and the loss of functional capacity and is a major cause of disability, mortality, and other adverse health outcomes [16].

Not many studies have examined the impact of psychological distress and sleep quality on balance confidence and function, and muscle strength in older people, which, in many cases, have shown inconclusive results and have focused on sleep duration or insomnia. Based on all of the above, the objective of this study was to evaluate the associations of psychological distress and sleep quality with the risk of falling according to balance confidence, functional balance, and muscle strength among community-dwelling middle-aged and older individuals.

2. Experimental Section

2.1. Study Design and Participants

An analytical cross-sectional study was conducted, to which end 315 community-dwelling middle-aged and older people were initially contacted and 304 finally took part. Recruitment was performed by contacting several senior centers from the Eastern Andalusia region. Prior to the beginning of the study, all participants provided their written informed consent. The research was approved by the Research Ethics Committee of the University of Jaén, Spain (NOV.18/2.TES), and was conducted in accordance with the Declaration of Helsinki, good clinical practices, and all applicable laws and regulations.

Community-dwelling ambulatory adults aged 50 years and older, able to understand and complete the required questionnaires and willing to give written informed consent to participate in the study were included in the protocol. Exclusion criteria were: conditions that limit physical activity, chronic and/or severe medical disease or any neuropsychiatric disorder that could influence their responses to the questionnaires.

2.2. Study Parameters

2.2.1. Balance Confidence

The Activities-specific Balance Confidence scale (ABC) was used to assess balance confidence in the performance of activities of daily living [17]. This is a 16-item questionnaire that quantifies the level of confidence in performing a specific task without losing balance or becoming unsteady [18]. Each item score ranges from 0–100%, and the total score is obtained by summing the ratings (0–1600) and then dividing by 16. A higher percentage indicates a greater level of balance confidence. A score of <67% has been identified as a reliable means of predicting a future fall [19]. This cut-off was used to identify which participants were at high risk of falling.

2.2.2. Muscle Strength

Muscle strength was assessed with an analog dynamometer (TKK 5001, Grip-A, Takei, Tokyo, Japan). Participants were required to apply their maximum handgrip strength three times with the dominant hand, each separated by 30 s. The maximal measured effort was regarded as their handgrip strength [20].

2.2.3. Functional Balance

The Timed Up-and-Go (TUG) test [21] is a simple and valid method for predicting changes in functional balance in older adults [22]. It is a sensitive and specific measure for identifying community-dwelling adults who are at risk of falls [23]. In the TUG test, individuals rise from a seated position on a chair, walk three meters, turn around, return, and sit down again. The time required to complete this task was recorded.

2.2.4. Sleep Quality

Sleep quality was assessed using the Pittsburgh Sleep Quality Index (PSQI) [24,25]. It comprises 19 self-rated questions and 5 more (only used for clinical purposes) to be completed by bedmates or roommates. The 19 items (ranged from 0–3) generate a total score and seven different domains or subscales (subjective sleep quality, sleep latency, sleep duration, habitual sleep efficiency, sleep disturbance, use of sleeping medication, and daytime dysfunction). Higher scores indicate poorer subjective sleep quality.

2.2.5. Psychological Distress

The Hospital Anxiety and Depression Scale (HADS) is a self-administered questionnaire widely used to assess psychological distress in the general population [26,27]. This questionnaire contains 14 items, 7 related to anxiety symptoms, and 7 to depressive symptoms. Each item ranges from 0–3, and the total scores for both anxiety and depression range from 0 to 21, with higher scores indicating more severe symptoms.

2.2.6. Fatigue Severity

In order to assess fatigue severity during the last 7 days, the Fatigue Severity Scale was used [28]. This questionnaire consists of 9 items (rated from 1–7) and produces a total score where larger values imply greater fatigue.

2.2.7. Nutritional Status

The Mini Nutritional Assessment survey (MNA) was used to evaluate nutritional status [29,30]. It has 18 questions that include anthropometric measures, health status, dietary patterns, and subjective assessments of nutritional and health status. Higher scores indicate better nutritional status.

2.2.8. Physical Activity Level

Physical activity level was assessed with the International Physical Activity Questionnaire-Short Form (IPAQ-SF) [31]. It consists of seven items that measure physical activity within three intensity levels (walking, moderate, and vigorous) during an average week. Physical activity was evaluated by combining the activity score of both moderate and vigorous-intensity activity (min/day) for each work and recreational activity domain. Responses were converted to Metabolic Equivalent Task minutes per week (MET-min / week) according to the scoring protocol.

2.3. Sample Size Calculation

For sample size calculation, at least 20 subjects per variable are required in the linear regression model [32], while a minimum of 10 subjects per variable was needed in the logistic regression model [33].

Since 15 possible predicting variables were considered (7 domains plus the total score of the PSQI, anxiety, depression, as well as physical activity level, nutritional status, fatigue, sex, and age as possible confounders), over 300 subjects were required for the purposes of our analysis. The final number of participants was 304.

2.4. Statistical Analysis

Continuous variables were described using means and standard deviations, and for categorical variables frequencies and percentages were used. The Kolmogorov–Smirnov test was performed to evaluate the normal distribution of the data. To analyze the differences between participants with and without risk of falling (ABC), Student's t test (continuous independent variables), and the Chi-squared test (sex) were used. In order to analyze the independent associations, a multivariate logistic regression was performed. Those variables with significant individual associations ($p < 0.05$) were selected for the stepwise logistic regression model. The odds ratio (OR) can be considered as significant when the 95% confidence interval (CI) does not include 1.00. The Chi-squared and Hosmer–Lemeshow tests were conducted to assess the overall goodness-of-fit for each of the steps of the model, as well as for the final model. To explore the possible individual associations of muscle strength and functional balance with PSQI, HADS, FSS, MNA, and IPAQ-SF scores, as well as with age (independent variables), Pearson's correlation was used. As for the analysis of the independent associations, the same procedure was applied, but using a stepwise multivariate linear regression. Functional balance and muscle strength were individually introduced as dependent variables in separate models. We first looked into the bivariate correlation coefficients, and any independent variables with significant associations ($p < 0.05$) were included in the multivariate linear regression. Adjusted R^2 was used to calculate the effect size coefficient of multiple determination in the linear models. R^2 can be considered insignificant when <0.02, small if between 0.02 and 0.15, medium if between 0.15 and 0.35, and large if >0.35 [34]. A 95% confidence level was used ($p < 0.05$). Data management and analysis were performed using the SPSS statistical package for the social sciences for Windows (SPSS Inc., Chicago, IL, USA).

3. Results

A total of 304 participants (72.04 ± 7.88 years) took part in this study. When studying the ABC score (23.42 ± 7.25), 24.01% of participants were at risk of falling. The analysis revealed (Table 1) that participants with an ABC score < 67 were individually associated with the largest values of anxiety ($p = 0.002$), depression ($p = 0.001$), fatigue ($p = < 0.001$), increased age ($p < 0.001$), and worse nutritional status ($p = 0.002$).

Table 1. Individual differences according to the risk of falling.

		All Participants (*n* = 304)		**Risk of Falling (ABC)**				
				No (*n* = 231)		**Yes (*n* = 73)**		***p*-Value**
		Mean	SD	Mean	SD	Mean	SD	
PSQI	Sleep quality	1.01	0.82	1.00	0.80	1.04	0.87	0.738
	Sleep latency	1.18	1.09	1.16	1.08	1.26	1.11	0.475
	Sleep duration	1.00	0.97	1.00	0.98	1.01	0.94	0.890
	Sleep efficiency	0.95	1.10	0.97	1.11	0.90	1.08	0.658
	Sleep disturbances	1.23	0.58	1.22	0.57	1.27	0.61	0.461
	Use of sleeping medication	1.01	1.34	1.02	1.34	0.97	1.34	0.804
	Daytime dysfunction	0.49	0.63	0.46	0.61	0.59	0.68	0.130
	Total score	6.87	4.70	6.82	4.58	7.04	5.11	0.725

Table 1. *Cont.*

		All Participants (n = 304)		Risk of Falling (ABC)				
				No (n = 231)		Yes (n = 73)		p-Value
Anxiety		5.74	4.02	5.34	4.07	7.01	3.58	0.002
Depression		4.99	3.44	4.62	3.38	6.14	3.39	0.001
Physical activity level, MET-min/week		1367.96	2213.43	1310.16	1817.89	1549.29	3157.97	0.422
Nutritional status		26.31	2.08	26.52	1.99	25.64	2.22	0.002
Fatigue		21.33	15.25	18.87	13.96	29.14	16.58	<0.001
Age, years		72.04	7.88	70.99	7.27	75.38	8.82	<0.001
		n	%	n	%	n	%	
Sex	Male	255	83.88	37	16.02	12	16.44	0.932
	Female	49	16.12	194	83.98	61	83.56	

ABC: Activities-Specific Balance Confidence Scale. MET: Metabolic Equivalent of Task. PSQI: Pittsburgh Sleep Quality Index. SD: Standard Deviation.

The multivariate logistic regression that looked into the risk of falls as assessed with the ABC score revealed several significant results. Higher values of anxiety (OR = 1.10, 95% CI = 1.02–1.18), fatigue (OR = 1.04, 95% CI = 1.02–1.06), and older age (OR = 1.08, 95% CI = 1.04–1.12) were independently associated with ABC scores < 67%. The Hosmer–Lemeshow test showed a good fit of the model (Chi-squared = 2.403, p = 0.966), which was able to classify correctly 78.29% of all participants at high risk of suffering a future fall, according to the ABC score (Table 2).

Table 2. Multivariate logistic regression analyses for factors associated with the risk of falling (determined through the ABC score).

		OR	95% CI	p-Value
Risk of falling (ABC)	Anxiety	1.10	1.02–1.18	0.012
	Fatigue	1.04	1.02–1.06	0.000
	Age	1.08	1.04–1.12	0.000

ABC: Activities-Specific Balance Confidence Scale. CI: Confidence Interval. OR: Odds Ratio.

As for functional balance (9.86 ± 2.91 s) and muscle strength (19.43 ± 6.42 kg), the individual associations are shown in Table 3. Muscle strength was only associated with anxiety (p = 0.001), fatigue (p = 0.020), and nutritional status (p = 0.038), whereas poor functional balance was related to greater age (p < 0.001) and physical activity level (p = 0.035), as well as with the use-of-sleeping-medication domain in PSQI (p = 0.028). Regarding sex differences, men displayed greater muscle strength (both p < 0.001), but worse functional balance (p = 0.005).

Table 3. Pearson's correlations of functional balance and muscle strength, with PSQI scores and possible confounders.

		Muscle Strength		Functional Balance	
		r	p-Value	r	p-Value
PSQI	Sleep quality	0.06	0.264	0.03	0.654
	Sleep latency	0.07	0.231	0.00	0.950
	Sleep duration	0.05	0.427	0.02	0.790
	Sleep efficiency	−0.00	0.963	−0.02	0.747
	Sleep disturbances	0.01	0.808	−0.02	0.665
	Use of sleeping medication	0.03	0.602	0.13	0.028
	Daytime dysfunction	0.01	0.854	0.04	0.474
	Total score	0.05	0.416	0.04	0.464

Table 3. *Cont.*

	Muscle Strength		Functional Balance	
	r	*p*-Value	r	*p*-Value
Anxiety	−0.18	0.001	0.05	0.355
Depression	−0.08	0.191	0.08	0.174
Nutritional status	−0.12	0.038	−0.05	0.401
Fatigue	−0.14	0.017	0.06	0.281
Age, years	−0.104	0.070	0.33	0.000
Physical activity level (MET-min / week)	0.103	0.075	−0.12	0.035

MET: Metabolic Equivalent of Task. PSQI: Pittsburgh Sleep Quality Index. r: Pearson's Correlation Coefficient.

Lastly, the linear regression analysis (Table 4) revealed that greater muscle strength was independently associated with the male sex ($p < 0.001$) and a better nutritional status ($p = 0.001$), and the effect size was large (adjusted $R^2 = 0.392$). On the other hand, being older ($p < 0.001$) and the use of sleeping medication ($p = 0.033$) were linked to poorer functional balance, although the effect size was small (adjusted $R^2 = 0.115$).

Table 4. Multivariate linear regression analyses for functional balance and muscle strength.

		B	β	95% CI		*p*-Value
Muscle strength	Sex	−10.74	−0.62	−12.28	−9.21	<0.001
	Nutritional status	0.44	0.14	00.17	0.71	0.002
Functional balance	Age	0.12	0.34	−0.09	−0.16	<0.001
	Use of sleeping medication	0.27	0.12	0.04	0.50	0.023

B: Unstandardized Coefficient. β: Standardized Coefficient. CI: Confidence Interval. MET: Metabolic Equivalent of Task. PSQI: Pittsburgh Sleep Quality Index.

4. Discussion

The objective of this study was to evaluate the associations of psychological distress and sleep quality with balance confidence, functional balance, and muscle strength among community-dwelling middle-aged and older individuals. In our study, anxiety, fatigue, older age, and the use of sleeping medication were shown to be associated with the risk of falling and poorer functional balance. Muscle strength was associated with being male and nutritional status.

In general, balance confidence scores are able to predict perceived physical function and even mobility in older adults [35]. Similar to our own study, a previously published paper also employed regression models to find a significant association of anxiety with confidence in balance, while depression was shown to be associated with avoidance of activity [36]. A systematic review with meta-analysis found an association between balance confidence and anxiety [37], and a similar link was established between depression and level of physical activity [38]. Regarding the association of age with balance confidence, Medley et al. [39] reported that participants with low balance confidence were older than those who reported high balance confidence. In our study, only anxiety, age, and fatigue were independently associated with the balance confidence. To our knowledge, this is the first study to observe an association between confidence in balance and fatigue in healthy middle-aged and older people, although there are studies that demonstrate this association, but in people with some pathology [40,41].

Muscle strength plays an important role in the execution of many activities of daily living and is considered an indicator of functional decline among community-dwelling older adults [42]. Low grip strength is predictive of poor outcomes and indicative of prolonged hospital stays, increased functional limitations, poor quality of life, and death [43]. For example, it has been shown that people who have a high level of grip strength have a significantly lower fear of falling than those who show lower levels [44,45]. In addition, it has been observed that the strength of the abductor muscles can identify older adults at risk of falling [46]. A recent study looking into the association between falls and lower-limb strength failed to find any link at a one-year follow-up [47]. Our study found no associations whatsoever between muscle strength and sleep quality, and increased muscle strength was independently associated only with being male (as in previous studies by Buchman et al. [48]) and with improved nutritional status. Other authors have agreed before that a poor diet is significantly associated with lower muscle strength, but they also linked it to lower physical function, longer TUG test time, depression, and risk of falling [49], although the results of the present study should be interpreted with caution since they are correlations and a cause-effect relationship cannot be established. Some recent studies even recommend the intake of supplementary proteins given their significant effect in increasing muscle mass and strength among elderly people with sarcopenia [50]. We must consider, however, that disparities in the literature may be due to a variety of population ages, measurement methods, and educational and cultural levels, which may have a confounding effect.

Balance confidence contributes to functional mobility performance [39], and there seems to be a strong link between balance self-efficacy and function capabilities [51]. A study by Brandão et al. [52] identified an association between excessive daytime sleepiness and quality of life, and also characterized the profile of older adults with poor sleep quality. Sleep duration is associated with inflammation markers (serum interleukin-6, tumor necrosis factor α, and C-reactive protein) in older adults, and in turn with mortality [53]. Loss of functional balance, as measured by the TUG test, is known to be one of the first signs of aging and is considered a marker for general health that is strongly associated with the risk of mortality [54]. In our results, and as far as individual associations are concerned, higher age, poorer sleep quality (use of sleep medication), and decreased levels of physical activity were linked to lower TUG scores. However, in the multivariate analysis model, such associations only held for the first two variables (age and poor sleep quality). The results of a study conducted among women indicate that a shorter sleep duration increased wakefulness after sleep onset, and decreased sleep efficiency are risk factors for functional or physical impairment in older women [55].

There are some limitations to our study that must be acknowledged. Firstly, its cross-sectional design did not allow for the evaluation of causal relationships. Secondly, sleep quality was assessed using self-report methods, and therefore the influence of recall bias must be considered. Thirdly, our study was conducted among people from a specific geographic area, and any generalization of its results should be limited to individuals with characteristics similar to those of our population sample. Future studies should consider exploring prospective designs, employing objective sleep quality assessment methods (polysomnography or actigraphy), and applying them to a general population of older adults.

5. Conclusions

Among middle-aged and older Spanish people, greater levels of anxiety and fatigue, as well as older age were associated with an increased risk of falling (assessed with the Activities-specific Balance Confidence scale). No associations were found with sleep quality and depression. Greater muscle strength was associated with being male and having a better nutritional status. Finally, increased age and the use of sleeping medication were linked to poorer functional balance.

Author Contributions: Conceptualization: R.F.-C. and F.H.-C.; methodology: R.F.-C. and A.A.-A.; formal analysis: F.H.-C. and R.F.-C.; supervision: A.M.-A. and A.A.-A.; writing—original draft preparation: R.F.-C. and F.H.-C.; writing—review and editing: A.M.-A. and A.A.-A.; funding acquisition: A.M.-A. and F.H.-C. All authors have read and agreed to the published version of the manuscript.

References

1. Sulbrandt, C.J.; Pino, Z.P.; Oyarzún, G.M. Active and healthy aging. Research and policies for population aging. *Rev. Chil. Enferm. Respir.* **2012**, *28*, 269–271.
2. Dziechciaż, M.; Filip, R. Biological psychological and social determinants of old age: Bio-psycho-social

aspects of human aging. *Ann. Agric. Environ. Med.* **2014**, *21*, 835–838. [CrossRef] [PubMed]
3. Alvarado, A.M.; Salazar, A.M. Aging concept analysis. *Gerokomos* **2014**, *25*, 57–62.
4. Wen, Y.; Liu, C.; Liao, J.; Yin, Y.; Wu, D. Incidence and risk factors of depressive symptoms in 4 years of follow-up among mid-aged and elderly community-dwelling Chinese adults: Findings from the China Health and Retirement Longitudinal Study. *BMJ Open* **2019**, *9*, e029529. [CrossRef] [PubMed]
5. Hohls, J.K.; Köning, H.H.; Raynik, Y.I.; Hajek, A. A systematic review of the association of anxiety with health care utilization and costs in people aged 65 years and older. *J. Affec. Disord.* **2018**, *232*, 163–176. [CrossRef]
6. Cybulski, M.; Cybulski, L.; Krajewska-Kulak, E.; Orzechowska, M.; Cwalina, U.; Kowalczuk, K. Sleep disorders among educationally active elderly people in Bialystok, Poland: A cross-sectional study. *BMC Geriatr.* **2019**, *19*, 225. [CrossRef] [PubMed]
7. Neikrug, A.B.; Ancoli-Israel, S. Sleep disorders in the older adult—A mini-review. *Gerontology* **2010**, *56*, 181–189. [CrossRef]
8. Tinetti, M.E. Clinical practice. Preventing falls in elderly persons. *N. Engl. J. Med.* **2003**, *348*, 42–49. [CrossRef]
9. Sun, D.Q.; Huang, J.; Varadhan, R.; Agrawal, Y. Race and fall risk: Data from the National Health and Aging Trends Study (NHATS). *Age Ageing* **2016**, *45*, 120–127. [CrossRef]
10. Deandrea, S.; Lucenteforte, E.; Bravi, F.; Foschi, R.; La Vecchia, C.; Negri, E. Risk Factors for Falls in Community-Dwelling Older People: A Systematic Review and Meta-Analysis. *Epidemiology* **2010**, *21*, 658–668. [CrossRef]
11. Scheffer, A.C.; Schuurmans, M.J.; Van Dijk, N.; Van der Hooft, T.; De Rooij, S.E. Fear of falling: Measurement strategy, prevalence, risk factors and consequences among older persons. *Age Ageing* **2008**, *37*, 19–24. [CrossRef] [PubMed]
12. Jácome, C.; Cruz, J.; Gabriel, R.; Figueiredo, D.; Marques, A. Functional Balance in Older Adults with Chronic Obstructive Pulmonary Disease. *J. Aging Phys. Act.* **2014**, *22*, 357–363. [CrossRef]
13. Cruz-Jentoft, A.J.; Bahat, G.; Bauer, J.; Boirie, Y.; Bruyère, O.; Cederholm, T.; Cooper, C.; Landi, F.; Rolland, Y.; Sayer, A.A.; et al. Sarcopenia: Revised European consensus on definition and diagnosis. *Age Ageing* **2019**, *48*, 16–31. [CrossRef]
14. Siparsky, P.N.; Kirkendall, D.T.; Garrett, W.E., Jr. Muscle changes in aging: Understanding sarcopenia. *Sports Health* **2014**, *6*, 36–40. [CrossRef] [PubMed]
15. Mitchell, W.K.; Williams, J.; Atherton, P.; Larvin, M.; Lund, J.; Narici, M. Sarcopenia, dynapenia, and the impact of advancing age on human skeletal muscle size and strength; a quantitative review. *Front. Physiol.* **2012**, *3*, 260. [CrossRef] [PubMed]
16. Dhillon, R.J.; Hasni, S. Pathogenesis and Management of Sarcopenia. *Clin. Geriatr. Med.* **2017**, *33*, 17–26. [CrossRef] [PubMed]
17. Powell, L.E.; Myers, A.M. The Activities-specific Balance Confidence (ABC) Scale. *J. Gerontol. A Biol. Sci. Med. Sci.* **1995**, *50A*, M28–M34. [CrossRef]
18. Montilla-Ibáñez, A.; Martínez-Amat, A.; Lomas-Vega, R.; Cruz-Díaz, D.; Torre-Cruz, M.J.; Casuso-Pérez, R.; Hita-Contreras, F. The Activities-specific Balance Confidence scale: Reliability and validity in Spanish patients with vestibular disorders. *Disabil. Rehabil.* **2017**, *39*, 697–703. [CrossRef]
19. Lajoie, Y.; Gallagher, S.P. Predicting falls within the elderly community: Comparison of postural sway, reaction time, the Berg balance scale and the Activities-specific Balance Confidence (ABC) scale for comparing fallers and non-fallers. *Arch. Gerontol. Geriatr.* **2004**, *38*, 11–26. [CrossRef]
20. Beaudart, C.; Rolland, Y.; Cruz-Jentoft, A.J.; Bauer, J.M.; Sieber, C.; Cooper, C.; Al-Daghri, N.; Araujo de Carvalho, I.; Bautmans, I.; Bernabei, R.; et al. Assessment of Muscle Function and Physical Performance in Daily Clinical Practice: A position paper endorsed by the European Society for Clinical and Economic Aspects of Osteoporosis, Osteoarthritis and Musculoskeletal Diseases (ESCEO). *Calcif. Tissue Int.* **2019**, *105*, 1–14. [CrossRef]
21. Podsiadlo, D.; Richardson, S. The timed "Up & Go": A test of basic functional mobility for frail elderly persons. *J. Am. Geriatr. Soc.* **1991**, *39*, 142–148. [PubMed]
22. Benavent-Caballer, V.; Sendín-Magdalena, A.; Lisón, J.F.; Rosado-Calatayud, P.; Amer-Cuenca, J.J.; Salvador-Coloma, P.; Segura-Ortí, E. Physical factors underlying the Timed "Up and Go" test in older adults. *Geriatr. Nurs.* **2016**, *37*, 122–127. [CrossRef] [PubMed]
23. Shumway-Cook, A.; Brauer, S.; Woollacott, M. Predicting the probability for falls in community-dwelling older adults using the Timed Up & Go Test. *Phys. Ther.* **2000**, *80*, 896–903. [PubMed]

24. Buysse, D.J.; Reynolds, C.F., 3rd; Monk, T.H.; Berman, S.R.; Kupfer, D.J. The Pittsburgh Sleep Quality Index: A new instrument for psychiatric practice and research. *Psychiatry Res.* **1989**, *28*, 193–213. [CrossRef]
25. Hita-Contreras, F.; Martínez-López, E.; Latorre-Román, P.A.; Garrido, F.; Santos, M.A.; Martínez-Amat, A. Reliability and validity of the Spanish version of the Pittsburgh Sleep Quality Index (PSQI) in patients with fibromyalgia. *Rheumatol. Int.* **2014**, *34*, 929–936. [CrossRef]
26. Zigmond, A.S.; Snaith, P.R. The hospital anxiety and depression scale. *Acta Psychiatr. Scand.* **1983**, *67*, 361–370. [CrossRef]
27. Herrero, M.J.; Blanch, J.; Peri, J.M.; De Pablo, J.; Pintor, L.; Bulbena, A. A validation study of the hospital anxiety and depression scale (HADS) in a Spanish population. *Gen. Hosp. Psychiatry* **2003**, *25*, 277–283. [CrossRef]
28. Krupp, L.B.; LaRocca, N.G.; Muir-Nash, J.; Steinberg, A.D. The fatigue severity scale. Application to patients with multiple sclerosis and systemic lupus erythematosus. *Arch. Neurol.* **1989**, *46*, 1121–1123. [CrossRef] [PubMed]
29. Vellas, B.; Guigoz, Y.; Garry, P.J.; Nourhashemi, F.; Bennahum, D.; Lauque, S.; Albarede, J.L. The Mini Nutritional Assessment (MNA) and its use in grading the nutritional state of elderly patients. *Nutrition* **1999**, *15*, 116–122. [CrossRef]
30. Muñoz Díaz, B.; Molina-Recio, G.; Romero-Saldaña, M.; Redondo Sánchez, J.; Aguado Taberné, C.; Arias Blanco, C.; Molina-Luque, R.; Martínez De La Iglesia, J. Validation (in Spanish) of the Mini Nutritional Assessment survey to assess the nutritional status of patients over 65 years of age. *Fam. Pract.* **2019**, *36*, 172–178. [CrossRef]
31. Craig, C.L.; Marshall, A.L.; Sjöström, M.; Bauman, A.E.; Booth, M.L.; Ainsworth, B.E.; Pratt, M.; Ekelund, U.; Yngve, A.; Sallis, J.F.; et al. International physical activity questionnaire: 12-country reliability and validity. *Med. Sci. Sports Exerc.* **2003**, *35*, 1381–1395. [CrossRef]
32. Concato, J.; Peduzzi, P.; Holford, T.R.; Feinstein, A.R. Importance of events per independent variable in proportional hazards analysis. I. Background, goals, and general strategy. *J. Clin. Epidemiol.* **1995**, *48*, 1495–1501. [CrossRef]
33. Ortega Calvo, M.; Cayuela Domínguez, A. Unconditioned logistic regression and sample size: A bibliographic review. *Rev. Esp. Salud Publica* **2002**, *76*, 85–93. [CrossRef] [PubMed]
34. Cohen, J. A power primer. *Psychol. Bull.* **1992**, *112*, 155–159. [CrossRef] [PubMed]
35. Torkia, C.; Best, K.L.; Miller, W.C.; Eng, J.J. Balance Confidence: A Predictor of Perceived Physical Function, Perceived Mobility, and Perceived Recovery 1 Year After Inpatient Stroke Rehabilitation. *Arch. Phys. Med. Rehabil.* **2016**, *97*, 1064–1071. [CrossRef] [PubMed]
36. Hull, S.L.; Kneebone, I.I.; Farquharson, L. Anxiety, Depression, and Fall-Related Psychological Concerns in Community-Dwelling Older People. *Am. J. Geriatr. Psychiatry* **2013**, *21*, 1287–1291. [CrossRef] [PubMed]
37. Payette, M.C.; Bélanger, C.; Léveille, V.; Grenier, S. Fall-Related Psychological Concerns and Anxiety among Community-Dwelling Older Adults: Systematic Review and Meta-Analysis. *PLoS ONE* **2016**, *11*, e0152848. [CrossRef]
38. Hughes, C.C.; Kneebone, I.I.; Jones, F.; Brady, B.A. Theoretical and Empirical Review of Psychological Factors Associated with Falls-Related Psychological Concerns in Community-Dwelling Older People. *Int. Psychogeriatr.* **2015**, *27*, 1071–1087. [CrossRef]
39. Medley, A.; Thompson, M. Contribution of age and balance confidence to functional mobility test performance: Diagnostic accuracy of L test and normal-paced timed up and go. *J. Geriatr. Phys. Ther.* **2015**, *38*, 8–16. [CrossRef]
40. Miller, K.K.; Combs, S.A.; Puymbroeck, M.V.; Altenburger, P.A.; Kean, J.; Dierks, T.A.; Schmid, A.A. Fatigue and Pain: Relationships with Physical Performance and Patient Beliefs after Stroke. *Top. Stroke Rehabil.* **2013**, *20*, 347–355. [CrossRef]
41. Abasiyanik, Z.; Özdoğar, A.T.; Sağıcı, Ö.; Baba, C.; Ertekin, Ö.; Özakbaş, S. Explanatory factors of balance confidence in persons with multiple sclerosis: Beyond the physical functions. *Mult. Scler. Relat. Disord.* **2020**, *43*, 102239. [CrossRef] [PubMed]
42. Hicks, G.E.; Shardell, M.; Alley, D.E.; Miller, R.R.; Bandinelli, S.; Guralnik, J.; Lauretani, F.; Simonsick, E.M.; Ferruci, L. Absolute strength and loss of strength as predictors of mobility decline in older adults: The InCHIANTI study. *J. Gerontol. A Biol. Sci. Med. Sci.* **2012**, *67*, 66–73. [CrossRef] [PubMed]
43. Ibrahim, K.; May, C.; Patel, H.P.; Baxter, M.; Sayer, A.A.; Roberts, H. A feasibility study of implementing grip

strength measurement into routine hospital practice (GRImP): Study protocol. *Pilot Feasibility Stud.* **2016**, *2*, 27. [CrossRef] [PubMed]

44. Kim, Y.S.; Lee, O.; Lee, J.H.; Kim, J.H.; Choi, B.Y.; Kim, M.J.; Kim, T.G. The Association between Levels of Muscle Strength and Fear of Falling in Korean Olders. *Korean J. Sports Med.* **2013**, *31*, 13–19. [CrossRef]
45. Silveira, T.; Pegorari, M.; Castro, S.; Ruas, G.; Novais-Shimano, S.; Patrizzi, L. Association of falls, fear of falling, handgrip strength and gait speed with frailty levels in the community elderly. *Medicina (Ribeirao Preto)* **2015**, *48*, 549–556. [CrossRef]
46. Gafner, S.C.; Germaine Bastiaenen, C.H.; Ferrari, S.; Gold, G.; Trombetti, A.; Terrier, P.; Hikfiker, R.; Allet, L. The Role of Hip Abductor Strength in Identifying Older Persons at Risk of Falls: A Diagnostic Accuracy Study. *Clin. Interv. Aging* **2020**, *15*, 645–654. [CrossRef]
47. Mello, J.P.; Cangussu-Oliveira, L.M.; Campos, R.C.; Tavares, F.V.; Capato, L.L.; García, B.M.; Carvalho de Abreu, D.C. Relationship Between Lower Limb Muscle Strength and Future Falls Among Community-Dwelling Older Adults with No History of Falls: A Prospective 1-Year Study. *J. Appl. Gerontol.* **2020**. online ahead of print. [CrossRef]
48. Buchmann, N.; Spira, D.; Norman, K.; Demuth, I.; Eckardt, R.; Steinhagen-Thiessen, E. Sleep, Muscle Mass and Muscle Function in Older People. *Dtsch. Arztebl. Int.* **2016**, *113*, 253–260.
49. Van Rijssen, N.M.; Rojer, A.G.M.; Trappenburg, M.C.; Reijnierse, E.M.; Meskers, C.G.M.; Maier, A.B.; van der Schueren, M.A.E. Is being malnourished according to the ESPEN definition for malnutrition associated with clinically relevant outcome measures in geriatric outpatients? *Eur. Geriatr. Med.* **2018**, *9*, 389–394. [CrossRef]
50. Gielen, E.; Beckwée, D.; Delaere, A.; De Breucker, S.; Vandewoude, M.; Bautmans, I. Sarcopenia Guidelines Development Group of the Belgian Society of Gerontology and Geriatrics (BSGG). Nutritional interventions to improve muscle mass, muscle strength, and physical performance in older people: An umbrella review of systematic reviews and meta-analyses. *Nutr. Rev.* **2020**, nuaa011. [CrossRef]
51. Kafri, M.; Hutzler, Y.; Korsensky, O.; Laufer, Y. Functional Performance and Balance in the Oldest-Old. *J. Geriatr. Phys. Ther.* **2019**, *42*, 183–188. [CrossRef] [PubMed]
52. Brandão, G.S.; Camelier, F.W.R.; Callou Sampaio, A.A.; Brandão, G.A.; Silva, A.S.; Freitas Gomes, G.S.B.; Donner, C.F.; Franco Oliveira, L.V.; Camelier, A.A. Association of sleep quality with excessive daytime somnolence and quality of life of elderlies of community. *Multidiscip. Respir. Med.* **2018**, *13*, 8. [CrossRef] [PubMed]
53. Hall, M.H.; Smagula, S.F.; Boudreau, R.M.; Ayonayon, H.N.; Goldman, S.E.; Harris, T.B.; Naydeck, B.L.; Rubin, S.M.; Samuelsson, L.; Satterfield, S.; et al. Association between Sleep Duration and Mortality Is Mediated by Markers of Inflammation and Health in Older Adults: The Health, Aging and Body Composition Study. *Sleep* **2015**, *38*, 189–195. [CrossRef] [PubMed]
54. Dommershuijsen, L.J.; Isik, B.M.; Darweesh, S.K.L.; van der Geest, J.N.; Ikram, M.K.; Ikram, M.A. Unravelling the association between gait and mortality—One step at a time. *J. Gerontol. A Biol. Sci. Med. Sci.* **2020**, *75*, 1184–1190. [CrossRef] [PubMed]
55. Spira, A.P.; Covinsky, K.; Rebok, G.W.; Punjabi, N.M.; Stone, K.L.; Hillier, T.A.; Ensrud, K.E.; Yaffe, K. Poor sleep quality and functional decline in older women. *J. Am. Geriatr. Soc.* **2012**, *60*, 1092–1098. [CrossRef]

12

Respiratory Muscle Strengths and their Association with Lean Mass and Handgrip Strengths in Older Institutionalized Individuals

Francisco Miguel Martínez-Arnau [1,2], Cristina Buigues [2,3], Rosa Fonfría-Vivas [2,3] and Omar Cauli [2,3,*]

1 Department of Physiotherapy, University of Valencia, 46010 Valencia, Spain; Francisco.m.martinez@uv.es
2 Frailty and Cognitive Impairment Research Group (FROG), University of Valencia, 46010 Valencia, Spain; cristina.buigues@uv.es (C.B.); rosa.fonfria@uv.es (R.F.-V.)
3 Department of Nursing, University of Valencia, 46010 Valencia, Spain
* Correspondence: Omar.Cauli@uv.es

Abstract: The study of reduced respiratory muscle strengths in relation to the loss of muscular function associated with ageing is of great interest in the study of sarcopenia in older institutionalized individuals. The present study assesses the association between respiratory muscle parameters and skeletal mass content and strength, and analyzes associations with blood cell counts and biochemical parameters related to protein, lipid, glucose and ion profiles. A multicenter cross-sectional study was performed among patients institutionalized in nursing homes. The respiratory muscle function was evaluated by peak expiratory flow, maximal respiratory pressures and spirometry parameters, and skeletal mass function and lean mass content with handgrip strength, walking speed and bioimpedance, respectively. The prevalence of reduced respiratory muscle strength in the sample ranged from 37.9% to 80.7%. Peak expiratory flow significantly ($p < 0.05$) correlated to handgrip strength and gait speed, as well as maximal inspiratory pressure ($p < 0.01$). Maximal expiratory pressure significantly ($p < 0.01$) correlated to handgrip strength. No correlation was obtained with muscle mass in any of parameters related to reduced respiratory muscle strength. The most significant associations within the blood biochemical parameters were observed for some protein and lipid biomarkers e.g., glutamate-oxaloacetate transaminase (GOT), urea, triglycerides and cholesterol. Respiratory function muscle parameters, peak expiratory flow and maximal respiratory pressures were correlated with reduced strength and functional impairment but not with lean mass content. We identified for the first time a relationship between peak expiratory flow (PEF) values and GOT and urea concentrations in blood which deserves future investigations in order to manage these parameters as a possible biomarkers of reduced respiratory muscle strength.

Keywords: spirometry; urea; fatigue; respiratory system; skeletal muscles; lipids; transaminases

1. Introduction

Sarcopenia is a geriatric syndrome that according to the European Working Group on Sarcopenia in Older People (EWGSOP) guidelines, is defined as a progressive and generalized loss of skeletal muscle mass and strength, with a risk of adverse outcomes, such as functional capacity impairment, dependence, falls and fractures, negative impact on quality of life, hospitalization and death [1]. In older individuals, sarcopenia has a widespread effect on all skeletal muscles throughout the body, but the features of sarcopenia in the respiratory muscles and its relationship with established sarcopenia parameters such as reduced lean mass, poor muscular strength and functional impairment [1,2] have been less widely investigated in older individuals [3,4], and no studies have been performed in nursing home residents, a significant population in western societies with a huge burden of comorbidities, including sarcopenia [5–8]. Besides the loss of muscular mass and strength, aging leads to proteolysis of elastic fiber and an increase in collagen in the pulmonary parenchyma, which coupled with an increase in the rigidity of the chest wall generates a mechanical disadvantage, and weakness of the respiratory muscles over time [9,10]. These changes results in a diminished respiratory muscle strength (RMS), referred to as sarcopenia of the respiratory muscle or reduced respiratory muscle strength as just it is analysed by quantifying the decline in respiratory function [3]. Respiratory muscles are also responsible of producing a proper pressure difference between inspiration and expiration to generate a correct airway flow rate, which guarantees a good respiratory function [11]. Other respiratory parameters, such as vital capacity (VC), forced vital capacity (FVC), forced expiratory volume in 1 s (FEV1), and peak expiratory flow rate (PEF) are also affected as a result of changes in elastic recoil and thorax compliance associated with aging [3,11,12]. RMS is therefore related to FEV1, FVC, and PEF. Even in patients without airway obstruction, these functions may decline due to age-induced weakness of the respiratory muscles. PEF measurements were recommended over RMS measurements for the assessment of respiratory function in the EWGSOP consensus report published in 2010 [2]. However, the EWGSOP report also indicated that PEF measurements should be used in association with other assessments, because there is a limited evidence about the relationship between PEF and skeletal muscle mass/sarcopenia in older adults. A previous study revealed that PEF is a significant predictor of mortality in older adults [13,14]. Further studies have demonstrated that sarcopenia is related to an increased incidence of pulmonary complications after surgery [15–17] and aspiration pneumonia mortality [18]. Izawa et al. [19] evaluated the relationship between maximal inspiratory pressure (MIP) and physical function as a measure of sarcopenia in older patients with heart disease, and found that sarcopenic patients presented lower values of MIP which also correlated with reduced skeletal muscle mass index, gait speed and hand grip strength. There is a lack of studies demonstrating the association between respiratory muscle weakness and sarcopenia parameters (reduced lean mass and muscular strength and low physical performance) in older institutionalized individuals. Moreover, no studies about the relationship of respiratory muscle function and blood analytical parameters in sarcopenic individuals have been performed. The objectives in this study were therefore to compare respiratory muscle function with lean mass content, handgrip strength and functional impairment (walking speed) in order to assess whether there is an association between respiratory muscle parameters such as the maximum respiratory pressures and peak expiratory flow and parameters of skeletal muscular function. Since skeletal sarcopenia have been associated to malnutrition and undernutrition, which in turn is accompanied by several alterations detectable in blood regarding both blood cell counts and biochemical metabolic markers [20–23] we also evaluated the associations between the parameters related to respiratory muscle strength and skeletal sarcopenia with blood cell counts and biochemical parameters related to protein, lipid, glucose and indirectly with energy production (glucose, creatinine, transaminases, and ions concentrations).

2. Materials and Methods

2.1. Design and Study Population

A cross-sectional study was conducted in individuals institutionalized in nursing homes and long-stay centers for the older individuals in the province of Valencia, Spain (GeroResidencias La Saleta, Valencia). We selected nursing home residents of both genders. Participants were excluded if they were unable to understand the content of questionnaires (moderate-severe cognitive impairment), had a poorly controlled major psychiatric disease (schizophrenia, bipolar disorders, etc.), acute infections, or a known cancer condition. According to the requirements of the Declaration of Helsinki, written consent was obtained from all of the selected subjects before beginning the study, after informing them about the procedures involved and the purpose of the research. The entire study protocol was approved by the local ethical committee at the University of Valencia (H1524420647893, approved 5 July 2018).

2.2. Sociodemographic and Clinical Variables

Socio-demographic variables and medical conditions were recorded, including the number of medications taken, the type and number of any comorbidities using the Charlson index, and several hematological and biochemical parameters. The Charlson index was used to assess comorbidity (with a Cronbach's Alpha of 0.78) [24]. This index assesses 16 diseases that are explicitly defined and scored by a continuous variable from 0 to 31. With this index, the 10-year survival prediction is estimated for patients with comorbidity [25].

2.3. Measurement of Respiratory Muscle Function

The assessment of respiratory function was carried out through two different tests, the assessment of lung volumes and flows by performing a forced spirometry, and the assessment of the maximum respiratory pressures that the respiratory muscles are capable of generating at mouth level as a result of maximum effort.

The spirometric assessment followed the standardized recommendations of the European Respiratory Society [26]. The patient was placed in a seated position, with his back supported by the backrest and with nasal clamps to avoid air leakage. The maneuver was explained in detail to the patient to minimize errors, requesting an initial maximum inspiration to reach total lung capacity, which allows the subsequent performance of a forced maximum expiration for at least 6 s, until the limit of expiration is reached. At least three manoeuvres are performed, with a rest of 1 min between each one, and the highest value of the three repetitions is recorded.

By carrying out this test, the following volumes and forced pulmonary capacities in absolute and relative values were obtained: forced vital capacity (FVC), forced expiratory volume in the first second (FEV1), FEV1/FVC, forced expiratory volume in smaller than 1mm diameter tracks (FEV2575) and peak expiratory flow (PEF). At least three repetitions of the maneuver were performed (with a maximum of 8 repetitions) to achieve the correct execution of the test, discarding those spirometric maneuvers with artifacts in their performance or variations of more than 0.150 L between the highest FEV1 and/or FVC values, as recommended by the ATS/ERS [26].

For the assessment of respiratory muscle strength, maximum static respiratory pressures in the mouth, inspiratory (MIP) and expiratory (MEP) were measured. These parameters allow us to know in a simple way the global force that the respiratory muscles are capable of exerting. The tests require the collaboration of the patient to perform a maximum isometric effort. The standardized regulations for this test were followed [27,28]. To evaluate the MIP, the patient was instructed to start from the residual volume and for the MEP to start from the total lung capacity, so that the maximum value of the three maneuvers could be collected, with a variation of less than 10% between them and a 1-min pause between each of the repetitions. This excluded those attempts where there was more than 10% variation between them, as recommended by Laveneziana, et al. [28].The proposed cut-off points for PEF and maximum respiratory pressures (MIP and MEP) were used to establish the existence of respiratory sarcopenia. The cut-off point for PEF was set at 4.40 L/s for men and 3.21 L/s for women [22]. The cut-off point for MIP was set at less than or equal to 55 H_2O cm for men and less than or equal to 45 H_2O cm for women, while for MEP it was set at less than or equal to 60 H_2O cm for men and less than or equal to 50 H_2O cm for women [4]. Before the test was conducted, the steps for correctly performing the test were carefully explained to the participants. Once explained, a test of all the steps to be followed was carried out, without demanding maximum effort from the participants to avoid accumulated fatigue. Afterwards, the tests were carried out in accordance with international standards [28].

The older institutionalized population has a high prevalence of cognitive impairment, which could make this type of testing difficult. However, we excluded patients with moderate and severe cognitive impairment, so that the collaboration of patients included was adequate to perform these tests. In addition, an adaptation procedure was carried out on the study subjects before the definitive test, excluding from the sample those subjects who presented poor coordination and, therefore, difficulty in carrying out the test at the discretion of the evaluator. In all the centres, assessments were made in the morning between 8 and 11 am and in the same period of time. To avoid inter-observer errors, all measurements were taken by the same trained investigator.

In addition, to analyze reliability, we assessed the stability of the measure obtaining values of intraclass correlation coefficient (ICC; one-way, mixed-effects model) between PEF values in the three centers of 0.71, what was indicative of moderate to good reliability.

2.4. Measurement of Sarcopenia

Muscle skeletal sarcopenia was assessed by indirect measures of muscle function and muscle mass, such as handgrip strength assessed by hand-dynamometry, walking speed and bioimpedance respectively. Hand-dynamometer was assessed in the dominant hand by means of a JAMAR dynamometer (Lafayette Instrument Company, Lafayette, IN, USA) as previously described [29]. The subject was placed in a standard position: in a sitting position, with the shoulder at 0° of flexion, the elbow attached to the body at 90° of flexion and the forearm in a neutral position. After the subject is positioned appropriately, the examiner asks the patient to squeeze as hard as possible for 3 s and then relax. Three attempts were made, with 1 min rest in between. The mean value obtained was recorded. The cut-offs for handgrip strength were ≤30 kg/m^2 for men and ≤20 kg/m^2 for women [2]. The walking speed was assessed using the 4-m walking test [30]. The patient was asked to walk at usual pace and from a standing start and using their usual walking aid. The time required to cover this distance was recorded and, based on this, the walking speed in m/s was calculated. The cut-off for low walking speed was ≤0.8 m/s walking through 4 m [2]. The body composition was assessed by bioelectrical impedance analysis (BIA) with a BF-300 device (Tanita, Tokyo, Japan) as previously described [31,32]. The BIA measure was performed with a standard technique using a single frequency of 50 KHz and 550 mA, and the placement of four electrodes in a distal position (four electrodes at feet) while participant was in a standing position. BIA measurements were carried out in the early morning following the next considerations: (1) No physical exercise in the previous hours; (2) 2–3 h of fasting, including drinking plenty of water or alcohol; (3) urination 30 min before the test; (4) no metal parts at the time of the test. The values of reactance and resistance were then recorded once the patient was stabilized. The repeatability and accuracy of the resistance and reactance measurements enabled the smallest changes to be recorded to a resolution of 0.1 Ω. Muscle mass was calculated using the formula of Janssen et al. [31]: muscle mass (kg) = $[(\text{height}^2/R \times 0.401) + (3.825 \times \text{sex}) + (-0.701 \times \text{age}) + 5.102]$ where height is expressed in cm, R in Ω, age in years and female sex has a value of zero and males a value of one. The muscle mass index (MMI) is defined as the muscle mass a person has, corrected by body surface area (muscle mass/height^2). The bioimpedance test was performed early in the morning while the patient is at rest, after overnight fasting (food and drink) and removing all metal elements. The cut-off for the loss of muscle mass assessed by bioimpedance of the whole body were ≤5.5 kg/m^2 for women and ≤7.25 kg/m^2) for men [2]. These muscle mass values are adjusted with the cut-off values for the Spanish population being 8.31 kg/m^2 for men and 6.68 kg/m^2 for women [33]. In order to minimize the influence of physical performance across the time of the day, all measurements were always conducted between 8–11 a.m.

2.5. Haemogram and Analytical Parameters

To obtain the analytical determinations, the usual blood controls carried out in residential centers were used. Thus, blood samples were collected from each subject at approximately 8 am (after 8–10 h fasting). 10 mL of blood plasma was collected into Vacutainer tubes (BD, Franklin Lakes, NJ, USA) containing EDTA.

Clinical laboratories belonging to local public health centers were used to analyze the different hematological parameters (white blood cells, hemoglobin, erythrocytes, and platelets) and biochemical parameters (glucose, urea, urate, cholesterol, triglycerides, creatinine, glutamic oxaloacetic transaminase [GOT], and serum glutamic pyruvic transaminase [GPT], sodium ions [Na^+], potassium ions [K^+], and Calcium [Ca^{++}]). Within public health centers, the variation range of metabolites in plasma sample varies between 0.4–1.1% dependent on the metabolite.

2.6. Statistical Analysis

Quantitative variables were analysed using descriptive statistics, specifically central tendency measures (means), standard error of the mean (SEM), 95% confidence interval and ranges. Frequencies and percentages were used to describe the qualitative variables. The normal distribution of the variables, in order to determine whether to carry out parametric or non-parametric tests, was analysed using the Shapiro-Wilk test. Outliers were identified on the boxplot drawn in SPSS program which uses a step of 1.5 × IQR (Interquartile range). No outliers were identified and all data were included in the statistical analysis. Differences in quantitative variables between the two groups were analyzed with the two-tailed tests e.g., parametric Student t-test or the nonparametric Mann-Whitney U-test. To analyze the correlation between quantitative variables, the parametric Pearson test or the non-parametric Spearman's test was used depending on their distribution. Statistical significance was considered at $p < 0.05$. SPSS version 25.0 statistical package (SPSS Inc., Chicago, IL, USA) was used to perform the statistical analyses.

3. Results

3.1. Sociodemographic and Clinical Parameters of the Study Sample

A total of 58 subjects (67.2% female) living in three nursing care centers located in the province of Valencia (Spain) were enrolled in the study (Table 1). All the participants were Caucasian. Their age ranged from 55 to 93 years, and the mean age was 78.6 ± 8.9 years. 63.8% of the subjects were independent in their walking ability (they did not require external aids such as a cane or walker). Smokers were 15.5% (n = 9) of the sample. A percentage of 21.1% (n = 12) in the study sample used bronchodilators as a usual treatment. Among individuals using bronchodilators, n = 6 used bronchodilator therapy containing glucocorticoids. Regarding the use of common medications affecting the muscular system, none of the individuals received oral glucocorticoid treatment, 37.9% (n = 22) used statins to lower cholesterol levels and 5.2% (n = 3) used muscle relaxant drugs. Mean body mass index was 28.8 ± 5.8 (Range 18.7–50.2). The Charlson comorbidity index score adjusted for age was 5.4 ± 1.9 (Range 1.0–11.0). The occurrence of the most common comorbidities are indicated in Table 1.

Respiratory function assessment showed an absence of respiratory failure related to oxyhemoglobin saturation, with 95.9 ± 1.9% (range 91.0–99.0). Respiratory functional exploration showed spirometric values within normal ranges for a population of these characteristics (FVC at 84.0 ± 23.6% (Range 23.0–149.0) and FEV1 at 83.3 ± 28.3% (Range 20.0–160.0)), except for a small reduction in the permeability of the smaller diameter airway, with an FEV2575 at 54.5 ± 25.7% (Range 12.0–149.0). Respiratory muscle strength was diminished, at both inspiratory (36.5 ± 17.4 H_2O cm) and expiratory (58.9 ± 23.7 H_2O cm) levels. The maximal respiratory pressures (MIP and MEP) and spirometric parameter values (FVC, FEV1, FEV1/FVC, FEV2575 and PEF) are shown in Table 2.

A positive correlation was found between oxyhemoglobin saturation and FVC (r = 0.287 p = 0.034, Pearson test) and oxyhemoglobin saturation and FEV1 (r = 0.269 p = 0.047, Pearson test). No correlations were found between heart rate and any other respiratory parameters.

Table 1. Characteristics of the study sample.

Clinical and Demographic Characteristics of Participants	Mean Value ± SD (Range) or Percentage
Age (years)	78.6 ± 8.9 (55–93)
Sex	Male 32.8%Female 67.2%
IBM (kg/m^2)	28.9 ± 6.1 (18.7–50.2)
Smokers	15.5%
Use of bronchodilators as a usual treatment	21.1%
Walking ability	Independent 63.8%Can 3.4%Walker 32.8%
Comorbidities (Charlson index)	5.4 ± 1.9 (1–11)
Diabetes	31.0%
Chronic obstructive pulmonary disease	17.2%
Hypertension	32.8%
Hypercholesterolemia	37.9%
Congestive heart failure	10.3%
Renal failure	12.1%
Osteoporosis	20.7%
Depression	19.0%

Table 2. Respiratory function parameters.

Respiratory Parameters	Mean Value (± SD)	Range
$SatO_2$ (%)	95.9 ± 1.9	91.0–99.0
Heart rate (bpm)	77.1 ± 14.2	49.0–114.0
FVC (L/s)	1.8 ± 0.7	0.3–4.4
FEV1(L/s)	1.3 ± 0.5	0.3–2.9
FEV1/FVC (%)	76.5 ± 12.1	45.9–100.0
FEV25-75 (L/s)	1.2 ± 0.5	0.3–3.1
PEF (L/s)	2.8 ± 1.2	0.7–5.7
MIP (H_2O cm)	36.5 ± 17.4	7.0–77.0
MEP (H_2O cm)	58.9 ± 23.7	10.0–99.0

A positive correlation can be found between the various parameters that describe the spirometric function by analyzing the correlation between the different parameters of respiratory function. There was a significant correlation between FVC percentage values and FEV1 percentage values (r = 0.894, $p < 0.001$, Pearson test), FEV2575 percentage values (r = 0.473, $p < 0.001$, Pearson test) and PEF (r = 0.281 $p = 0.033$, Pearson test). Significant correlations were also found between FEV1 percentage values and FEV2575 percentage values (r = 0.689, $p < 0.001$, Pearson test). There was a correlation between PEF and maximum respiratory pressures, with both MIP (r = 0.419, $p < 0.001$, Pearson test) and with MEP (r = 0.575, $p < 0.001$, Pearson test), and the maximum respiratory pressures between them (r = 0.559, $p < 0.001$, Pearson test).

Based on the PEF cut-off points established by Kera et al., (22), the prevalence of respiratory sarcopenia in the sample studied was 70.7%. On the other hand, if the values of MIP and MEP established by Ohara et al., (4) are taken as the benchmark, the prevalence of respiratory sarcopenia was 80.7% and 37.9%, respectively.

3.2. Evaluation of Skeletal Muscle Mass and Function

According to the EWGSOP guidelines, 17.6% of the subjects were classified as sarcopenic, with 17.6% meeting the criteria of reduced lean mass, 65.4% meeting the criteria of low physical performance and 84.5% meeting the criteria of reduced muscle strength. The mean values of each criterion were skeletal muscle-mass index of 9.21 ± 2.793 kg/m^2, walking speed of 0.66 ± 0.331 m/s and handgrip strength of 17.90 ± 8.506 kg. The data from the anthropometric characteristics of all the participants in this study are summarized in Table 3.

Table 3. Anthropometric analysis and sarcopenia parameters.

Anthropometric Analysis	Mean Value (± SD)	Range	% of Individuals Fulfilling the EWGSOP Criterion for Sarcopenia
Muscle mass (Janssen)	22.8 ± 8.2	13.2–49.5	Reduced lean mass: 17.6%
Skeletal muscle mass index (Janssen)	9.2 ± 2.8	5.5–20.1	Reduced lean mass: 17.6%
Hand grip in dominant hand (Kg)	17.9 ± 8.5	6.5–42.0	Muscle strength (dominant hand): 84.5%
Hand grip in non-dominant hand (Kg)	16.5 ± 7.6	3.3–36.7	Muscle strength (non-dominant hand): 84.5%
Walking speed (m/s)	0.6 ± 0.3	0.1–1.5	Physical performance: 65.4%

3.3. Evaluation of the Relationship between Muscle Skeleñata Parameters (Mass and Function) and Muscle Respiratory Function

There was a significant and positive correlation between physical performance and PEF absolute values (r = 0.563, $p < 0.001$, Spearman's test), PEF percentage values (r = 0.440, $p = 0.001$, Pearson test) and MIP values (r = 0.354, $p = 0.011$, Spearman's test). No correlation between physical performance and MEP was found (r = 0.268, $p = 0.268$, Spearman's test). No significant correlation was found between the other parameters of respiratory function and physical performance ($p > 0.05$ in all cases).

There was a significant and positive correlation between handgrip strength and MIP values (r = 0.599, $p < 0.001$, Spearman's test), MEP values (r = 0.465, $p < 0.001$, Spearman's test) and PEF absolute values (r = 0.375, $p = 0.004$, Spearman's test). There was also a significant but negative correlation between handgrip strength and FEV1 percentage values (r = −0.307, $p = 0.019$, Spearman's test). No significant correlation was found between other parameters of respiratory function and handgrip strength ($p > 0.05$ in all cases) (Figure 1).

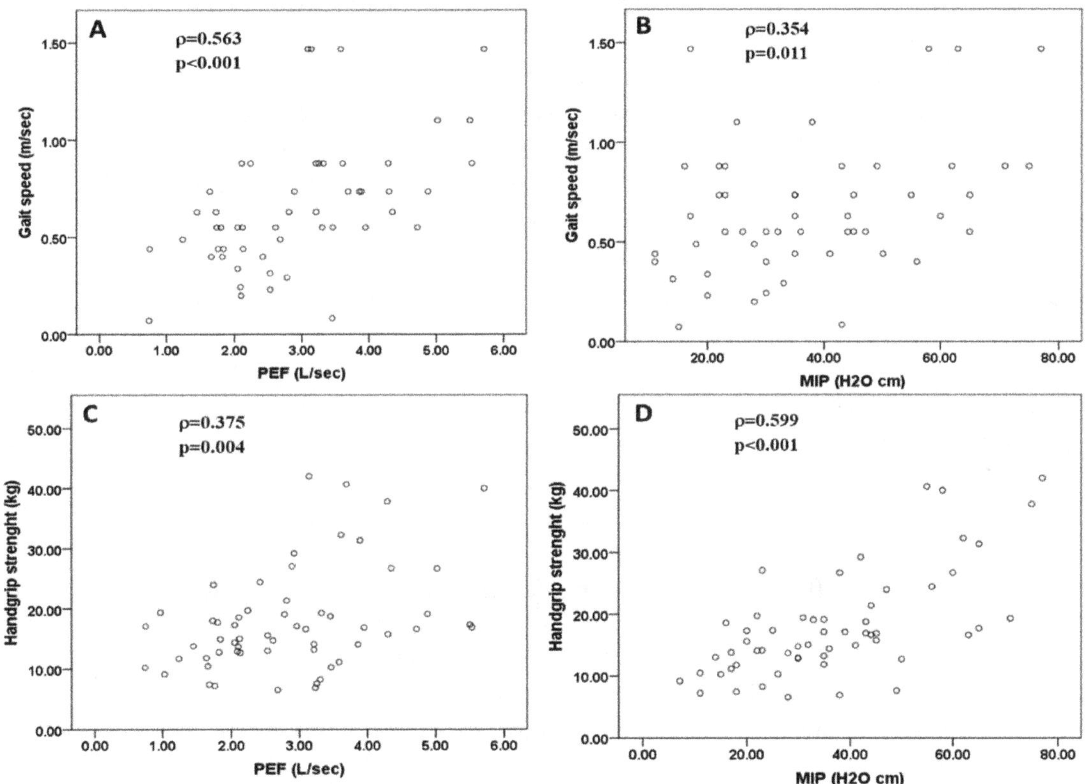

Figure 1. Representation of the significant correlations between skeletal and respiratory muscle sarcopenia parameters. Significant correlations between gait speed and PEF (**A**) or MIP (**B**) and between handgrip strength and PEF (**C**) or MIP (**D**).

No significant correlations were found between skeletal muscle mass index and respiratory function parameters, in relation to either PEF absolute values (r = 0.252, $p = 0.074$, Spearman's test), or MIP (r = 0.143, $p = 0.322$, Spearman's test), or MEP (r = 0.225, $p = 0.112$, Spearman's test).

We categorized patients based on cut-off scores for skeletal sarcopenia (see Methods section) and we evaluated whether there were any differences in the respiratory parameters and respiratory muscle parameters (Figure 2).

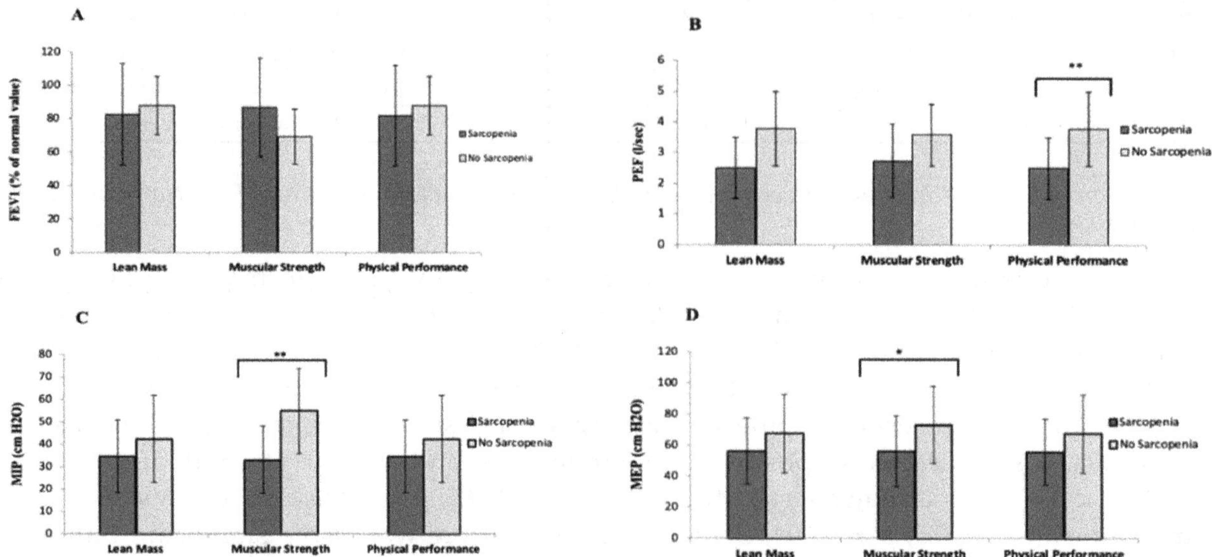

Figure 2. Mean difference of respiratory parameters ((**A**): FEV1; (**B**): PEF; (**C**): MIP; (**D**): MEP) according to the presence or not of the three cut-off values for sarcopenia parameters * $p < 0.05$; ** $p < 0.001$.

As for physical performance, differences were observed in both PEF (NS = 3.78 vs. S = 2.49, MeanDiff = 1.29 [95%CI: 0.67–1.91], $p < 0.001$) and PEF% (NS = 64.11 vs. S = 47.21, MeanDiff = 16.90 [95%CI: 6.59–27.22], $p = 0.002$).

For the handgrip strength, different maximal respiratory pressures were observed in both groups, MIP (NS = 54.89 vs. S = 33.06, MeanDiff = 21.83 [95%CI: 10.48–33.18], $p < 0.001$) and MEP (NS = 73.22 vs. S = 56.69, MeanDiff = 16.92 [95%CI: 0.13–37.70], $p = 0.048$). When analyzing the PEF we observed no statistically significant differences, although a trend was observed in them (NS = 3.57 vs. S = 2.74, MeanDiff = 0.86 [95%CI: −0.006–1.72], $p = 0.052$)

No significant differences for lean mass content were observed for any of the comparisons ($p > 0.05$) (Figure 2).

We also categorized patients based on respiratory muscle sarcopenia according to Kera et al. (22) and Ohara et al. (4) (see methods), and we evaluated whether there were any differences in the somatic sarcopenia parameters, such as skeletal muscle mass index, handgrip strength and gait speed (Figure 3).

For MIP, differences were observed in both gait speed (NS = 0.89 vs. S = 0.59, MeanDiff = 0.30 [95%CI: 0.51–0.85], $p = 0.007$) and handgrip strength (NS = 27.35 vs. S = 15.64, MeanDiff = 11.71 [95%CI: 4.75–18.66], $p = 0.003$). No differences were found for skeletal muscle mass index ($p = 0.844$).

As regards MEP, a different maximal handgrip strength were observed in both groups, (NS = 20.31 vs. S = 13.96, MeanDiff = 6.35 [95%CI: 2.59–10.11], $p = 0.001$). No statistically significant differences were found in gait speed or skeletal muscle mass index ($p = 0.156$ and $p = 0.214$, respectively).

For PEF, differences were observed in gait speed (NS = 0.82 vs. S = 0.58, MeanDiff = 0.24 [95%CI: 0.32–0.45], $p = 0.025$), but not in handgrip strength (NS = 17.90 vs. S = 17.90, MeanDiff = 0.01 [95%CI: −4.99–4.98], $p = 0.997$) (Figure 3).

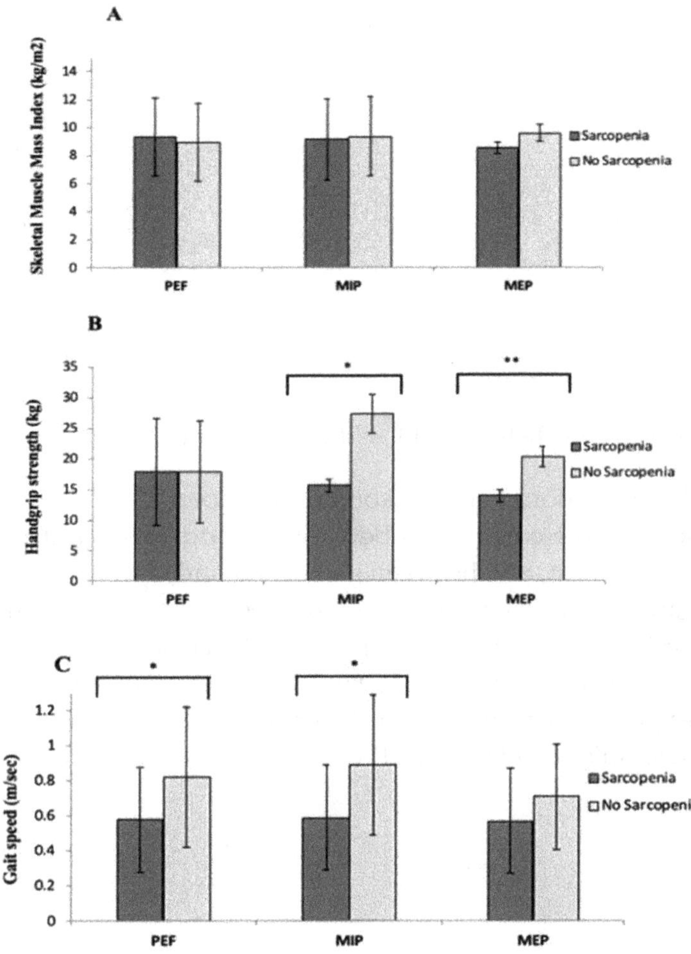

Figure 3. Mean difference of muscle mass (**A**), Handgrip strength (**B**) and gait speed (**C**) according to the presence of each respiratory muscle sarcopenia criteria. * $p < 0.05$; ** $p < 0.001$.

3.4. Evaluation of the Relationship between Sarcopenia Parameters and Blood Analytical Markers

No significant associations were found when analyzing the possible correlations between the parameters of the hemogram (white blood cells, hemoglobin, erythrocytes, and platelets) and the parameters of respiratory sarcopenia and somatic sarcopenia ($p > 0.05$ in all cases).

The relationship between respiratory sarcopenia parameters and biochemical parameters (glucose, urea, urate, cholesterol, triglycerides, creatinine, glutamic oxaloacetic transaminase [GOT], and serum glutamic pyruvic transaminase [GPT], sodium ions [Na^+], potassium ions [K^+], Calcium [Ca^{++}]) was subsequently studied. There was a significant and positive correlation between PEF values and GOT (r = 0.387, $p = 0.004$, Spearman's test) and a significant and negative correlation between PEF values and urea (r = −0.366, $p = 0.007$, Pearson test) (Figure 4). No significant correlation was found between other parameters of biochemical markers and respiratory sarcopenia parameters values ($p > 0.05$ in all cases, Pearson's and Spearman's correlation test).

We also categorized patients based on criteria of respiratory sarcopenia according to Kera et al. (22) and Ohara et al. (4) (see methods) and we evaluated whether there were any differences on blood analytical markers.

Significant differences were found in urea values for the presence of sarcopenia estimated by PEF (NS = 32.58 vs. S = 46.70, MeanDiff = 14.12 [95%CI: −23.59–4.64], $p = 0.005$) but not in GOT values (NS = 18.50 vs. S = 14.97, MeanDiff = 3.53 [95%CI: −1.18–8.23], $p = 0.132$).

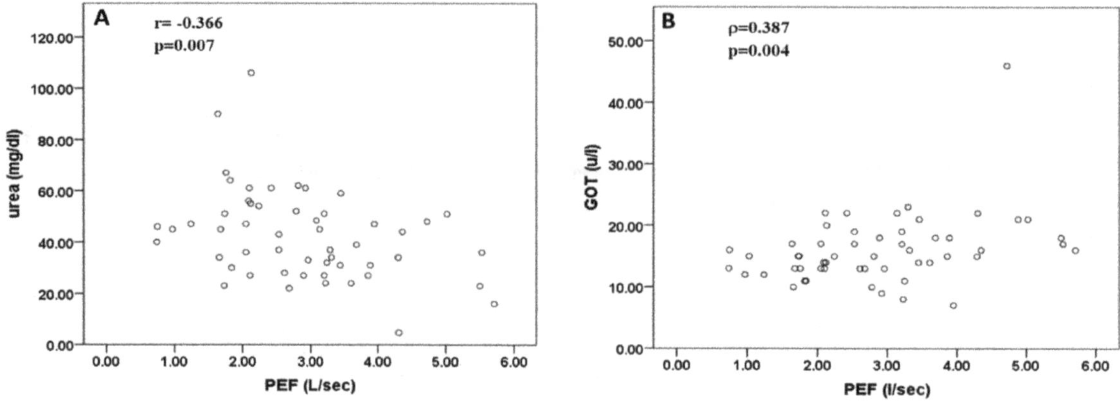

Figure 4. Correlation between PEF and urea (**A**) and GOT (**B**) concentration.

Studying the possible correlations between somatic sarcopenia values and biochemical parameters showed a significant and positive correlation between handgrip strength and urate concentration (r = 0.279, $p = 0.041$, Spearman's test) and between gait speed and GOT (r = 0.390, $p = 0.006$, Spearman's test). There was also a significant and negative correlation between skeletal muscle mass index and total cholesterol (r = −0.405, $p = 0.004$, Spearman's test) and triglycerides (r = −0.357, $p = 0.017$, Spearman's test), and between urea and gait speed (r = −0.36, $p = 0.012$, Spearman's test). No significant correlation was found between other parameters of biochemical markers and muscle mass and function values ($p > 0.05$ in all cases, Spearman's correlation test) (Figure 5).

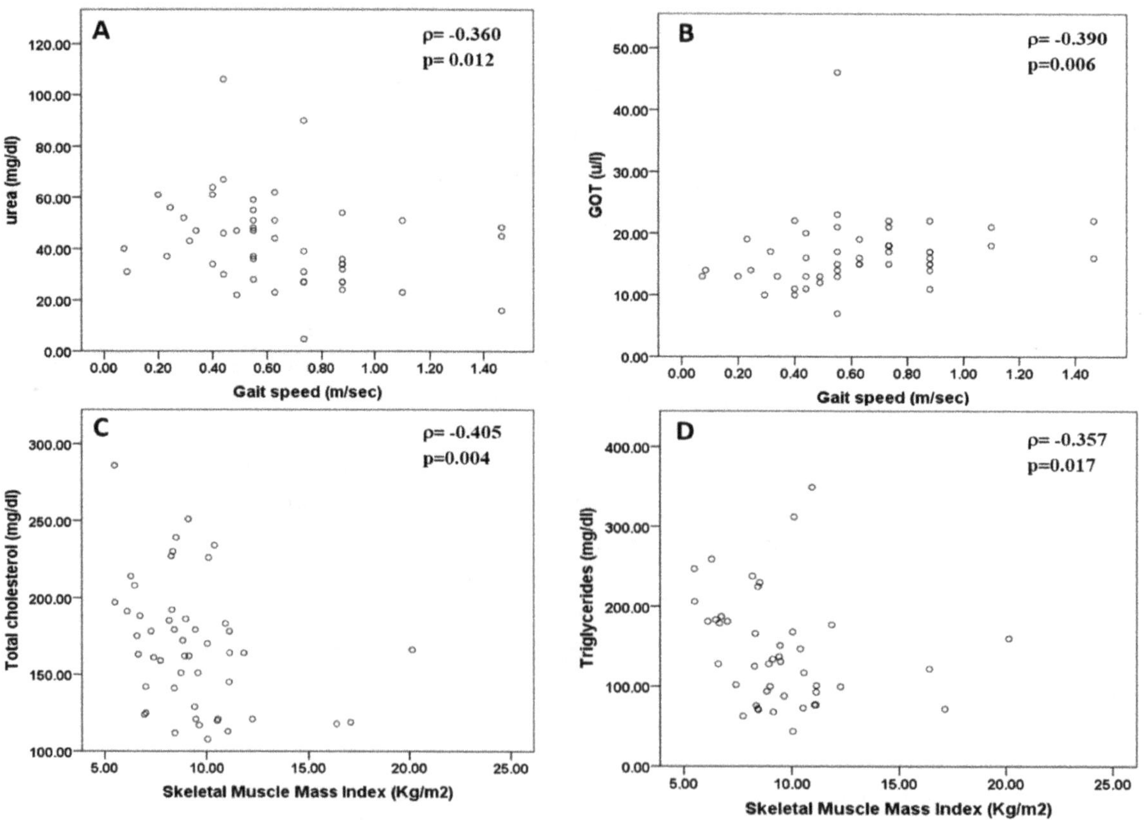

Figure 5. Correlation between skeletal muscle sarcopenia parameters and urea (**A**), GOT (**B**) and lipids ((**C**): total cholesterol; (**D**): triglycerides) concentration in blood.

We also categorized the patients based on the cut-off scores of the three parameters studied for the evaluation of sarcopenia (see Methods section) and evaluated if there were any differences in blood analytical markers.

For the gait speed, there were statistically significant differences in urea values (NS = 34.72 vs. S = 45.82, MeanDiff = 11.10 [95%CI: −20.44–1.76], p = 0.042) but not in GOT values (NS = 17.0 vs. S = 16.42, MeanDiff = 0.58 [95%CI: −2.31–3.48], p = 0.685).

For the presence of sarcopenia according to lean mass content, there were statistically significant differences in total cholesterol values (NS = 162.29 vs. S = 199.13, MeanDiff = 36.83 [95%CI:−71.58—2.08], p = 0.04) but not in tryglicerides (NS = 135.92 vs. S = 180.75, MeanDiff = 44.83 [95%CI: −99.94–10.27], p = 0.101)

As for handgrip strength, no differences were observed in urate values between groups (NS = 4.74 vs. S = 4.79, MeanDiff = 0.05 [95%CI: −0.94–0.85], p = 0.807).

4. Discussion

This study, which analyzes sarcopenia parameters in older people living in nursing homes, shows the direct relationship between respiratory muscle function and skeletal muscle function, especially with regard to the muscular strength and walking speed, and we report on the correlation between sarcopenia parameters and several biochemical markers obtained in routine blood analysis. This is the first study, to our knowledge, that considers the relationship between respiratory muscle strength and blood biochemical markers, finding a relationship between peak expiratory flow (PEF) values and glutamate-oxaloacetate transaminase (GOT) and urea concentration. We also observed associations between musculoskeletal parameters of sarcopenia with some blood markers, e.g., muscle mass and total cholesterol and triglyceride values, walking speed and urea and GOT values and handgrip strength and urate values. We discuss these new findings below.

The prevalence of sarcopenia in the sample of nursing home residents, following the EWGSOP criteria [2] and adjusting the skeletal muscle mass index to the Spanish population according to the cut-off points proposed by Masanés and coworkers [33], was 17.6%. These data are lower than those previously proposed for the Spanish institutionalized population [8], 41.4% applying the same assessment criteria, but are consistent with those described in a literature review that includes studies in several countries of patients residing in long-term care homes [6], like the population of our study. It is possible that the exclusion of patients who were not able to understand the content of the questionnaires influences the prevalence of the sample in the present study, since the presence of cognitive impairment increases the rates of sarcopenia [34].

The relationship between respiratory function parameters and somatic sarcopenia in community-dwelling older people has been studied in recent years, given the objectivity of these parameters and the ease and speed of assessment, but no studies in nursing home residents displaying higher levels of functional impairment and comorbidity burdens have been reported. Three parameters of respiratory function that have been established in the literature as determinants of respiratory sarcopenia, PEF [35] and maximum inspiratory (MIP) and expiratory (MEP) respiratory pressures [4].

Prevalence scores of respiratory sarcopenia according to PEF values were 70.7%, while maximum respiratory pressures were 80.7% according for MIP and 37.9% for MEP. The highest prevalence values of respiratory sarcopenia were obtained for both MIP and PEF, as in the study by Bahat et al. [36]. This may be due to the fact that loss of respiratory muscle strength occurs first in the inspiratory muscles, and is related to deterioration of type IIx and/or IIb muscle fibers of the diaphragm [3]. Loss of inspiratory muscle strength (MIP) leads to a reduced volume of inspired air prior to glottal closure and contraction of the expiratory muscle, preventing effective maximal expiration (PEF) [37,38]. In addition, it implies an inability to fully inflate the lungs, which is necessary to achieve the optimization of the length-tension relationship of the expiratory muscles, stimulate lung surfactant production and distribution, and open the collapsed peripheral airways that often accompany the hypoventilation processes associated with age and the aging process [39–41].

Furthermore, the greater relevance of the inspiratory muscles in the deterioration of the peripheral muscles was also justified by the decline in handgrip strength (84.5% of the sample studied) and the decline in walking speed (65.4% of the sample studied), as established in previous studies [4,19].

PEF was considered the most relevant parameter for establishing respiratory sarcopenia by Kera et al. [35,42] due to the involvement of the respiratory muscles in its execution and the minimal impact of the deterioration of the airway on its values, since it is measured at the beginning of forced expiration, and is not affected by the modifications in elastic recoil and thorax compliance associated with age [43]. The authors highlighted their preference for this test over respiratory muscle strength because of the lesser effort required and to avoid maneuvers that involve an increase in intracranial pressure, with the risks that this entails [35].

The results of this study confirm the results obtained by Kera et al. [42] in community-dwelling older people, but obtain higher values of correlation than Kera in the criterion of strength (handgrip strength) ($r = 0.375$ vs. $r = 0.283$) and in the criterion of functional performance (gait speed) ($r = 0.563$ vs. $r = 0.167$). No correlation was obtained in this study with the index of musculoskeletal mass, with muscle function more relevant than the amount of existing lean muscle mass in sarcopenic older individuals. In turn, Kera et al. [35] obtained differences between patients categorized as respiratory sarcopenic for the three determining variables of somatic sarcopenia, which were always higher in non-sarcopenic patients, while these differences were only obtained for gait speed in this study, possibly due to the high rates of sedentarism among nursing home residents and their more limited independence in their basic activities of daily life. In our study, no associations were found between respiratory muscle function and lean mass content and it could be explained in part by the obesity paradox [44]. The body mass index in the study sample widely varies among the participants enrolled in the study (range 18.7–50.2) and one third of patients have overweight and obesity grade I. This paradoxical benefit of a medically unfavorable phenotype is particularly strong in the overweight and class I obesity, and less pronounced in the more severe or morbidly obese populations (class II–III and greater). Rather than an obesity paradox, it is possible that this phenomenon may represent a "lean paradox", in which individuals classified as normal weight or underweight may have a reduced lean mass, as a result of a progressive catabolic state and lean mass loss [45–47] whereas overweight and obese patients maintain an adequate lean mass content compared to under and normo-weight individuals [44,48]. Likely, the reduced respiratory muscle strength in overweight and obese individuals could be explained by other pathophysiological factors related to excessive fat accumulation in the thoracic-abdominal region which limits the chest wall expansion and diaphragm contraction, lengthens abdominal muscles, reduces the upper airway calibre, modifies airway configuration, and increases in intra-abdominal pressure and these effects may reduce respiratory muscle function independently on lean mass content [49–51]. Alternatively the reduced muscular function in obese individuals may be also related to chronic low-grade inflammation characterized by the predominance of interleukin-1β, interleukin-6, and tumor necrosis factor-α (TNF-α) observed in obese patients [52]. Further studies with larger sample should evaluate in details the comparison the effects of underweight, obesity with or without sarcopenia on respiratory muscle strengths in order to shed new lights on these apparent discrepancies between muscular strength and lean mass content.

Other reports suggested that valuable markers of reduced respiratory muscle strength are the values related to the maximum respiratory pressures (MIP and MEP), because these parameters are a more direct measurement of the maximum strength of respiratory muscles [4,19,36,53]. In our study, MIP correlated with both walking speed and handgrip strength ($r = 0.599$ and $r = 0.354$, respectively), while MEP correlated with handgrip strength ($r = 0.465$). This parameter, which is slightly more difficult to evaluate than the PEF due to its assessment procedure, is directly related to the loss of strength in the peripheral muscles, as seen in previous studies not only of older people living in the community [19,53] and in nursing homes [4], but also in healthy [54] and hospitalized young adults [55]. On the other hand, no relationship could be found between skeletal muscle mass index and maximum respiratory pressures, like those reported in previous studies of healthy older patients [53] and older patients with cardiovascular diseases [19].

These parameters of maximum respiratory strength appear to be good indicators of reduced respiratory muscle strength in older institutionalized individuals, since patients who presented sarcopenia according to these cut-off values presented significantly lower values of gait speed and handgrip strength that were as good as those recently shown by community dwelling older adults [4].

We demonstrated that parameters related to reduced respiratory muscle strength, e.g., PEF values, are significantly associated with urea and GOT concentrations in blood, which have not been previously reported for the respiratory muscle function. GOT, also known as aspartate aminotransferase, is a mitochondrial and cytoplasmic enzyme, with an important role in cell energy production [56]. Alterations in GOT levels in blood are considered well-known markers of hepatic, myocardial and skeletal muscle cytolysis, while GPT also known as alanine aminotransferase, is mainly a hepatic cytoplasmic enzyme [57–59]. In our study, the lack of a significant association between PEF and GPT levels in blood suggests that the association between PEF and GOT levels is related to myocardial or skeletal muscle metabolism. High serum GOT with normal serum GPT is highly prevalent among community dwelling older individuals who are underweight, and might reflect skeletal muscle pathology [60]. Furthermore, high levels of GOT in serum are present in obese subjects, regardless of age, which may be associated with sarcopenic obesity, reduced muscle mass and overweight, in some of the subjects studied [61,62]. However, the processes involved in regulating blood GOT levels in both underweight and obese subjects remain unknown, but they seem to be related to low muscle mass and function, and in this respect we found a new association with PEF values. The role of cardiac diseases cannot be ruled out, since 30% of the sample presents a comorbidity of this type. However, due to the limited size of the sample of nursing home residents with preserved cognitive function necessary to perform spirometry analysis, it was impossible to study selective pathologies.

However, confirming the association between GOT levels and muscular metabolism and function, GOT levels were also found to be significantly associated with gait speed and almost significantly with grip strength ($p = 0.05$). PEF values were also inversely and significantly associated with urea concentration in blood. Elevated serum urea, a breakdown product of protein, is generally considered a marker of muscle wasting in several conditions [63,64]. Another possible explanation for increased urea levels could be an alteration in kidney function, but the creatinine levels in our study were not significantly associated with any of the sarcopenia parameters and the correlation between urea levels and PEF therefore suggested effects based on muscle metabolism. A recent study with a machine learning approach found that urea concentration is one of risk factors for the development of predictive models for patients with sarcopenia [65], and we also reported an association between urea levels and gait speed. In relation to the positive correlation between uric acid levels and muscle strength reported in our study, this finding replicates the association reported in community dwelling-older individuals in the "InCHIANTI" study [66], which observed that higher urate levels were significantly associated with higher measures of muscle strength, and concluded that high urate levels could create a protective reaction that would counteract the excessive production of free radicals that damage muscle proteins and reduce muscle strength. Likewise, Can et al. [67], focusing on markers of inflammation and oxidative stress, analyzed a sample of 72 geriatric patients confirmed that patients with sarcopenia had significantly lower levels of uric acid than non-sarcopenic patients. Moreover, high serum urate levels are a good positive predictor of grip strength in nonagenarian older individuals, and may delay the progression of sarcopenia [68]. The skeletal muscle criterion of lean mass content was the only criterion that was significantly (and inversely) correlated with blood lipid (cholesterol and triglycerides) concentration. The aging process stimulates the appearance of fat infiltration in muscle tissue, and obesity enhances fat deposits at visceral level, in the liver, heart, pancreas and skeletal muscle, which generates a negative effect on sarcopenia. These lipids cause a pro-inflammatory effect that secretes paracrine and cytokine hormones, promoting a feedforward cycle by producing intramyocellular lipids. This toxicity generated by fats hinders the contraction of muscle fibers and the synthesis of muscle proteins, favoring the development of sarcopenia [69,70].

A study by the South Korean KNHANES conducted an evaluation of sarcopenic obesity subjects and showed a link to an increased risk of dyslipemia in these patients [71]. Mesinovic et al. [72] recently determined the associations between metabolic syndrome and components of sarcopenia, including muscle mass and quality, absolute and relative strength, and physical performance, in 84 overweight and obese older adults, and demonstrated that triglyceride levels had a negative association with leg extension strength and lower-limb relative strength. Lu et al. [73] reported that serum triglycerides and high-density lipoprotein cholesterol were independently associated with sarcopenic obesity. All the biomarkers found to be significantly associated with sarcopenia indexes can be obtained in a routine blood analysis, as they can be rapidly, inexpensively, and reproducibly assayed. Future longitudinal investigations should test these biomarkers as a part of a valuable panel of metabolites to diagnose sarcopenia and monitor the efficacy of clinical interventions in sarcopenic individuals. This is the first study to demonstrate an independent relationship between respiratory muscle strength and some aspects of body sarcopenia in institutionalized elderly people with high rates of comorbidities and polypharmacy. The fact that respiratory sarcopenia is associated with muscle strength and gait speed supports the beneficial effect of various exercises and rehabilitation interventions on breathing muscles [74–76]. New randomized clinical trial should evaluate the effects of such interventions not only for skeletal sarcopenia but also to improve respiratory muscle strength thus allowing a better respiratory function which can influence many respiratory tract diseases since the impairment of (inspiratory and expiratory) respiratory muscles is a common clinical finding, not only in patients with neuromuscular disease but also in those with respiratory diseases affecting the lung parenchyma or airways [77–79]. We provided further evidence for the use of suitable cut-off points for respiratory muscle strength which can be tested in future researches prior its proposal as indicator of muscle respiratory function in clinical settings. Loss of mass and function of the respiratory muscles could be prevented by properly applying these exercises. More studies on sarcopenia and its effects on respiratory muscle strength are needed to improve life expectancy and quality of life in the older institutionalized individuals.

Author Contributions: Conceptualization, F.M.M.-A., C.B., R.F.-V., O.C.; Methodology, F.M.M.-A., C.B., R.F.-V., O.C.; formal analysis, F.M.M.-A., O.C.; investigation, F.M.M.-A., C.B., R.F.-V., O.C.; data curation, F.M.M.-A., C.B., R.F.-V., O.C.; writing—Original draft preparation, F.M.M.-A., O.C.; writing—Review and editing, F.M.M.-A., C.B., R.F.-V., O.C. All authors have read and agreed to the published version of the manuscript.

Abbreviations

95% CI	95% Confidence interval
EDTA	Ethylenediaminetetraacetic acid
EWGSOP	European Working Group for Sarcopenia in Older People
FEV1	Forced Expiratory Volume in first second
FEV2575	Mesoexpiratory volume
FVC	Forced vital capacity
GOT	Glutamic oxaloacetic transaminase
GPT	Glutamic pyruvic transaminase
MEP	Maximal expiratory pressure
MIP	Maximal inspiratory pressure
NS	Non-sarcopenic individuals
PEF	Peak expiratory flow
RMS	Respiratory muscle strength
S	Sarcopenic individuals
Sat O_2	Oxyhemoglobinic saturation
SD	Standard deviation
VC	Vital capacity

References

1. Cruz-Jentoft, A.J.; Bahat, G.; Bauer, J.; Boirie, Y.; Bruyère, O.; Cederholm, T.; Cooper, C.; Landi, F.; Rolland, Y.; Sayer, A.A.; et al. Sarcopenia: Revised {European} consensus on definition and diagnosis. *Age Ageing* **2019**, *48*, 16–31. [CrossRef] [PubMed]
2. Cruz-Jentoft, A.J.; Baeyens, J.P.; Bauer, J.M.; Boirie, Y.; Cederholm, T.; Landi, F.; Martin, F.C.; Michel, J.P.; Rolland, Y.; Schneider, S.M.; et al. Sarcopenia: European consensus on definition and diagnosis. *Age Ageing* **2010**, *39*, 412–423. [CrossRef] [PubMed]
3. Elliott, J.E.; Greising, S.M.; Mantilla, C.B.; Sieck, G.C. Functional impact of sarcopenia in respiratory muscles. *Respir. Physiol. Neurobiol.* **2016**, *226*, 137–146. [CrossRef] [PubMed]
4. Ohara, D.G.; Pegorari, M.S.; Oliveira dos Santos, N.L.; de Fátima Ribeiro Silva, C.; Monteiro, R.L.; Matos, A.P.; Jamami, M. Respiratory Muscle Strength as a Discriminator of Sarcopenia in Community-Dwelling Elderly: A Cross-Sectional Study. *J. Nutr. Health Aging* **2018**, *22*, 952–958. [CrossRef] [PubMed]
5. Papadopoulou, S.K.; Tsintavis, P.; Potsaki, G.; Papandreou, D. Differences in the Prevalence of Sarcopenia in Community-Dwelling, Nursing Home and Hospitalized Individuals. A Systematic Review and Meta-Analysis. *J. Nutr. Heal. Aging* **2020**, *24*, 83–90. [CrossRef]
6. Rodríguez-Rejón, A.I.; Ruiz-López, M.D.; Wanden-Berghe, C.; Artacho, R. Prevalence and Diagnosis of Sarcopenia in Residential Facilities: A Systematic Review. *Adv. Nutr.* **2019**, *10*, 51–58. [CrossRef]
7. Shen, Y.; Chen, J.; Chen, X.; Hou, L.S.; Lin, X.; Yang, M. Prevalence and Associated Factors of Sarcopenia in Nursing Home Residents: A Systematic Review and Meta-analysis. *J. Am. Med. Dir. Assoc.* **2019**, *20*, 5–13. [CrossRef]
8. Bravo-José, P.; Moreno, E.; Espert, M.; Romeu, M.; Martínez, P.; Navarro, C. Prevalence of sarcopenia and associated factors in institutionalised older adult patients. *Clin. Nutr. ESPEN* **2018**, *27*, 113–119. [CrossRef]
9. Kovacs, E.; Lowery, E.; Kuhlmann, E.; Brubaker, A. The aging lung. *Clin. Interv. Aging* **2013**, *8*, 1489. [CrossRef]
10. Skloot, G.S. The Effects of Aging on Lung Structure and Function. *Clin. Geriatr. Med.* **2017**, *33*, 447–457. [CrossRef]
11. Conn, P.M. *Handbook of Models for Human Aging*; Elsevier Academic Press: Cambridge, MA, USA, 2006; ISBN 9780080460062.
12. Sharma, G.; Goodwin, J. Effect of aging on respiratory system physiology and immunology. *Clin. Interv. Aging* **2006**, *1*, 253–260. [CrossRef]
13. Vaz Fragoso, C.A.; Gahbauer, E.A.; Van Ness, P.H.; Concato, J.; Gill, T.M. Peak Expiratory Flow as a Predictor of Subsequent Disability and Death in Community-Living Older Persons. *J. Am. Geriatr. Soc.* **2008**, *56*, 1014–1020. [CrossRef]
14. Roberts, M.H.; Mapel, D.W. Limited Lung Function: Impact of Reduced Peak Expiratory Flow on Health Status, Health-Care Utilization, and Expected Survival in Older Adults. *Am. J. Epidemiol.* **2012**, *176*, 127–134. [CrossRef] [PubMed]
15. Ida, S.; Watanabe, M.; Yoshida, N.; Baba, Y.; Umezaki, N.; Harada, K.; Karashima, R.; Imamura, Y.; Iwagami, S.; Baba, H. Sarcopenia is a Predictor of Postoperative Respiratory Complications in Patients with Esophageal Cancer. *Ann. Surg. Oncol.* **2015**, *22*, 4432–4437. [CrossRef] [PubMed]
16. Zhang, S.; Tan, S.; Jiang, Y.; Xi, Q.; Meng, Q.; Zhuang, Q.; Han, Y.; Sui, X.; Wu, G. Sarcopenia as a predictor of poor surgical and oncologic outcomes after abdominal surgery for digestive tract cancer: A prospective cohort study. *Clin. Nutr.* **2018**. [CrossRef] [PubMed]
17. Nishigori, T.; Okabe, H.; Tanaka, E.; Tsunoda, S.; Hisamori, S.; Sakai, Y. Sarcopenia as a predictor of pulmonary complications after esophagectomy for thoracic esophageal cancer. *J. Surg. Oncol.* **2016**, *113*, 678–684. [CrossRef]
18. Maeda, K.; Akagi, J. Muscle Mass Loss Is a Potential Predictor of 90-Day Mortality in Older Adults with Aspiration Pneumonia. *J. Am. Geriatr. Soc.* **2017**, *65*, e18–e22. [CrossRef]
19. Izawa, K.P.; Watanabe, S.; Oka, K.; Kasahara, Y.; Morio, Y.; Hiraki, K.; Hirano, Y.; Omori, Y.; Suzuki, N.; Kida, K.; et al. Respiratory muscle strength in relation to sarcopenia in elderly cardiac patients. *Aging Clin. Exp. Res.* **2016**, *28*, 1143–1148. [CrossRef]
20. Omran, M.L.; Morley, J.E. Assessment of protein energy malnutrition in older persons, part II: Laboratory evaluation. *Nutrition* **2000**, *16*, 131–140. [CrossRef]

21. Zhang, Z.; Pereira, S.L.; Luo, M.; Matheson, E.M. Evaluation of blood biomarkers associated with risk of malnutrition in older adults: A systematic review and meta-analysis. *Nutrients* **2017**, *9*, 829. [CrossRef]
22. Li, S.; Zhang, J.; Zheng, H.; Wang, X.; Liu, Z.; Sun, T. Prognostic Role of Serum Albumin, Total Lymphocyte Count, and Mini Nutritional Assessment on Outcomes After Geriatric Hip Fracture Surgery: A Meta-Analysis and Systematic Review. *J. Arthroplast.* **2019**, *34*, 1287–1296. [CrossRef] [PubMed]
23. Shakersain, B.; Santoni, G.; Faxén-Irving, G.; Rizzuto, D.; Fratiglioni, L.; Xu, W. Nutritional status and survival among old adults: An 11-year population-based longitudinal study. *Eur. J. Clin. Nutr.* **2016**, *70*, 320–325. [CrossRef] [PubMed]
24. Zelada Rodríguez, M.A.; Gómez-Pavón, J.; Sorando Fernández, P.; Franco Salinas, A.; Mercedes Guzmán, L.; Baztán, J.J. Fiabilidad interobservador de los 4 índices de comorbilidad más utilizados en pacientes ancianos. *Rev. Esp. Geriatr. Gerontol.* **2012**, *47*, 67–70. [CrossRef]
25. Charlson, M.E.; Pompei, P.; Ales, K.L.; MacKenzie, C.R. A new method of classifying prognostic comorbidity in longitudinal studies: Development and validation. *J. Chronic Dis.* **1987**, *40*, 373–383. [CrossRef]
26. Miller, M.R.; Hankinson, J.; Brusasco, V.; Burgos, F.; Casaburi, R.; Coates, A.; Crapo, R.; Enright, P.; van der Grinten, C.P.M.; Gustafsson, P.; et al. Standardisation of spirometry. *Eur. Respir. J.* **2005**, *26*, 319–338. [CrossRef] [PubMed]
27. American Thoracic Society. ATS/ERS Statement on respiratory muscle testing. *Am. J. Respir. Crit. Care Med.* **2002**, *166*, 518–624. [CrossRef]
28. Laveneziana, P.; Albuquerque, A.; Aliverti, A.; Babb, T.; Barreiro, E.; Dres, M.; Dubé, B.P.; Fauroux, B.; Gea, J.; Guenette, J.A.; et al. ERS statement on respiratory muscle testing at rest and during exercise. *Eur. Respir. J.* **2019**, *53*. [CrossRef]
29. Roberts, H.C.; Denison, H.J.; Martin, H.J.; Patel, H.P.; Syddall, H.; Cooper, C.; Sayer, A.A. A review of the measurement of grip strength in clinical and epidemiological studies: Towards a standardised approach. *Age Ageing* **2011**, *40*, 423–429. [CrossRef]
30. Studenski, S.; Perera, S.; Patel, K.; Rosano, C.; Faulkner, K.; Inzitari, M.; Brach, J.; Chandler, J.; Cawthon, P.; Connor, E.B.; et al. Gait speed and survival in older adults. *JAMA J. Am. Med. Assoc.* **2011**, *305*, 50–58. [CrossRef]
31. Janssen, I.; Heymsfield, S.B.; Baumgartner, R.N.; Ross, R. Estimation of skeletal muscle mass by bioelectrical impedance analysis. *J. Appl. Physiol.* **2000**, *89*, 465–471. [CrossRef]
32. Martínez-Arnau, F.M.; Fonfría-Vivas, R.; Buigues, C.; Castillo, Y.; Molina, P.; Hoogland, A.J.; van Doesburg, F.; Pruimboom, L.; Fernández-Garrido, J.; Cauli, O. Effects of leucine administration in sarcopenia: A randomized and placebo-controlled clinical trial. *Nutrients* **2020**, *12*, 932. [CrossRef] [PubMed]
33. Masanés, F.; Rojano i Luque, X.; Salvà, A.; Serra-Rexach, J.A.; Artaza, I.; Formiga, F.; Cuesta, F.; López Soto, A.; Ruiz, D.; Cruz-Jentoft, A.J. Cut-off points for muscle mass—not grip strength or gait speed—determine variations in sarcopenia prevalence. *J. Nutr. Heal. Aging* **2017**, *21*, 825–829. [CrossRef]
34. Liu, X.; Hou, L.; Xia, X.; Liu, Y.; Zuo, Z.; Zhang, Y.; Zhao, W.; Hao, Q.; Yue, J.; Dong, B. Prevalence of sarcopenia in multi ethnics adults and the association with cognitive impairment: Findings from West-China health and aging trend study. *BMC Geriatr.* **2020**, *20*. [CrossRef] [PubMed]
35. Kera, T.; Kawai, H.; Hirano, H.; Kojima, M.; Watanabe, Y.; Motokawa, K.; Fujiwara, Y.; Ihara, K.; Kim, H.; Obuchi, S. Definition of Respiratory Sarcopenia With Peak Expiratory Flow Rate. *J. Am. Med. Dir. Assoc.* **2019**, *20*, 1021–1025. [CrossRef] [PubMed]
36. Bahat, G.; Tufan, A.; Ozkaya, H.; Tufan, F.; Akpinar, T.S.; Akin, S.; Bahat, Z.; Kaya, Z.; Kiyan, E.; Erten, N.; et al. Relation between hand grip strength, respiratory muscle strength and spirometric measures in male nursing home residents. *Aging Male* **2014**, *17*, 136–140. [CrossRef]
37. Schramm, C.M. Current concepts of respiratory complications of neuromuscular disease in children. *Curr. Opin. Pediatr.* **2000**, *12*, 203–207. [CrossRef] [PubMed]
38. Kang, S.W.; Bach, J.R. Maximum insufflation capacity: Vital capacity and cough flows in neuromuscular disease. *Am. J. Phys. Med. Rehabil.* **2000**, *79*, 222–227. [CrossRef] [PubMed]
39. Lowery, E.M.; Brubaker, A.L.; Kuhlmann, E.; Kovacs, E.J. The aging lung. *Clin. Interv. Aging* **2013**, *8*, 1489–1496. [PubMed]
40. Lalley, P.M. The aging respiratory system-Pulmonary structure, function and neural control. *Respir. Physiol. Neurobiol.* **2013**, *187*, 199–210. [CrossRef]

41. Schmidt-Nowara, W.W.; Altman, A.R. Atelectasis and neuromuscular respiratory failure. *Chest* **1984**, *85*, 792–795. [CrossRef]
42. Kera, T.; Kawai, H.; Hirano, H.; Kojima, M.; Fujiwara, Y.; Ihara, K.; Obuchi, S. Relationships among peak expiratory flow rate, body composition, physical function, and sarcopenia in community-dwelling older adults. *Aging Clin. Exp. Res.* **2018**, *30*, 331–340. [CrossRef] [PubMed]
43. Janssens, J.P.; Pache, J.C.; Nicod, L.P. Physiological changes in respiratory function associated with ageing. *Eur. Respir. J.* **1999**, *13*, 197–205. [CrossRef] [PubMed]
44. Elagizi, A.; Kachur, S.; Lavie, C.J.; Carbone, S.; Pandey, A.; Ortega, F.B.; Milani, R.V. An Overview and Update on Obesity and the Obesity Paradox in Cardiovascular Diseases. *Prog. Cardiovasc. Dis.* **2018**, *61*, 142–150. [CrossRef] [PubMed]
45. Do, J.G.; Park, C.H.; Lee, Y.T.; Yoon, K.J. Association between underweight and pulmonary function in 282,135 healthy adults: A cross-sectional study in Korean population. *Sci. Rep.* **2019**, *9*, 14308. [CrossRef] [PubMed]
46. Jeon, Y.K.; Shin, M.J.; Kim, M.H.; Mok, J.H.; Kim, S.S.; Kim, B.H.; Kim, S.J.; Kim, Y.K.; Chang, J.H.; Shin, Y.B.; et al. Low pulmonary function is related with a high risk of sarcopenia in community-dwelling older adults: The Korea National Health and Nutrition Examination Survey (KNHANES) 2008–2011. *Osteoporos. Int.* **2015**, *26*, 2423–2429. [CrossRef] [PubMed]
47. Park, C.H.; Yi, Y.; Do, J.G.; Lee, Y.T.; Yoon, K.J. Relationship between skeletal muscle mass and lung function in Korean adults without clinically apparent lung disease. *Medicine* **2018**, *97*. [CrossRef]
48. Yanek, L.R.; Vaidya, D.; Kral, B.G.; Dobrosielski, D.A.; Moy, T.F.; Stewart, K.J.; Becker, D.M. Lean Mass and Fat Mass as Contributors to Physical Fitness in an Overweight and Obese African American Population. *Ethn Dis.* **2015**, *25*, 214–219.
49. Carbone, S.; Billingsley, H.E.; Rodriguez-Miguelez, P.; Kirkman, D.L.; Garten, R.; Franco, R.L.; Lee, D.-C.; Lavie, C.J. Lean Mass Abnormalities in Heart Failure: The Role of Sarcopenia, Sarcopenic Obesity, and Cachexia. *Curr. Probl. Cardiol.* **2019**, 100417. [CrossRef]
50. Magnani, K.L.; Cataneo, A.J.M. Respiratory muscle strength in obese individuals and influence of upper-body fat distribution. *Sao Paulo Med. J.* **2007**, *125*, 215–219. [CrossRef]
51. Lin, C.K.; Lin, C.C. Work of breathing and respiratory drive in obesity. *Respirology* **2012**, *17*, 402–411. [CrossRef]
52. Lima, T.R.L.; Almeida, V.P.; Ferreira, A.S.; Guimarães, F.S.; Lopes, A.J. Handgrip strength and pulmonary disease in the elderly: What is the link? *Aging Dis.* **2019**, *10*, 1109–1129. [CrossRef] [PubMed]
53. iee Shin, H.; Kim, D.K.; Seo, K.M.; Kang, S.H.; Lee, S.Y.; Son, S. Relation between respiratory muscle strength and skeletal muscle mass and hand grip strength in the healthy elderly. *Ann. Rehabil. Med.* **2017**, *41*, 686–692. [CrossRef] [PubMed]
54. Sawaya, Y.; Ishizaka, M.; Kubo, A.; Sadakiyo, K.; Yakabi, A.; Sato, T.; Shiba, T.; Onoda, K.; Maruyama, H. Correlation between skeletal muscle mass index and parameters of respiratory function and muscle strength in young healthy adults according to gender. *J. Phys. Ther. Sci.* **2018**, *30*, 1424–1427. [CrossRef]
55. Peterson, S.J.; Park, J.; Zellner, H.K.; Moss, O.A.; Welch, A.; Sclamberg, J.; Moran, E.; Hicks-McGarry, S.; Becker, E.A.; Foley, S. Relationship Between Respiratory Muscle Strength, Handgrip Strength, and Muscle Mass in Hospitalized Patients. *J. Parenter. Enter. Nutr.* **2019**. [CrossRef] [PubMed]
56. Chowdhury, M.S.I.; Rahman, A.Z.; Haque, M.; Nahar, N.; Taher, A. Serum Aspartate Aminotransferase (AST) and Alanine Aminotransferase (ALT) Levels in Different Grades of Protein Energy Malnutrition. *J. Bangladesh Soc. Physiol.* **1970**, *2*, 17–19. [CrossRef]
57. Karaphillis, E.; Goldstein, R.; Murphy, S.; Qayyum, R. Serum alanine aminotransferase levels and all-cause mortality. *Eur. J. Gastroenterol. Hepatol.* **2017**, *29*, 284–288. [CrossRef]
58. Nathwani, R.A.; Pais, S.; Reynolds, T.B.; Kaplowitz, N. Serum alanine aminotransferase in skeletal muscle diseases. *Hepatology* **2005**, *41*, 380–382. [CrossRef]
59. Malakouti, M.; Kataria, A.; Ali, S.K.; Schenker, S. Elevated Liver Enzymes in Asymptomatic Patients—What Should I Do? *J. Clin. Transl. Hepatol.* **2017**, *5*, 1–10. [CrossRef]
60. Shibata, M.; Nakajima, K.; Higuchi, R.; Iwane, T.; Sugiyama, M.; Nakamura , T. Nakamura High Concentration of Serum Aspartate Aminotransferase in Older Underweight People: Results of the Kanagawa Investigation of the Total Check-Up Data from the National Database-2 (KITCHEN-2). *J. Clin. Med.* **2019**, *8*, 1282. [CrossRef]

61. Zamboni, M.; Mazzali, G.; Fantin, F.; Rossi, A.; Di Francesco, V. Sarcopenic obesity: A new category of obesity in the elderly. *Nutr. Metab. Cardiovasc. Dis.* **2008**, *18*, 388–395. [CrossRef]
62. Stenholm, S.; Harris, T.B.; Rantanen, T.; Visser, M.; Kritchevsky, S.B.; Ferrucci, L. Sarcopenic obesity: Definition, cause and consequences. *Curr. Opin. Clin. Nutr. Metab. Care* **2008**, *11*, 693–700. [CrossRef] [PubMed]
63. Haines, R.W.; Zolfaghari, P.; Wan, Y.; Pearse, R.M.; Puthucheary, Z.; Prowle, J.R. Elevated urea-to-creatinine ratio provides a biochemical signature of muscle catabolism and persistent critical illness after major trauma. *Intensive Care Med.* **2019**, *45*, 1718–1731. [CrossRef] [PubMed]
64. Lattanzi, B.; D'Ambrosio, D.; Merli, M. Hepatic Encephalopathy and Sarcopenia: Two Faces of the Same Metabolic Alteration. *J. Clin. Exp. Hepatol.* **2019**, *9*, 125–130. [CrossRef] [PubMed]
65. Kang, Y.J.; Yoo, J.I.; Ha, Y.C. Sarcopenia feature selection and risk prediction using machine learning: A cross-sectional study. *Medicine* **2019**, *98*, e17699. [CrossRef]
66. Macchi, C.; Molino-Lova, R.; Polcaro, P.; Guarducci, L.; Lauretani, F.; Cecchi, F.; Bandinelli, S.; Guralnik, J.M.; Ferrucci, L. Higher circulating levels of uric acid are prospectively associated with better muscle function in older persons. *Mech. Ageing Dev.* **2008**, *129*, 522–527. [CrossRef]
67. Can, B.; Kara, O.; Kizilarslanoglu, M.C.; Arik, G.; Aycicek, G.S.; Sumer, F.; Civelek, R.; Demirtas, C.; Ulger, Z. Serum markers of inflammation and oxidative stress in sarcopenia. *Aging Clin. Exp. Res.* **2017**, *29*, 745–752. [CrossRef]
68. Molino-Lova, R.; Sofi, F.; Pasquini, G.; Vannetti, F.; Del Ry, S.; Vassalle, C.; Clerici, M.; Sorbi, S.; Macchi, C. Higher uric acid serum levels are associated with better muscle function in the oldest old: Results from the Mugello Study. *Eur. J. Intern. Med.* **2017**, *41*, 39–43. [CrossRef]
69. Batsis, J.A.; Villareal, D.T. Sarcopenic obesity in older adults: Aetiology, epidemiology and treatment strategies. *Nat. Rev. Endocrinol.* **2018**, *14*, 513–537. [CrossRef]
70. Carnio, S.; LoVerso, F.; Baraibar, M.A.; Longa, E.; Khan, M.M.; Maffei, M.; Reischl, M.; Canepari, M.; Loefler, S.; Kern, H.; et al. Autophagy Impairment in Muscle Induces Neuromuscular Junction Degeneration and Precocious Aging. *Cell Rep.* **2014**, *8*, 1509–1521. [CrossRef]
71. Baek, S.J.; Nam, G.E.; Han, K.D.; Choi, S.W.; Jung, S.W.; Bok, A.R.; Kim, Y.H.; Lee, K.S.; Han, B.D.; Kim, D.H. Sarcopenia and sarcopenic obesity and their association with dyslipidemia in Korean elderly men: The 2008-2010 Korea National Health and Nutrition Examination Survey. *J. Endocrinol. Investig.* **2014**, *37*, 247–260. [CrossRef]
72. Mesinovic, J.; McMillan, L.; Shore-Lorenti, C.; De Courten, B.; Ebeling, P.; Scott, D. Metabolic Syndrome and Its Associations with Components of Sarcopenia in Overweight and Obese Older Adults. *J. Clin. Med.* **2019**, *8*, 145. [CrossRef] [PubMed]
73. Lu, C.W.; Yang, K.C.; Chang, H.H.; Lee, L.T.; Chen, C.Y.; Huang, K.C. Sarcopenic obesity is closely associated with metabolic syndrome. *Obes. Res. Clin. Pract.* **2013**, *7*. [CrossRef] [PubMed]
74. Buchman, A.S.; Boyle, P.A.; Wilson, R.S.; Leurgans, S.; Shah, R.C.; Bennett, D.A. Respiratory muscle strength predicts decline in mobility in older persons. *Neuroepidemiology* **2008**, *31*, 174–180. [CrossRef] [PubMed]
75. Kim, J.; Davenport, P.; Sapienza, C. Effect of expiratory muscle strength training on elderly cough function. *Arch. Gerontol. Geriatr.* **2009**, *48*, 361–366. [CrossRef]
76. Kim, J.; Sapienza, C.M. Implications of expiratory muscle strength training for rehabilitation of the elderly: Tutorial. *J. Rehabil. Res. Dev.* **2005**, *42*, 211–223. [CrossRef]
77. Laghi, F.; Tobin, M.J. Disorders of the respiratory muscles. *Am. J. Respir. Crit. Care Med.* **2003**, *168*, 10–48. [CrossRef]
78. Meek, P.M.; Schwartzstein, R.M.; Adams, L.; Altose, M.D.; Breslin, E.H.; Carrieri-Kohlman, V.; Gift, A.; Hanley, M.V.; Harver, A.; Jones, P.W.; et al. Dyspnea: Mechanisms, assessment, and management: A consensus statement. *Am. J. Respir. Crit. Care Med.* **1999**, *159*, 321–340.
79. Caruso, P.; De Albuquerque, A.L.P.; Santana, P.V.; Cardenas, L.Z.; Ferreira, J.G.; Prina, E.; Trevizan, P.F.; Pereira, M.C.; Iamonti, V.; Pletsch, R.; et al. Métodos diagnósticos para avaliação da força muscular inspiratória e expiratória. *J. Bras. Pneumol.* **2015**, *41*, 110–123. [CrossRef]

13

Rehabilitation Strategies for Patients with Femoral Neck Fractures in Sarcopenia

Marianna Avola [1], Giulia Rita Agata Mangano [1], Gianluca Testa [2,*], Sebastiano Mangano [2], Andrea Vescio [2], Vito Pavone [2] and Michele Vecchio [1]

1 Department of Biomedical and Biotechnological Sciences, Section of Pharmacology, University Hospital Policlinico-San Marco University of Catania, 95123 Catania, Italy; mariannaavola.md@gmail.com (M.A.); giuliarita.mangano@gmail.com (G.R.A.M.); michele.vecchio@unict.it (M.V.)

2 Department of General Surgery and Medical Surgical Specialties, Section of Orthopaedics and Traumatology, University Hospital Policlinico-San Marco, University of Catania, 95123 Catania, Italy; sebymangano@hotmail.com (S.M.); andreavescio88@gmail.com (A.V.); vitopavone@hotmail.com (V.P.)

* Correspondence: gianpavel@hotmail.com

Abstract: Sarcopenia is defined as a syndrome characterized by progressive and generalized loss of skeletal muscle mass and strength. It has been identified as one of the most common comorbidities associated with femoral neck fracture (FNF). The aim of this review was to evaluate the impact of physical therapy on FNF patients' function and rehabilitation. The selected articles were randomized controlled trials (RCTs), published in the last 10 years. Seven full texts were eligible for this review: three examined the impact of conventional rehabilitation and nutritional supplementation, three evaluated the effects of rehabilitation protocols compared to new methods and a study explored the intervention with erythropoietin (EPO) in sarcopenic patients with FNF and its potential effects on postoperative rehabilitation. Physical activity and dietary supplementation are the basic tools of prevention and rehabilitation of sarcopenia in elderly patients after hip surgery. The most effective physical therapy seems to be exercise of progressive resistance. Occupational therapy should be included in sarcopenic patients for its importance in cognitive rehabilitation. Erythropoietin and bisphosphonates could represent medical therapy resources.

Keywords: sarcopenia; elderly; frailty; fractures; ageing fractures; complications; recovery; rehabilitation; nutritional supplements; physical therapy

1. Introduction

Sarcopenia is defined as a syndrome characterized by progressive and generalized loss of skeletal muscle mass and strength, with risk of adverse outcomes such as physical disability, poor quality of life and death. [1] Prevalence of sarcopenia varies among age groups, geographic regions and evaluated context. Estimated prevalence is 1% to 29% in community-dwelling older people, 14% to 33% in long-term care and 10% in acute hospital care populations [2,3]. Starting from 40 years of age, each ten years, healthy adults lose approximately 8% of their muscle mass. Moreover, between 40 and 70 years old, healthy adults lose an average of 24% of muscle, which accelerates to 15% per decade past the age of 70. [4] The diagnosis of sarcopenia should be based on concomitant presence of low muscle mass and low muscle function [4,5].

The European Working Group on Sarcopenia in Older People (EWGSOP) defined sarcopenia as an acute or chronic disease based on low levels three measured parameters: muscle strength, muscle quantity/quality and physical performance, as an indicator of its severity [1,6].

Early sarcopenia is characterized by size reduction in muscle. Gradually, it also occurs as a decrease in the quality of muscle tissue, which leads to loss of functionality and fragility [7,8]. The assessment of sarcopenia requires objective measurements of muscle strength and muscle mass. Several methods of evaluation for sarcopenia considered walking speed, the circumference of the calf, the analysis of bioimpedance, grip strength and DEXA imaging methods. However, none of these measurements are sufficiently sensitive or specific [8–10]. Sarcopenia has been identified as one of the most common comorbidities associated with femoral neck fracture (FNF) patients [11]. Among these different comorbidities, apart from Sarcopenia, protein-energy malnutrition has been reported in 20 to 85 % of cases, depending on age and gender [12,13]. Besides the age-related loss of muscle mass, trauma mechanism, and consequent associated immobilization, cause negative adjustment in body composition. Bed confinement, and the reduced mobility of hospitalized older patients, are associated with loss of muscle mass, muscle function and bone mineral density from the 10th day, and up to two months, after the fracture [13,14]. During the first year from fracture, about 5–6% of muscle mass may be lost [15,16]. It was reported that 28% of patients who were outpatients before hip fracture were unable to walk 12 months after surgery, while as many as 25–30% of patients were unable to return to their previous situation. [16–18].

Treatment of sarcopenia is mainly nonpharmacological. First, an adequate nutrition to ensure the intake of micronutrients and macronutrients is needed. Calories should be 24 to 36 kcal/kg per day; a minimum daily protein intake of 1.0 g/kg body weight, up to 1.5 g spread equally over three meals and maintenance of serum vitamin D levels to 100 nmol/L (40 ng/mL) from vitamin D–rich diet or vitamin D supplementation. Supplementation with creatine monohydrate, antioxidants, amino acid metabolites, omega-3 fatty acids and other compounds are being studied [3]. A crucial role is played by physical activity, especially resistance training, which is the key element for increasing muscle strength and physical performance. Currently, the strategy of combined nutrition supplementation and exercise appears encouraging in the management of sarcopenia.

The aim of this review is to evaluate the impact of rehabilitation with or without other interventions, including nutritional supplementation and pharmacological therapy, on indicators of sarcopenia for FNF (femoral neck fracture) patients.

2. Experimental Section

2.1. Literature Search Strategy

To find clinical trials involving the rehabilitation of sarcopenia and FNF, two authors (M.A, G.R.A.M.) searched in three medical databases (PubMed, Cochrane Library and PEDro) during the month of June 2020. The terms used for the research were sarcopenia and hip fracture and rehabilitation.

2.2. Selection Criteria

The selected articles had to be published in the last 10 years, written in the English language and had to be randomized controlled trials (RCT), observational studies or cases reports published in peer reviewed journals. The authors excluded articles written in other languages, studies with no results or subjects involved and reviews about the topic. Papers with no accessible data, or no available full texts, were also excluded. M.A. and G.R.A.M. selected the studies independently, resolving any discrepancies about the selection by discussion. The senior investigator (M.V.) was consulted to revise the selection process.

3. Results

3.1. Search Progress and Data Extraction

A total of 74 articles were selected based on their titles. Excluding doubles, 63 articles were screened upon their titles. At the end of this screening, 14 abstracts were selected and read independently by the two authors. Five abstracts were excluded: three were not trials, two were reviews and one did not assess sarcopenia in the subjects studied. The authors screened and read eight full texts, one of which was excluded, being a rehabilitation protocol without results on patients.

Every full text was examined, and characteristics of the study, study sample, type of rehabilitation and treatment, outcome measures and results were extracted from the full text and summarized in Table 1.

Table 1. Characteristics of examined studies.

Author	Study Type	Treatment	Type of Fracture	Sample Size	Outcome Measures	Results/Conclusions
Flodin et al. 2015	Randomized controlled study	40 g of protein and 600 kcal combined with risedronate and calcium 1 g and vit D 800 IE (group N); risedronate and calcium 1 g and vit D 800 IE (group B); calcium 1 g and vit D 800 IE (group C). All groups received conventional rehabilitation	Femoral neck or Trochanteric fracture	79 patients: 56 women (71 %), 23 men (29 %); Mean age 79 (SD 9, range 61–96 years)	Body composition, Hand grip strength (HGS), Health-related quality of life (HRQoL)	No differences among the groups regarding change in fat-free mass index (FFMI), HGS, or HRQoL. Intra-group analyses showed improvement of HGS between baseline and six months in the N group ($p = 0.04$). HRQoL decreased during the first year in the C and B groups ($p = 0.03$ and $p = 0.01$, respectively) but not in the nutritional supplementation N group ($p = 0.22$).
Invernizzi et al. 2018	Randomized controlled study	Two groups (A and B). Both groups performed a physical exercise rehabilitative program and received dietetic counseling; only group A was supplemented with two sachets of 4 g/day of essential amino acids.	Osteoporotic hip fracture	32 patients aged more than 65 years (mean aged 79.03 ± 7.80 years) divided in two groups. Patients in both groups were divided into sarcopenic and nonsarcopenic.	Hand grip strength test (HGS), Timed Up and Go test (TUG), Iowa Level of Assistance scale (ILOA), Nutritional assessment, Health-related quality of life (HRQoL). All the outcome measures were assessed at baseline (T0) and after two months of treatment (T1)	Sarcopenic patients in group A showed statistically significant differences in all the outcomes at T1 ($p < 0.017$), whereas sarcopenic patients in group B showed a significant reduction of ILOA only. In nonsarcopenic patients, no differences at T1 in all outcome measures.
Lim et al. 2018	Prospective Observational Study	FIRM (Fragility Fracture Integrated Rehabilitation Management)	Femoral neck, Intertrochanteric, or Subtrochanteric fracture.	68 patients; M = 15, F = 53 Sarcopenia (n = 32): Age 81.66 ± 7.49; Nonsarcopenia (n = 36): Age 79.81 ± 5.95	KOVAL, FAC, (primary) MMRI, BBS, MMSE, K-GDS, EQ-5D, K-MBI, K-IADL, K-FRAIL scale (secondary)	The primary outcomes improved significantly in both sarcopenic and nonsarcopenic patients. Mobility, balance, cognitive functioning and quality of life improved in both groups, K-IADL ($p = 0.029$) and K-FRAIL ($p = 0.023$) scores were significantly improved in only the nonsarcopenia group after rehabilitation.

Table 1. *Cont.*

Author	Study Type	Treatment	Type of Fracture	Sample Size	Outcome Measures	Results/Conclusions
Lim et al. 2019	Prospective Observational Study	FIRM (Fragility Fracture Integrated Rehabilitation Management)	Femoral neck, Intertrochanteric, or Subtrochanteric fracture.	80 patients; M = 18, F = 62 Sarcopenia (n = 35): Age 82.8 ± 7.5 Nonsarcopenia (n = 45): Age 79.7 ± 6.5	KOVAL, FAC, (primary) MMRI, BBS, MMSE, K-GDS, EQ-5D, K-MBI, K-IADL, K-FRAIL scale, HGS (secondary)	Koval and FAC scores improved over time ($p < 0.001$). The two groups did not differ in terms of the time course of improvement in Koval scores. There was no difference between the groups regarding the time course for improvement in FAC scores after discharge. All secondary functional outcomes, except for HGS, significantly improved over time in both the sarcopenia and nonsarcopenia groups, even though the functional status of the sarcopenia group was lower at both the three- and six month follow-up evaluations. However, the two groups did not differ significantly in terms of final functional status
Malafarina et al. 2017	Multicentre randomized trial	Standard diet (1500 kcal, 23.3% protein (87.4 g/day), 35.5% fat (59.3 g/day) and 41.2% carbo- hydrates (154.8 g/day) plus oral nutritional supplementation (ONS) enriched with CaHMB 0.7 g/100 mL, 25(OH)D 227 IU/100 mL and 227 mg/100 mL of calcium. (Intervention Group (IG); Standard diet only (Control group CG). All patients received Physical therapy	Various type of hip fracture	107 patients aged 65 years and over (mean age 85.4 ± 6.3, 74% female)	Body composition, Hand grip strength (HGS), Mini Nutritional Assessment—Short Form (MNA-SF), Barthel index (BI), Functional Ambulation Categories (FAC) score	BMI and lean mass were stable in IG patients, while decreased in the CG. The concentration of proteins and vitamin D increased more in the IG than in the CG. The recovery of ADL was more common in the IG (68%) than in the CG (59%) ($p = 0.261$)

Table 1. *Cont.*

Author	Study Type	Treatment	Type of Fracture	Sample Size	Outcome Measures	Results/Conclusions
Min-Kyun et al. 2020	Randomized Control Double-Blinded Trial	Antigravity Treadmill (Cxperimental Group) Conventional Rehabilitation (Control Group)	Femoral neck, Intertrochanteric, or Subtrochanteric fracture.	38 Patients; M = 12, F = 26 65–90 years old;	KOVAL (primary), FAC, BBS, Korean version of MMSE, EQ-5D, K-MBI, HGS (secondary)	Higher and longer improvement in KOVAL, FAC score, BBS, EQ-5D, and K-MBI in experimental group. The comparison of change scores in BBS between the two groups revealed a between-group difference of 11.63 (95% CI: 5.85, 17.40; p for trend = 0.001), 9.00 (95% CI: 2.28, 15.71; p for trend = 0.006), and 11.05 (95% CI: 3.62, 18.48; p for trend = 0.006), respectively. In the EQ-5D and KMBI, the experimental group showed an improvement of 0.49 and 32.63 scores, respectively, compared with 0.23 and 16.00, respectively, by the control group in the three weeks. The comparison of change scores in EQ-5D and K-MBI between the two groups revealed a between-group difference of 0.25 (95% CI: 0.10, 0.41; p for trend = 0.005) and 16.63 (95% CI: 4.80, 28.45; p for trend = 0.009), respectively.
Zhang et al. 2020	Randomized Control Trial	Recombinant Human Erythropoietin	Femoral Intertrochanteric fracture	141 patients; M = 64 (mean age 76.21 years, SD 7.90 years), F = 77 (mean age 79.16 years, SD 6.65 years)	Handgrip strength, ASM (appendicular skeletal muscle) index and post-operative stay and infection	In females, the handgrip strength during week one (13.9 ± 3.327 kg) became significantly higher in the intervention group than in the control group (9.30 ± 2.812 kg), and the difference was statistically significant ($p < 0.05$). During week two (13.212 ± 3.071) and week four (14.742 ± 3.375), the handgrip strength was consistently higher in the intervention group than in the control group ($p \leq 0.05$).

Table 1. *Cont.*

Author	Study Type	Treatment	Type of Fracture	Sample Size	Outcome Measures	Results/Conclusions
						At the fourth week after EPO intervention, the ASM increment in the female and male intervention group (0.56 ± 0.43 kg,) was significantly higher than the ASM increment (0.24 ± 0.38 kg) in the control group over the fourth week.($p < 0.001$). Infection rate in intervention group was significantly inferior and hospitalization state was significantly shorter.

KOVAL = walking ability scale; FAC = Functional Ambulatory Category; MMRI = modified Rivermead mobility index; BBS = Berg Balance Scale; MMSE = Mini-Mental State Examination; K-GDS = Korean version of the geriatric depression scale; EQ-5D = Euro quality-of-life questionnaire 5-dimensional classification; K-MBI = Korean modified Barthel index; K-IADL = the Korean instrumental activity of daily living.

Upon the seven full texts eligible for this review, three examined the impact of conventional rehabilitation and nutritional supplementation, based on food richness of proteins and aminoacids, on patients affected by sarcopenia following FNF [16,19,20] Three papers evaluated the effects of rehabilitation protocols only, especially comparing new methods to conventional rehabilitation and evaluating the impact of sarcopenia on rehabilitation progress [21–23]. A study explored the intervention with erythropoietin (EPO) in sarcopenic patients with femoral intertrochanteric fractures and its potential effects on postoperative rehabilitation. [24]

3.2. Sarcopenia Diagnosis

Various definitions of sarcopenia have been developed by different international consensus panels, (the Asian Working Group on Sarcopenia (AWGS), the European Working Group on Sarcopenia in Older People (EWGSOP) and the Foundation of the National Institute of Health, International Working Group on Sarcopenia) each defining cut-off values from mobility limitation measures (appendicular skeletal mass index, grip strength and physical performance). In our review, the authors specifically used the diagnostic criteria included in the AWGS [21–25] and EWGSOP [1,16,19,20].

The EWGSOP defines sarcopenia when ASM is less than 20 kg for men and 15 kg for women, ASM/height^2 is less than 7.0 kg/m^2 for men and 5.0 kg/m^2 for women (muscle quantity), grip strength is less than 27 kg for men and 16 kg for women, chair stand > 15 s for five rises (muscle strength), gait speed is no more than 0.8 m/s, short Ppysical performance battery (SPPB) is less than 8 points, timed up and go (TUG) test is less than 20 s and 400 m walk test is completed in more than 6 min or not completed at all (physical performance) [1].

AWGS criteria include decreased handgrip strength (males < 28 kg, females < 18 kg), physical performance evaluated with gait speed ≤ 0.8 m/s or 5-time chair stand test: ≥12 s or short physical performance battery: ≤9, and loss of muscle mass, indexed by appendicular skeletal muscle mass (ASM) divided by height squared evaluated through dual-energy X-ray absorptiometry (M: <7.0 kg/m2, F: <5.4 kg/m^2) or bioelectrical impedance analysis (M: <7.0 kg/m^2, F: <5.7 kg/m^2) [25].

3.3. New Rehabilitation Protocols

In Study 1 (Table 1), the functional outcomes of a new integrated rehabilitation management (FIRM) were assessed in sarcopenic and nonsarcopenic inpatients [21]. Sixty-eight patients (32 Sarcopenic and 36 nonsarcopenic) who had undergone surgery for fragility FNF were included.

FIRM included intensive physical and occupational therapy, fall prevention education with discharge planning and referral to community-based care. After surgery, the patients stayed in hospital with 10 days of physical therapy with two sessions per day and four days of occupational therapy. Physical therapy consisted of weight bearing exercises, strengthening exercises, gait training and aerobic exercise, and functional training progressed gradually based on the individual's functional level. Occupational therapy aimed to train the patients in ADL (transfer, sit to stand, bed mobility, dressing, self-care retraining and using adaptive equipment).

The outcome measures used in the eligible studies were walking ability through two scales: the KOVAL walking ability scale [26] and the functional ambulatory category (FAC) [27]; general mobility; balance and fall risk; cognitive functioning; quality of life; mood; ADL; frailty and handgrip strength of the patients; modified Rivermead mobility index [28]; Berg balance scale [29]; MMSE [30]; Korean version of the geriatric depression scale [31]; the Euro quality-of-life questionnaire 5-dimensional classification [32]; the Korean modified Barthel index [33]; the Korean instrumental ADL [34] and the Korean version of the fatigue, resistance, ambulation, illnesses and loss of weight (FRAIL) scale [35]) at admission to the in-hospital rehabilitation unit and at discharge.

KOVAL and FAC were significantly improved in both sarcopenic and nonsarcopenic patients. Prefacture ambulatory functioning, rather than the presence of sarcopenia, was significantly correlated with short-term recovery of ambulatory functioning. Mobility, balance, cognitive functioning and quality of life improved in both groups, demonstrating the clinical effectiveness of FIRM in sarcopenic patients. In contrast, K-IADL ($p = 0.029$) and K-FRAIL ($p = 0.023$) scores were significantly improved in only the nonsarcopenia group after rehabilitation.

Limitations of this study were the short time after which the outcomes were evaluated (after two weeks of interventions) and the exclusion of several patients before the start of the treatment. The use of the sarcopenia classification itself may have affected the group allocation. Even though the results of Study 1 suggest that FIRM was effective for short-term functional recovery in older patients with or without sarcopenia who have suffered fragility hip fracture, further research comparing FIRM with conventional therapy is needed.

Study 2 (Table 1) [22] evaluated the FIRM program in a prospective observational investigation of 80 patients (35 Sarcopenic and 45 nonsarcopenic) older than 65 after FNF surgery. The author, unlike the previous study, ruled out gait speed from the diagnostic criteria for sarcopenia in the sample evaluated because this result could not be estimated before the fracture or surgery. The FIRM program was administered during two weeks of hospital stay after surgery. All functional outcomes (KOVAL, FAC, EQ-5D, K-IADL, and K-FRAIL) were assessed on admission for rehabilitation, at discharge, and at the three and six months follow-up visits after surgery (or with a telephone interview). In the considered sample, patients with sarcopenia had impairment in cognitive function in a significantly superior percentage than the nonsarcopenic group. Both groups had improvement in the primary outcome (KOVAL) and functional outcome (FAC score) after discharge. Other evaluations, excluded HGS, significantly improved in both groups with no significant difference. Even though sarcopenia was not a predictor of poorer results in ambulatory independence, at six months from surgery, the type of operation and high HGS (handgrip strength) were significantly correlated.

Study 2 [22] demonstrated that ambulation and functional outcomes were improved in patients with or without sarcopenia suffering from fragility after FNF surgery, due to a complete multidisciplinary rehabilitation. Limitations were caused by the assessment of sarcopenia in patients soon after the surgery, namely the time of follow-up that in fragile patients may have been longer, and the lack of a control group following conventional rehabilitation.

Study 3 [23] compared the efficacy of an antigravity treadmill (AGT) combined with conventional physical therapy, and physical therapy alone, in a double-blinded (to outcome) study. Selected patients were 65–90 years old, who had undergone surgery for FNF associated with sarcopenia, according to the AWGS recommendation [25]. Thirty-eight patients included in the primary analysis were treated. One group ($n = 19$) had only standardized rehabilitation treatment for 30 min per day for 10 days, the other ($n = 19$) received standardized treatment plus AGT for 20 min per day. Standardized therapy consisted in passive hip and knee mobilization, strengthening of the hip abductor and extensor muscles, transfer, and gait training on the floor and stairs.

The outcomes evaluated were the same as Studies 1 and 2 [21,22], except for the absence of the I-ADL measurement. The experimental group experienced higher and longer therapeutic effects, with improvement in all outcomes. However, in both groups, KOVAL and FAC scores were slightly improved and then decreased from 3 three to 6 months. This study provided evidence not only that AGT with CR is more effective than only CR for sarcopenic patients, but also that there is a strong association between muscle mass and bone mass, supporting the theory that muscle forces mediate mechanical loading effects on bones [36]. Limitations of Study 3 were the high amount of drop outs after hospital discharge, it was carried out in only one center, and the number of the sample was not sufficient to significantly represent subgroups with different cognitive function, hip fracture and hip operation type.

3.4. *Nutritional Supplements and Physical Therapy*

Study 4 (Table 1) [16] was a randomized controlled study evaluating the effects of combined therapy with bisphosphonate, protein-rich nutritional supplementation and conventional rehabilitation in 79 sarcopenic patients after FNF [16]. Measured parameters were body composition, hand grip strength (HGS) and health-related quality of life (HRQoL). Patients were randomized into three treatment groups. All patients received calcium 1 g and vitamin D 800 I.E. divided into two daily doses for 12 months. The nutritional supplementation group (protein + energy = N group, $n = 26$) received a 200 mL package twice daily, each containing 20 g of protein and 300 kcal. This supplement was given for the first six months after FNF, combined with 35 mg risedronate once weekly for 12 months. The second group (B, $n = 28$) received risedronate alone, 35 mg once weekly for 12 months. The controls (C, $n = 25$) received only calcium and vitamin D for 12 months. Treatment began as soon as the patients were medically stable after surgery, able to take orally administered medications and able to sit upright for one hour after intaking bisphosphonates.

Energy supplementation combined with bisphosphonate, vitamin D and calcium had no positive effect on hand-grip strength, HRQoL, or lean mass, when compared to administration of bisphosphonate along with vitamin D and calcium supplementation, or just vitamin D and calcium supplementation, after FNF. Protein and energy supplementation combined with conventional rehabilitation was not able to preserve lean mass after a hip fracture better than vitamin D and calcium alone or combined with bisphosphonates. There were no intergroup differences concerning effects on HGS or HRQoL, but intragroup improvement in HGS, and a positive effect on HRQoL, were seen in the nutritional supplementation group. A limitation of this study was the small sample size.

In Study 5 (Table 1) [19], 32 patients (23 Sarcopenic, nine nonsarcopenic) aged more than 65 years were enrolled three months after osteoporotic FNF and treated with total hip replacement. The authors evaluated the impact of a two months rehabilitative protocol, combined with dietetic counseling with or without essential aminoacid supplementation, on functioning. Patients were divided into two groups. Patients in group A ($n = 16$, 11 Sarcopenic, five nonsarcopenic) were treated for two months with essential aminoacid supplementation sachets of 4 g per day. Furthemore, patients performed a concomitant specific physical exercise rehabilitative program consisting of five sessions of 40 min each per week for two weeks with the supervision of an experienced physiotherapist, and received dietetic counseling. The physical activity included walking training, resistance and stretching exercises and balance exercises. After these two two weeks, all participants performed a home-based exercise protocol up to the end of the study period, two months from intervention. Patients in group B ($n = 16$, 12 Sarcopenic and four nonsarcopenic) performed the same physical exercise rehabilitative program as group A and received concomitant dietetic counseling alone, without essential amino acid supplementation.

Outcome measures were the hand grip strength test (HGS), physical performance, using the timed up and go test (TUG) [37], level of assistance measured by the Iowa level of assistance scale (ILOA) [38], nutritional assessment, with evaluation of daily caloric intake and daily protein intake, and the health-related quality of life (HRQoL) evaluation. All outcome measures were assessed at baseline (T0) and after two months of treatment (T1). Patients in both groups were divided into sarcopenic and nonsarcopenic patients. All patients in both groups showed statistically significant differences in all primary outcome measures (HGS, TUG, ILOA) at the T1 evaluation ($p < 0.017$). Sarcopenic patients in group A showed statistically significant differences in all primary outcomes (HGS, TUG, ILOA) at T1 ($p < 0.017$), whereas sarcopenic patients in group B showed a significant reduction of ILOA at the end of treatment. On the other hand, in nonsarcopenic patients, they found no differences at T1 in the TUG test and level of assistance test. In both groups, there were no differences at T1 in all other outcome measurements. Furthermore, there were no differences between groups in all outcome measuresments both at baseline and after two months of treatment.

Even though it was performed on a small sample size, data emerging from this study showed a good impact of this combined intervention on function and disability in hip fracture patients after two months of treatment. Essential amino acid supplementation induced considerable improvements in the sarcopenic subpopulation of the study.

Study 6 (Table 1) [20] was a multicentric randomized trial evaluating a nutritional supplement, enriched with β-hydroxy-β-methylbutyrate (HMB), calcium (Ca) and 25-hydroxy-vitamin D (25(OH)D) during rehabilitation therapy to improve muscle mass and, thereby, functional recovery. It included 107 sarcopenic patients aged more than 65 years old with FNF. There were 15 drop-outs during the study. This was the first study to evaluate the effects of HMB in sarcopenic patients with hip fractures. Patients in the intervention group (IG, $n = 49$) received a standard diet plus oral nutritional supplementation enriched with 0.7 g/100 mL of HMB, 227 IU/100 mL of 25(OH)D and 227 mg/100 mL of Ca, while those in the control group (CG, $n = 43$) received a standard diet only. Physical therapy was based on moving patients early, using technical aids, and rehabilitation of activities of daily living including exercises to strengthen the lower limbs, balance exercises and walking retraining in individual or group 50 minute sessions, once a day five days a week. Outcomes measured were gait speed, hand grip strength, appendicular lean mass (aLM, kg/height^2), nutritional assessment carried out by the Mini Nutritional Assessment-Short Form (MNA-SF) [39] and patients' functional situation using the Barthel index (BI) [40] and the functional ambulation categories (FAC) score [27].

The outcome variable was the difference between aLM upon discharge and aLM upon admission (Δ-aLM). BMI and aLM were stable in intervention group (IG) patients, whilst these parameters decreased in the control group (CG). The concentration of proteins ($p = 0.007$) and vitamin D (p.001) increased more in the IG than the CG. A positive effect of oral nutritional supplementation was reported on recovery of ADL. The recovery of ADL was more common in the intervention group (68%) than in the control group (59%) ($p = 0.261$).

This study had a number of limitations. Patients received rehabilitation five days a week. It would be interesting to see whether participation in a program of resistance exercises during the patients' stay at a rehabilitation center improved the functional results reported. The authors could not do any follow-up of patients after discharge to assess whether the benefits obtained were maintained. Furthermore, diagnostic criteria for sarcopenia proposed by the EWGSOP were difficult to apply in patients with hip fractures admitted to rehabilitation units, because most of the patients were unable to walk when they arrived. Despite these limitations, this research had some important strengths. Due to the characteristics of the patients included, this study could be representative of the geriatric population admitted to rehabilitation centers.

3.5. Other Treatments

Study 7 (Table 1) [24] assessed the effects of recombinant human erythropoietin (EPO), already used in in sarcopenic patients for perioperative recovery, in patients with femoral intertrochanteric fracture and sarcopenia, to investigate its potential benefits on postoperative rehabilitation. EPO, through the activation of the signaling cascades in hematopoietic cells, may stimulate proliferation and differentiation of skeletal muscle myoblasts, making the skeletal muscle a potential target [41,42].

The effects of EPO were analyzed in 141 sarcopenic patients older than 60 years with intertrochanteric femoral fracture, randomly divided in intervention and control groups and examined by sex. The intervention group ($n = 83$) received recombinant human erythropoietin via intravenous injection once per day for 10 days after surgery. All patients, including the control group ($n = 58$) received adequate nutrition and exercise for recovery. The outcomes evaluated were: handgrip strength, appendicular skeletal muscle (ASM) index and postoperative hospitalization and infection. The intervention group, especially in female patients, had significant improvement in handgrip strength during the first week after the surgery. The improvement was consistent in the following three weeks. Even the ASM index was improved, with a more important improvement, but not significant, in the intervention group. The rate of post-operative infection and length of hospitalization were significantly decreased in patients who received EPO intervention.

4. Discussion

In this review, we considered seven studies of older adults (>60 years) in which both rehabilitation and nutrition, alone or combined, were used to improve recovery after hip fracture surgery in terms of walking independence, muscle strength, mobility, live activity and fragility. The studies included participants with different degrees of general, cognitive and mobility functions, who had experienced different types of fracture and undergone various surgery methods. The rehabilitation and supplementation strategies, as well as study designs (duration and setting) were different.

The main finding was that sarcopenia, being a multifactor disease, needs a treatment that cannot rely on a single drug. The treatment should be a combination of methods including nutritional intervention, intervention of functional exercise and medications [24]. Physical inactivity was negatively linked to losses of muscle mass and strength, suggesting that increasing levels of physical activity should have protective effects. Also, muscle strength is a critical component of walking, and its decrease in the elderly contributed to a high prevalence of falls [6,43]. Furthermore, early ambulation after hip fracture had beneficial effects on functioning, readmission rate and multidisciplinary rehabilitation reducing the risk of poor outcomes, such as death and admission to nursing homes following FNF [44].

To strengthen muscle and physical function, progressive resistance exercise training is a commonly used tool [21–23]. Ambulatory independence is a crucial outcome to examine in patients after hip-surgery, and it must be evaluated before and after the surgery intervention and rehabilitation protocol. In Study 1 [21], it was found that ambulatory independence is more associated with individual ambulatory function before the fracture than in the presence of sarcopenia. However, Study 2 [22] considered poor ambulatory independence as predictive factor for worse results in the evaluated outcome.

Progressive resistance training, associated with occupational therapy, in the above-mentioned studies, resulted in important improvements in walking ability, strength and general mobility, especially in the short-term rehabilitation of sarcopenic patients. Occupational therapy may also have an important role in cognitive function. Cognitive function is a crucial factor, affecting the rehabilitation outcomes after FNF in patients. When occupational therapy was not involved, there was no significant difference in outcome measurements between the two groups at all follow-ups in K-MMSE [21,22].

Type and intensity of exercise is an important variable that significantly influences functional outcomes in FNF patients. Study 3 [23], compared the effects of antigravity treadmill rehabilitation with conventional rehabilitation and conventional rehabilitation alone, and which did not include progressive resistance training and was uncertain in terms of compliance, found an important and significant improvement in the ability to walk, ambulatory function, general mobility, balance and quality of life in the experimental group. The antigravity treadmill, in fact, allowed a task-specific repetitive approach, facilitating the practice of numerous complex gait cycles, which were not possible in the control group.

In the literature, less is reported about the role of diet in older age, although there is evidence that improvements in diet among older adults at risk of developing sarcopenia may have the potential both to prevent, or delay, age-related losses of muscle mass and function, as well as being potential management strategies for sarcopenic patients. However, existing evidence from nutrient supplementation studies is mixed [2,6].

In our review, the effects of provision of additional amino acids, protein, bisphosphonates, calcium, Vitamin D and HMB, in combination with a standardized diet and exercise training, were reported. The supplements differed in type, dose, frequency and delivery among the patients, as did the results and improvement in patients. The sample was somewhat evenlydistributed in terms of age, sex and type of fracture. All three studies (Studies 4, 5 and 6) showed that supplemental nutrition improved functional results in patients with sarcopenic FNF. However, some findings must be discussed. Study 4 [16] did not confirm any hypothesis because the improvements were not significant between the different groups. However, in the nutritional supplementation group, analysis did show a positive effect on quality of life and handgrip strength. In the other two studies, significant improvement was seen in ADLs, in particular, and in HGS and walking ability in the intervention groups [19,20]. Moreover, Study 5 [19] found that sarcopenic patients with amino acid intake had important improvements in ADLs, compared to other groups. The same difference did not occur in the nonsarcopenic patients. The improvement disappeared after two months when the intake was suspended. This may prove the importance of amino-acid supplementation, especially in sarcopenic patients after hip surgery, beinmg maintained for a longer period in older adults.

As for medical therapy, no drugs are specifically designed for the treatment of sarcopenia. Testosterone, growth hormone and beta-adrenergic receptor agonists are commonly used to improve sarcopenia [45], but more research is needed because they do not always improve muscle function [46].

Study 7 [24] tried to include EPO as a drug to treat sarcopenia when used as a perioperative red blood cell mobilization drug in patients with FNF. The authors found that EPO improved the muscle strength of female patients with sarcopenia during the perioperative period, increased muscle mass of both women and men to a certain degree and significantly reduced the incidence of complications during the preoperative period. EPO may work as a new treatment option for patients with FNF in short-term postoperative rehabilitation.

5. Conclusions

Physical activity, in its various forms, and dietary supplementation, are the basic tools of prevention and rehabilitation of sarcopenia in elderly patients after hip surgery. Exercise training increases muscle mass in the elderly population with varying fragility and nutritional status, helping outpatient recovery, which is the primary outcome in these patients. The most effective physical therapy seems to be exercise of progressive resistance. However, occupational therapy should be included in sarcopenic patients for its importance in cognitive rehabilitation, especially in older adults, to help their return to normal daily activities. Nutritional support, combined with task-specific repetitive exercises, is supported by accumulating evidence for improving sarcopenia and preventing disability. Protein-rich dietary supplementation should primarily include amino acids for a long period in elderly patients. Treatment should include medical therapy, such as erythropoietin and bisphosphonates, which are increasingly important resources, even though they need further research for their validation.

Author Contributions: Conceptualization, G.R.A.M. and M.A.; methodology, M.A.; software, A.V.; validation, G.T., V.P. and M.V.; formal analysis, S.M.; investigation, G.R.A.M.; resources, M.A.; data curation, A.V.; writing—original draft preparation, G.R.A.M.; writing—review and editing, M.A.; visualization, A.V.; supervision, G.T.; project administration, M.V.; funding acquisition, V.P. All authors have read and agreed to the published version of the manuscript.

References

1. Cruz-Jentoft, A.J.; Bahat, G.; Bauer, J.; Boirie, Y.; Bruyère, O.; Cederholm, T.; Cooper, C.; Landi, F.; Rolland, Y.; Sayer, A.A.; et al. Sarcopenia: Revised European consensus on definition and diagnosis. *Age Ageing* **2019**, *48*, 16–31. [CrossRef] [PubMed]
2. Cruz-Jentoft, A.J.; Landi, F.; Schneider, S.; Zúñiga, C.; Arai, H.; Boirie, Y.; Chen, L.-K.; Fielding, R.A.; Martin, F.C.; Michel, J.-P.; et al. Prevalence of and interventions for sarcopenia in ageing adults: A systematic review. Report of the International Sarcopenia Initiative (EWGSOP and IWGS). *Age Ageing* **2014**, *43*, 748–759. [CrossRef] [PubMed]
3. Woo, J. Sarcopenia. *Clin. Geriatr. Med.* **2017**, *33*, 305–314. [CrossRef]
4. Marzetti, E.; on behalf of the SPRINTT Consortium; Calvani, R.; Tosato, M.; Cesari, M.; Di Bari, M.; Cherubini, A.; Collamati, A.; D'Angelo, E.; Pahor, M.; et al. Sarcopenia: An overview. *Aging Clin. Exp. Res.* **2017**, *29*, 11–17. [CrossRef] [PubMed]
5. Goodpaster, B.H.; Park, S.W.; Harris, T.B.; Kritchevsky, S.B.; Nevitt, M.; Schwartz, A.V.; Simonsick, E.M.; Tylavsky, F.A.; Visser, M.; Newman, A.B.; et al. The Loss of Skeletal Muscle Strength, Mass, and Quality in Older Adults: The Health, Aging and Body Composition Study. *J. Gerontol. Ser. A Boil. Sci. Med. Sci.* **2006**, *61*, 1059–1064. [CrossRef]
6. Robinson, S.; Denison, H.; Cooper, C.; Sayer, A.A. Prevention and optimal management of sarcopenia: A review of combined exercise and nutrition interventions to improve muscle outcomes in older people. *Clin. Interv. Aging* **2015**, *10*, 859–869. [CrossRef]
7. Ryall, J.G.; Schertzer, J.D.; Lynch, G.S. Cellular and molecular mechanisms underlying age-related skeletal muscle wasting and weakness. *Biogerontology* **2008**, *9*, 213–228. [CrossRef]

8. Dhillon, R.J.; Hasni, S.A. Pathogenesis and Management of Sarcopenia. *Clin. Geriatr. Med.* **2017**, *33*, 17–26. [CrossRef]
9. Cesari, M.; Fielding, R.A.; Pahor, M.; Goodpaster, B.; Hellerstein, M.; Van Kan, G.A.; Anker, S.D.; Rutkove, S.; Vrijbloed, J.W.; Isaac, M.; et al. Biomarkers of sarcopenia in clinical trials-recommendations from the International Working Group on Sarcopenia. *J. Cachex Sarcopenia Muscle* **2012**, *3*, 181–190. [CrossRef]
10. Van Kan, G.A.; Cedarbaum, J.M.; Cesari, M.; Dahinden, P.; Fariello, R.G.; Fielding, R.A.; Goodpaster, B.H.; Hettwer, S.; Isaac, M.; Laurent, D.; et al. Sarcopenia: Biomarkers and imaging (International Conference on Sarcopenia research). *J. Nutr. Heal. Aging* **2011**, *15*, 834–846. [CrossRef]
11. Bell, J.J.; Bauer, J.; Capra, S.; Pulle, C.R. Barriers to nutritional intake in patients with acute hip fracture: Time to treat malnutrition as a disease and food as a medicine? *Can. J. Physiol. Pharm.* **2013**, *91*, 489–495. [CrossRef] [PubMed]
12. Di Monaco, M.; Castiglioni, C.; Vallero, F.; Di Monaco, R.; Tappero, R. Sarcopenia is more prevalent in men than in women after hip fracture: A cross-sectional study of 591 inpatients. *Arch. Gerontol. Geriatr.* **2012**, *55*, e48–e52. [CrossRef] [PubMed]
13. Hida, T.; Ishiguro, N.; Shimokata, H.; Sakai, Y.; Matsui, Y.; Takemura, M.; Terabe, Y.; Harada, A. High prevalence of sarcopenia and reduced leg muscle mass in Japanese patients immediately after a hip fracture. *Geriatr. Gerontol. Int.* **2012**, *13*, 413–420. [CrossRef] [PubMed]
14. Vellas, B.; Fielding, R.; Miller, R.; Rolland, Y.; Bhasin, S.; Magaziner, J.; Bischoff-Ferrari, H. Designing drug trials for sarcopenia in older adults with hip fracture—A task force from the international conference onfrailty and sarcopenia research (icfsr). *J. Frailty Aging* **2014**, *3*, 199–204. [PubMed]
15. Fox, K.M.; Magaziner, J.; Hawkes, W.G.; Yu-Yahiro, J.; Hebel, J.R.; Zimmerman, S.I.; Holder, L.; Michael, R. Loss of Bone Density and Lean Body Mass after Hip Fracture. *Osteoporos. Int.* **2000**, *11*, 31–35. [CrossRef] [PubMed]
16. Flodin, L.; Cederholm, T.; Sääf, M.; Samnegård, E.; Ekström, W.; Al-Ani, A.N.; Hedström, M. Effects of protein-rich nutritional supplementation and bisphosphonates on body composition, handgrip strength and health-related quality of life after hip fracture: A 12-month randomized controlled study. *BMC Geriatr.* **2015**, *15*, 149. [CrossRef]
17. Al-Ani, A.N.; Flodin, L.; Söderqvist, A.; Ackermann, P.W.; Samnegård, E.; Dalen, N.; Sääf, M.; Cederholm, T.; Hedström, M. Does Rehabilitation Matter in Patients With Femoral Neck Fracture and Cognitive Impairment? A Prospective Study of 246 Patients. *Arch. Phys. Med. Rehabil.* **2010**, *91*, 51–57. [CrossRef]
18. Samuelsson, B.; Hedström, M.I.; Ponzer, S.; Söderqvist, A.; Samnegård, E.; Thorngren, K.-G.; Cederholm, T.; Sääf, M.; Dalen, N. Gender differences and cognitive aspects on functional outcome after hip fracture–a 2 years' follow-up of 2,134 patients. *Age Ageing* **2009**, *38*, 686–692. [CrossRef]
19. Invernizzi, M.; De Sire, A.; D'Andrea, F.; Carrera, D.; Renò, F.; Migliaccio, S.; Iolascon, G.; Cisari, C. Effects of essential amino acid supplementation and rehabilitation on functioning in hip fracture patients: A pilot randomized controlled trial. *Aging Clin. Exp. Res.* **2018**, *31*, 1517–1524. [CrossRef]
20. Malafarina, V.; Uriz-Otano, F.; Malafarina, C.; Martínez, J.A.; Zulet, M.A. Effectiveness of nutritional supplementation on sarcopenia and recovery in hip fracture patients. A multi-centre randomized trial. *Maturitas* **2017**, *101*, 42–50. [CrossRef]
21. Lim, S.-K.; Lee, S.Y.; Beom, J.; Lim, J.-Y. Comparative outcomes of inpatient fragility fracture intensive rehabilitation management (FIRM) after hip fracture in sarcopenic and non-sarcopenic patients: A prospective observational study. *Eur. Geriatr. Med.* **2018**, *9*, 641–650. [CrossRef]
22. Lim, J.-Y.; Beom, J.; Lee, S.Y.; Lim, J.-Y. Functional Outcomes of Fragility Fracture Integrated Rehabilitation Management in Sarcopenic Patients after Hip Fracture Surgery and Predictors of Independent Ambulation. *J. Nutr. Heal. Aging* **2019**, *23*, 1034–1042. [CrossRef] [PubMed]
23. Oh, M.-K.; Yoo, J.-I.; Byun, H.; Chun, S.-W.; Lim, S.-K.; Jang, Y.J.; Lee, C.H. Efficacy of combined antigravity treadmill and conventional rehabilitation after hip fracture in patients with sarcopenia. *J. Gerontol. Ser. A Boil. Sci. Med. Sci.* **2020**, 158. [CrossRef]
24. Zhang, Y.; Chen, L.; Wu, P.; Lang, J.; Chen, L. Intervention with erythropoietin in sarcopenic patients with femoral intertrochanteric fracture and its potential effects on postoperative rehabilitation. *Geriatr. Gerontol. Int.* **2019**, *20*, 150–155. [CrossRef] [PubMed]
25. Chen, L.-K.; Woo, J.; Assantachai, P.; Auyeung, T.-W.; Chou, M.-Y.; Iijima, K.; Jang, H.C.; Kang, L.; Kim, M.;

Kim, S.; et al. Asian Working Group for Sarcopenia: 2019 Consensus Update on Sarcopenia Diagnosis and Treatment. *J. Am. Med. Dir. Assoc.* **2020**, *21*, 300–307.e2. [CrossRef] [PubMed]

26. Koval, K.J.; Skovron, M.L.; Aharonoff, G.B.; Meadows, S.E.; Zuckerman, J.D. Ambulatory ability after hip fracture. A prospective study in geriatric patients. *Clin. Orthop. Relat. Res.* **1995**, *310*, 150–159.
27. Collen, F.M.; Wade, D.T.; Bradshaw, C.M. Mobility after stroke: Reliability of measures of impairment and disability. *Int. Disabil. Stud.* **1990**, *12*, 6–9. [CrossRef]
28. Lennon, S.; Johnson, L. The modified Rivermead Mobility Index: Validity and reliability. *Disabil. Rehabil.* **2000**, *22*, 833–839. [CrossRef]
29. Downs, S.; Marquez, J.; Chiarelli, P. The Berg Balance Scale has high intra- and inter-rater reliability but absolute reliability varies across the scale: A systematic review. *J. Physiother.* **2013**, *59*, 93–99. [CrossRef]
30. Kim, T.H.; Jhoo, J.H.; Park, J.H.; Kim, J.L.; Ryu, S.H.; Moon, S.W.; Choo, I.H.; Lee, N.W.; Yoon, J.C.; Do, Y.J.; et al. Korean Version of Mini Mental Status Examination for Dementia Screening and Its' Short Form. *Psychiatry Investig.* **2010**, *7*, 102–108. [CrossRef]
31. Jung, I.K.; Kwak, D.I.; Joe, S.H.; Lee, H.S. A study of standardization of Korean Form of Geriatric Depression Scale (KGDS). *Korean J. Geriatr. Psychiatry* **1997**, *1*, 61–72.
32. Group, The EuroQol. EuroQol—A new facility for the measurement of health-related quality of life. *Health Policy* **1990**, *16*, 199–208. [CrossRef]
33. Lee, K.W.; Kim, S.B.; Lee, J.H.; Lee, S.J.; Yoo, S.W. Effect of Upper Extremity Robot-Assisted Exercise on Spasticity in Stroke Patients. *Ann. Rehabil. Med.* **2016**, *40*, 961–971. [CrossRef] [PubMed]
34. Song, M.; Lee, S.H.; Jahng, S.; Kim, S.-Y.; Kang, Y. Validation of the Korean-Everyday Cognition (K-ECog). *J. Korean Med. Sci.* **2019**, *34*, e67. [CrossRef]
35. Jung, H.-W.; Yoo, H.-J.; Park, S.-Y.; Kim, S.-W.; Choi, J.-Y.; Yoon, S.-J.; Kim, C.-H.; Kim, K.-I. The Korean version of the FRAIL scale: Clinical feasibility and validity of assessing the frailty status of Korean elderly. *Korean J. Intern. Med.* **2016**, *31*, 594–600. [CrossRef]
36. Binder, E.F.; Storandt, M.; Birge, S.J. The relation between psychometric test performance and physical performance in older adults. *J. Gerontol. Ser. A Boil. Sci. Med. Sci.* **1999**, *54*, M428–M432. [CrossRef]
37. Podsiadlo, D.; Richardson, S. The TiMed. "Up & Go": A Test of Basic Functional Mobility for Frail Elderly Persons. *J. Am. Geriatr. Soc.* **1991**, *39*, 142–148. [CrossRef]
38. Soh, S.-E.; Stuart, L.; Raymond, M.; Kimmel, L.A.; Holland, A. The validity, reliability, and responsiveness of the modified Iowa Level of Assistance scale in hospitalized older adults in subacute care. *Disabil. Rehabil.* **2017**, *40*, 2931–2937. [CrossRef]
39. Rubenstein, L.Z.; Harker, J.O.; Salva, A.; Guigoz, Y.; Vellas, B. Screening for undernutrition in geriatric practice: Developing the short-form mini-nutritional assessment (MNA-SF). *J. Gerontol. Ser. A Boil. Sci. Med. Sci.* **2001**, *56*, M366–M372. [CrossRef]
40. Mahoney, F.I.; Barthel, D.W. Functional evaluation: The Barthel Index: A simple index of independence useful in scoring improvement in the rehabilitation of the chronically ill. *Md. State Med. J.* **1965**, *14*, 61–65.
41. Ogilvie, M.; Yu, X.; Nicolas-Metral, V.; Pulido, S.M.; Liu, C.; Ruegg, U.T.; Noguchi, C.T. Erythropoietin Stimulates Proliferation and Interferes with Differentiation of Myoblasts. *J. Boil. Chem.* **2000**, *275*, 39754–39761. [CrossRef] [PubMed]
42. Lamon, S.; Russell, A.P. The role and regulation of erythropoietin (EPO) and its receptor in skeletal muscle: How much do we really know? *Front. Physiol.* **2013**, *4*, 176. [CrossRef] [PubMed]
43. Liu, C.-J.; Latham, N.K. Progressive resistance strength training for improving physical function in older adults. *Cochrane Database Syst. Rev.* **2009**, *2009*, 002759. [CrossRef] [PubMed]
44. Siu, A.L.; Penrod, J.D.; Boockvar, K.S.; Koval, K.; Strauss, E.; Morrison, R.S. Early Ambulation after Hip Fracture. *Arch. Intern. Med.* **2006**, *166*, 766–771. [CrossRef]
45. West, D.W.D.; Phillips, S.M. Anabolic Processes in Human Skeletal Muscle: Restoring the Identities of Growth Hormone and Testosterone. *Physician Sportsmed.* **2010**, *38*, 97–104. [CrossRef]
46. Studenski, S.; Peters, K.W.; Alley, D.E.; Cawthon, P.M.; McLean, R.R.; Harris, T.B.; Ferrucci, L.; Guralnik, J.M.; Fragala, M.S.; Kenny, A.M.; et al. The FNIH sarcopenia project: Rationale, study description, conference recommendations, and final estimates. *J. Gerontol. Ser. A Boil. Sci. Med. Sci.* **2014**, *69*, 547–558. [CrossRef]

14

Effect of Aerobic Exercise Training and Deconditioning on Oxidative Capacity and Muscle Mitochondrial Enzyme Machinery in Young and Elderly Individuals

Andreas Mæchel Fritzen [1,2,*], Søren Peter Andersen [1], Khaled Abdul Nasser Qadri [1], Frank D. Thøgersen [1], Thomas Krag [1], Mette C. Ørngreen [1], John Vissing [1] and Tina D. Jeppesen [1]

1 Department of Neurology, Copenhagen Neuromuscular Center, Rigshospitalet, DK-2100 Copenhagen, Denmark; ggspa@greve-gym.dk (S.P.A.); khaled_qadri@hotmail.com (K.A.N.Q.); frank.thogersen@gmail.com (F.D.T.); thomas.krag@regionh.dk (T.K.); mette.cathrine.oerngreen.01@regionh.dk (M.C.Ø.); john.vissing@regionh.dk (J.V.); tina@dysgaard.dk (T.D.J.)

2 Molecular Physiology Group, Department of Nutrition, Exercise, and Sports, Faculty of Science, University of Copenhagen, DK-2100 Copenhagen, Denmark

* Correspondence: amfritzen@nexs.ku.dk.

Abstract: Mitochondrial dysfunction is thought to be involved in age-related loss of muscle mass and function (sarcopenia). Since the degree of physical activity is vital for skeletal muscle mitochondrial function and content, the aim of this study was to investigate the effect of 6 weeks of aerobic exercise training and 8 weeks of deconditioning on functional parameters of aerobic capacity and markers of muscle mitochondrial function in elderly compared to young individuals. In 11 healthy, elderly (80 ± 4 years old) and 10 healthy, young (24 ± 3 years old) volunteers, aerobic training improved maximal oxygen consumption rate by 13%, maximal workload by 34%, endurance capacity by 2.4-fold and exercise economy by 12% in the elderly to the same extent as in young individuals. This evidence was accompanied by a similar training-induced increase in muscle citrate synthase (CS) (31%) and mitochondrial complex I–IV activities (51–163%) in elderly and young individuals. After 8 weeks of deconditioning, endurance capacity (−20%), and enzyme activity of CS (−18%) and complex I (−40%), III (−25%), and IV (−26%) decreased in the elderly to a larger extent than in young individuals. In conclusion, we found that elderly have a physiological normal ability to improve aerobic capacity and mitochondrial function with aerobic training compared to young individuals, but had a faster decline in endurance performance and muscle mitochondrial enzyme activity after deconditioning, suggesting an age-related issue in maintaining oxidative metabolism.

Keywords: aerobic exercise training; mitochondria; sarcopenia; endurance; deconditioning; skeletal muscle; elderly

---

1. Introduction

Age-related loss of muscle mass and function, referred to as sarcopenia, is an inevitable process, affecting more than 40% of individuals above 80 years of age [1]. Sarcopenia and reduced aerobic capacity in elderly individuals are strong mediators of morbidity [2] and mortality [3,4]. The ability to perform activities of daily living in healthy individuals is progressively reduced with age, seemingly associated with a decrease in aerobic capacity [5]. Lower levels of aerobic capacity can contribute to a loss of independence, increased incidence of disability, frailty, and reduced quality of life in older people. Sarcopenia and age-related impaired aerobic capacity are related to a multitude of factors, including muscle mitochondrial degeneration [6,7].

It is well established that aerobic exercise training increases maximal aerobic exercise capacity (VO_{2peak}), accompanied by improvements in mitochondrial content, function, and enzyme expression in young, untrained individuals [8–11]. In elderly, findings have been equivocal. Some studies found that 6–16 weeks of intense aerobic exercise training improved aerobic capacity and mitochondrial enzyme activity [12–17], while others were not able to confirm significant effects of training in elderly [18–20]. Thus, it is unclear whether elderly have an attenuated response to training in aerobic capacity compared with young individuals [13,21,22]; in particular, it is not fully understood whether the plasticity for mitochondrial adaptations to aerobic training occurs to the same extent in young and elderly individuals.

A training-induced increase in muscle mitochondrial content and enzyme activity were shown to return to baseline with as little as 4–8 weeks of deconditioning in healthy, young individuals [23–27]. Thus, aerobic training and deconditioning are effective ways to provoke mitochondrial plasticity. In elderly, it could be hypothesized that the age-associated impairments in aerobic capacity and muscle mitochondrial function could relate to relatively faster loss of mitochondrial capacity with deconditiong, but the effect of deconditioning on mitochondrial content and enzyme activity has never been studied in elderly.

Mitochondria are important for many vital functions of the cell, including being a key initiator of programmed cell death (apoptosis). Studies in rats showed an increased apoptotic activity in the aging muscle, accompanied by a lowered expression of the mitochondrial outer membrane antiapoptotic B-cell lymphoma 2 (Bcl2) protein, which was reversed by 12 weeks of aerobic training [28–30]. Furthermore, cleavage of cysteine-dependent, aspartate-specific protease-3 (caspase-3), indicative of increased activation of caspase-3, is a key factor in induction of apoptosis, and it was found to be increased in skeletal muscle of 24-month-old compared to 12-month-old rats [31]. Collectively, these findings in rodents led to the idea that increased apoptotic activity driven by mitochondria could be a contributing mediator of age-related muscle loss in humans that can be reversed by exercise training [32]. These data imply that mitochondria-driven apoptosis could be a key factor behind age-related muscle function and mass loss. However, studies investigating mitochondrial and apoptotic biomarkers in skeletal muscle of elderly in response to aerobic training and deconditioning—and, thus, potential explanation for age-related muscle mass—are scarce.

The aim of this study was to investigate the effect of aerobic training and deconditioning on aerobic capacity and muscle mitochondrial function in elderly (>75 years old) and young healthy individuals (age < 30 years old). We hypothesized that elderly individuals would have indices of mitochondrial dysfunction, but that elderly would increase their aerobic and endurance capacity, as well as measures of mitochondrial content and function, to the same extent as the young individuals after aerobic training.

2. Materials and Methods

2.1. Individuals

The aim was to include a minimum of 10 elderly healthy individuals (age above 75 years old) and 10 healthy young individuals at the age of 20 to 30 years old. Exclusion criteria were nonsedentary, illness that required medication other than antihypertensive and antithrombotic treatment, severe musculoskeletal pain, neurological disorder, smoking, cardiovascular disease, attendance rate below 80% of total training sessions, additional training during the training phase, or failure to comply with instructions of inactivity during the deconditioning phase. Sedentary was defined as performing less than one hour of exercise a week at low to moderate intensity or a maximum of 5 km of cycling for transportation a day.

All participants completed a detailed medical history and electrocardiography, and all had a normal neurological examination before entering the study.

In total, 21 healthy individuals, 11 elderly (four women and seven men; 80 ± 4 years) and 10 young (five women and five men; 24 ± 3 years) individuals were included in the study. Every included participant completed the study in full.

All individuals gave oral and written consent to participate according to the Helsinki declaration. The study was approved by the Ethics Committee of the Capital Region (No. KF-293615). The individuals were all informed about the nature and risks of the study and gave written consent to participate before inclusion.

2.2. Study Design

The 11 elderly and 10 young participants completed a 6 week aerobic exercise training intervention on a bicycle ergometer followed by 8 weeks of deconditioning (Figure 1). Maximal aerobic exercise capacity (VO_{2peak}) and maximal workload were evaluated by an incremental test and aerobic endurance capacity evaluated by a time-to-exhaustion test at 80% of pretraining maximal workload before and after aerobic exercise training, and again after 4 and 8 weeks of deconditioning. Skeletal muscle biopsies were taken from vastus lateralis muscle before and after aerobic exercise training and after 8 weeks of deconditioning for measurement of mitochondrial and apoptotic markers. Dual-energy X-ray absorptiometry (DEXA) scanning of body composition was performed at baseline.

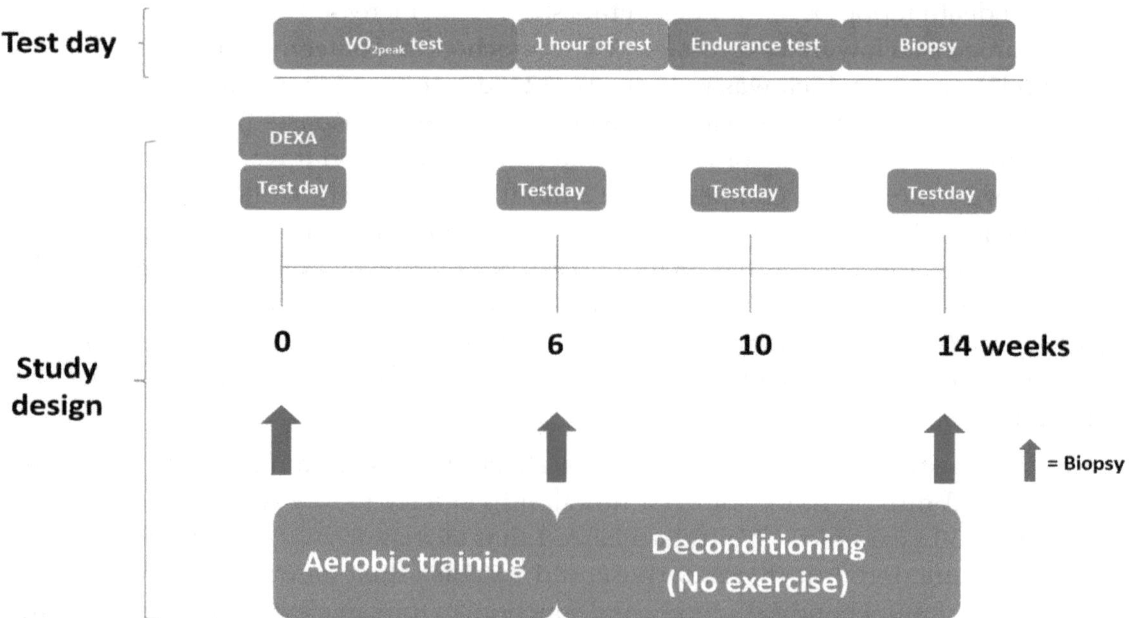

Figure 1. Study design overview. Twenty-one participants completed a 6 week aerobic exercise training intervention followed by 8 weeks of deconditioning (detraining—no exercise). Maximal aerobic exercise capacity and aerobic endurance capacity were evaluated using a maximal oxygen consumption rate test and an endurance time-to-exhaustion test, respectively, before and after aerobic exercise training and after subsequent 4 and 8 weeks of deconditioning. Skeletal muscle biopsies were taken from vastus lateralis muscle at baseline, after 6 weeks of aerobic training and after 8 weeks of deconditioning. DEXA: Dual-energy X-ray absorptiometry, VO_{2peak}: Peak oxygen consumption rate.

2.3. DEXA Scanning

A whole-body dual-energy X-ray absorptiometry (DEXA) scan (GE Medical Systems, Lunar, Prodigy, Chicago, IL) was performed prior to the intervention. Elderly and young individuals were instructed to drink 2.5 L of liquid and, hence, be well hydrated the day before the DEXA scan. They arrived overnight-fasted and were encouraged to empty their bladder prior to the scan.

They underwent the DEXA scan by lying straight and centered on the table with the hip region within two sets of hash marks on either side of the long edge of the table to ensure the entire body was within the scan area according to the manufacturer's instructions. The images were analyzed using enCORE™2004 Software (v.8.5) (GE Medical Systems, Lunar, Prodigy, Chicago, IL, USA). Reliability of this DEXA scanning procedure was recently described [33].

2.4. Maximal Oxygen Consumption Test

Before initial testing, individuals were familiarized with the equipment and test protocol on a separate day with a training session to reduce the impact that skill learning has on strength performance.

On each test day, individuals carried out an incremental cycling test to exhaustion on a stationary bicycle (Monark 939E, Sweden), and VO_2 was measured by pulmonary gas exchange with a breath-by-breath gas analyzer using an open-circuit online respirometer for indirect calorimetry measurements (Cosmed, Quark B2, Pavona, Italy). Load was set individually, increasing every other minute for the first 10 min, and thereafter every minute until exhaustion. Heart rate (HR) was measured during exercise, and the subject's self-assessed feeling of exertion, on a Borg scale, was assessed every minute. Maximal workload (Wmax) was the maximal power output (in Watt) achieved and sustained for at least 1 min during the incremental test.

2.5. Endurance Test

After the incremental test, individuals rested for 1 h before carrying out an endurance test on a stationary bicycle (Monark 939E, Sweden) evaluating time to exhaustion at 80% of pretraining Wmax, obtained under the test for maximal oxygen consumption. Exhaustion was achieved when individuals could not maintain a self-chosen pedal cadence rpm minus 10 rpm for 10 s (e.g., if a chosen rpm at 70 dropped to less than 60 rpm for more than 10 s, exhaustion was achieved). During this test, VO_2 was measured by pulmonary gas exchange as described above, and HR was also measured continuously throughout the test. Exercise economy during the endurance test was calculated as average VO_2 during the test divided by the workload (Watt).

2.6. Aerobic Exercise Training and Deconditioning Interventions

During the 6 week aerobic exercise training intervention, volunteers trained four times per week on a cycle ergometer. Each session lasted 35 min, and sessions alternated between continuous exercise bouts and intermittent exercise bouts. Continuous exercise sessions involved 35 min of continuous cycling at an intensity of 70% of the maximal heart rate (HRmax) reserve (the dynamic area between the resting HR (HRrest) and HRmax). Intermittent exercise consisted of 5 × 4 min intervals at an intensity of 95% of HRmax reserve, with 3 min of rest between intervals.

HRmax reserve has been shown to be well correlated to the intensity as percentage of VO_{2peak}. Heart rate intervals were estimated using the following formula, described by Swain et al. (2000) [34]:

$$\text{HR\% intensity} = (\text{HRmax} - \text{HRrest}) \times \text{Intensity (\%)} + \text{HRrest}.$$

Heart rate intervals were set to the calculated HR ± 5 bpm. Training was carried out in a progressive manner, with an increasing workload during the training period to achieve the determined HR intervals. All training sessions were supervised to ensure correct exercise intensity and were carried out on stationary bikes (Monark 939E, Sweden or Tunturi T6, Finland). Heart rate was recorded during exercise by a heart-rate monitor. After 6 weeks of aerobic training, participants stopped the training program and returned to their habitual sedentary lifestyle and were instructed not to initiate any new form of training for the following eight weeks. Individuals wore a step counter during the entire study, i.e., the training and deconditioning period, to ensure that the level of daily activity during the training period corresponded to the activity level of the deconditioning period. Step counters were checked once per week throughout the period to ensure that the physical activity level did not vary more than 10% on a weekly basis.

2.7. Skeletal Muscle Biopsies

A skeletal muscle biopsy was performed after the endurance test in vastus lateralis right leg muscle pre- and post-training and after 8 weeks of deconditioning within 15 min of the endurance test. The biopsy was performed as previously described using a 5 mm percutaneous Bergström needle [35]. Needle entry was at least 3 cm away from the previous insertion to avoid scar tissue and interference with data due to post-biopsy edema. Muscle samples were immediately frozen in liquid isopentane cooled by liquid nitrogen before storage at −80 °C for later analysis.

2.8. Mitochondrial Enzyme Activities

Citrate synthase (CS) and mitochondrial complex I–IV enzyme activities were determined as previously described [23,36]. Muscle tissue was homogenized in 19 volumes of ice-cold medium containing protease and phosphatase inhibitor cocktail. Enzyme assays for CS and complex I–IV were performed at 25 °C in a Lambda 16 spectrophotometer (Perkin Elmer) [37]. Complex I specific activity was measured by following the decrease in absorbance due to the oxidation of nicotinamide adenine dinucleotide (NADH) at 340 nm with 425 nm as the reference wavelength. Sample was added to a buffer containing 25 mM potassium phosphate (pH 7.2), 5 mM MgC12, 2 mM KCN, 2.5 mg/mL antimycin A, 0.13 mM NADH, 0.1 mg/mL sonicated phospholipids, and 75 μM decylubiquinone. Complex I activity was measured 3–5 min before addition of 2 μg/mL rotenone, after which the activity was measured for an additional 3 min. Complex I activity was the rotenone-sensitive activity [37,38]. Complex II specific activity was measured by following the reduction of 2,6-dichlorophenolindophenol (DCPIP) at 600 nm. Samples were preincubated in buffer containing 25 mM potassium phosphate (pH 7.2), 5 mM $MgCl_2$, and 20 mM succinate at 30 °C for 10 min. Antimycin A (2 μg/mL), 2 μg/mL rotenone, 2mM KCN, and 50 μM DCPIP were added, and a baseline rate was recorded for 3 min. The reaction was started with decylubiquinone (50 μM), and the enzyme-catalyzed reduction of DCPIP was measured for 3–5 min [37,38].

Complex III specific activity was determined in a reaction mixture containing the sample and 100 μM ethylenediaminetetraacetic acid (EDTA), 0.2% defatted bovine serum albumin (*w/v*), 3 mM/L sodium azide, and 60 μM/L ferricytochrome c in 50 mM/L potassium buffer (pH 8.0). The reaction was started by addition of 150 μM decylubiquinol in ethanol and monitored for 2 min at 550 nm [39]. Complex IV activity was measured by following the oxidation of cytochrome c (II) at 550 nm with 580 nm as the reference wavelength. The reaction buffer contained 20 mM potassium phosphate (pH 7.0) and 15 μM cytochrome c (II). Sample was added to the reaction buffer, and the initial activity was calculated from the apparent first-order rate constant after fully oxidizing cytochrome c [37,38].

CS activity was measured following the NADH changes at 340 nm at 25 °C by 50-fold dilution in a solution containing 100 μM acetoacetyl-CoA, 0.5 mM NAD (free acid), 1 mM sodium malate, 8 μg/mL malate dehydrogenase, 2.5 mM EDTA, and 10 mM Tris-HCl (pH 8.0). Samples were preincubated with 0.25% Triton X-100.

2.9. Western Blotting Analysis

Western blot analysis was performed as previously described [23,40]. For Western blotting, biopsies were sectioned on a cryostat (Microm HM550, Thermo Fisher Scientific, Waltham, MA, USA) at −20 °C and homogenized in ice-cold lysis buffer mixed with sample buffer. Proteins were separated on an SDS-PAGE gel, blotted to polyvinylidene difluoride (PVDF) membranes, and incubated in primary and secondary antibodies. Antibodies were directed toward Bcl2 (diluted 1:5000; Cell Signalling Technologies, Beverly, MA, USA) and alpha-tubulin (diluted 1:30.000; Abcam, UK, no 4074), with alpha-tubulin used as a loading control. Secondary goat anti-rabbit and goat anti-mouse antibodies coupled with horseradish peroxidase at a concentration of 1:10,000 were used to detect primary antibodies (DAKO, Glostrup, Denmark). Immunoreactive bands were detected by chemiluminescence using Clarity Max, (BioRad), quantified using a GBox XT16 darkroom, and GeneTools software was used to measure the intensities of immunoreactive bands (Syngene, Cambridge, UK). Immunoreactive band intensities were normalized to the intensity of the alpha-tubulin bands for each participant to correct for differences in total muscle protein loaded on the gel.

2.10. Bioplex Analysis

Muscle tissue was homogenized in the same way as described above (see Western blotting analysis). The prepared homogenates were diluted to a final protein concentration of 400 μg/mL. The Human Apoptosis 3-plex Panel (Invitrogen, CA, USA) was used for protein quantification of cleaved caspase-3 (cl. caspase-3) and a single-plex magnetic bead assay for beta-tubulin (loading control) (Millipore, Merck KGaA, Darmstadt, Germany). Then, 100 μL of prepared standards were added to separate wells and incubated at room temperature in the dark for 2 h. The plate was washed twice, before adding a 1× detection antibody to the wells, and then incubated for 1 h in darkness at room temperature. The plate was again washed twice, and 50 μL of streptavidin-R-Phycoerythrin (RPE) was added to the wells, followed by 30 min of incubation. The plate was washed three times, and 130 μL of wash solution was added to each well, upon reading the plate on a Luminex Bio-plex 200 system (Biorad, Hercules, CA, USA).

2.11. Statistical Analysis

All statistical analyses were carried out using SigmaPlot 11.0 and GraphPad PRISM 8 (GraphPad, La Jolla, CA, USA). All data are expressed as the mean ± standard error of mean (SE), except for baseline anthropometric characterization of participants shown as mean ± standard deviation (SD) (Table 1). A Shapiro–Wilk test was performed to test for normal distribution of data. The differences among groups were analyzed by a repeated-measures two-way analysis of variance (ANOVA) followed by Tukey's multiple comparison tests, when ANOVA revealed significant interactions. Baseline subject characteristics were evaluated with unpaired t-tests between young and elderly groups. Correlation analyses were performed with the Pearson's product-moment correlation coefficient. Differences were considered statistically significant when $p < 0.05$.

Table 1. General demographic data.

Demographic Parameter	Young Group	Elderly Group
Age, years	24 ± 3	80 ± 4 ***
Height, cm	175 ± 13	169 ± 9
Weight, kg	70 ± 14	76 ± 14
BMI, kg/m^2	22.5 ± 2.5	26.5 ± 3.5 *
FFM, kg	50.7 ± 14.3	48.4 ± 10.5
FM, kg	15.5 ± 6.0	26.0 ± 6.9 **
Body fat, %	24.2 ± 9.9	34.9 ± 7.7 *
$VO_{2\,peak}$, mL O_2/kg/min	37.5 ± 9.0	22.5 ± 6.1 ***

BMI, body mass index; FFM, fat-free mass; FM, fat mass, VO_{2peak}, maximal oxygen consumption rate. Data are shown as means ± SD. n = 10 in young and n = 11 in elderly. */**/*** Significantly different (p < 0.05/0.01/0.001) from young group.

3. Results

3.1. Anthropometry

Height, total body weight, and fat-free mass were similar among the young and the elderly individuals, whereas the elderly had a higher BMI (+15%), fat mass (+40%), and body fat% (+31%) and a lower VO_{2peak} (−40%) compared with the young individuals ($p < 0.05$; Table 1).

3.2. Functional Parameters of Aerobic Capacity

The elderly individuals had lower absolute values of VO_{2peak} (~40%) and Wmax (~60%) compared with the young individuals ($p < 0.001$; Figure 2A,B). Six weeks of aerobic training improved VO_{2peak} and Wmax by 13% and 34%, respectively, in elderly individuals ($p < 0.05$) and to the same extent by 9% and 26%, respectively, in young individuals ($p < 0.05$) (Figure 2A,B). VO_{2peak} was lowered by 13% already after 4 weeks of deconditioning in the elderly only ($p < 0.05$), and VO_{2peak} returned to baseline in both the elderly and the young individuals after 8 weeks of deconditioning (Figure 2A). In the elderly individuals, Wmax also returned to pretraining level after 8 weeks of deconditioning, while Wmax was still increased by 11% in the young individuals compared with pretraining level ($p < 0.05$; Figure 2B). Endurance capacity, measured as time to exhaustion on 80% of pretraining Wmax, was improved to a similar extent by 2.4- and 1.5-fold in elderly and young individuals ($p < 0.05$), respectively (Figure 2C). Endurance capacity was impaired by 20% and 25% in the elderly by 4 and 8 weeks of deconditioning, but remained at post-training levels in the young individuals during deconditioning (Figure 2C).

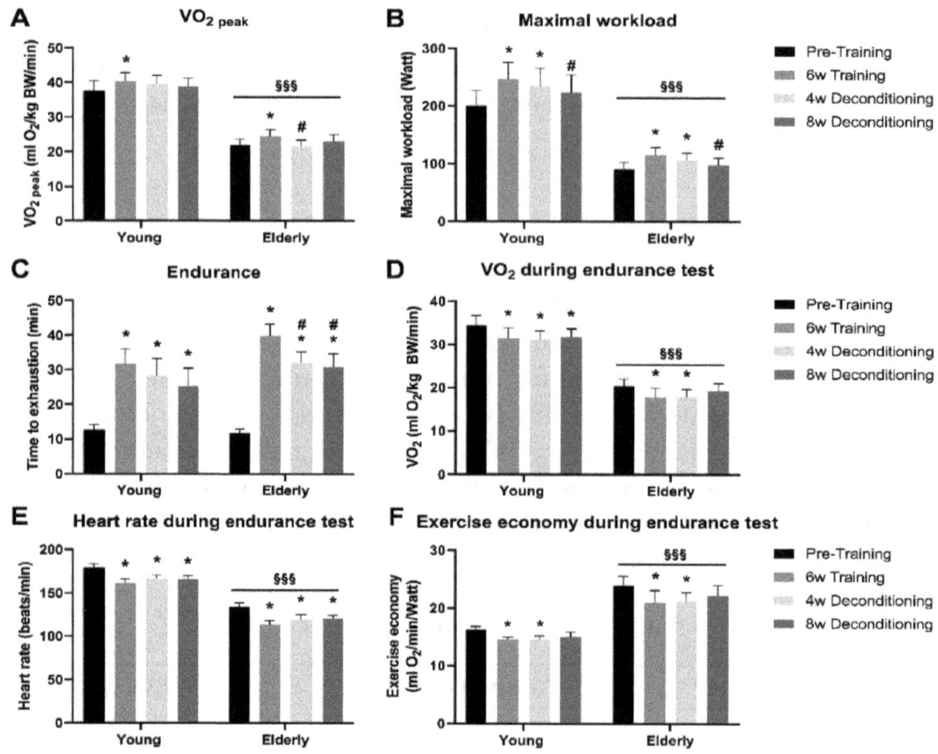

Figure 2. Functional parameters of aerobic capacity. (**A**) Maximal oxygen consumption rate (VO_{2peak}) and maximal workload (**B**) measured in an incremental bicycle test before and after 6 weeks of aerobic exercise training and after 4 and 8 weeks of subsequent deconditioning in elderly and young men and women. Time to exhaustion (**C**), average VO_2 (**D**), average heart rate (**E**), and exercise economy (**F**) during an endurance test on bicycle at 80% of maximal workload in elderly and young men and women. $n = 10$ in young and $n = 11$ elderly. * Significantly different ($p < 0.05$) from pretraining within age group. # Significantly different ($p < 0.05$) from 6 weeks of training within age group. §§§ Significantly different ($p < 0.001$) from young participants. All data are presented as means ± standard error (SE).

VO_2 (Figure 2D) and heart rate (Figure 2E) during the endurance test were overall ~30% lower in the elderly compared with the young individuals ($p < 0.001$). VO_2 (Figure 2D) and heart rate (Figure 2E) were ~15% decreased during the endurance test in both the elderly and the young subjects ($p < 0.05$) and remained so during 4 and 8 weeks of deconditioning. Exercise economy during the endurance test was improved by 12% and 10% in elderly and young individuals ($p < 0.05$), respectively, and remained improved after 4 weeks of deconditioning, but returned to pretraining levels after 8 weeks of deconditioning in both groups (Figure 2F). As a consequence of the relatively lower workload compared with oxygen use during the endurance test in the elderly, exercise economy during the endurance test was overall ~30% lower in the elderly compared with the young individuals ($p < 0.001$) (Figure 2F).

3.3. Mitochondrial Enzyme Activities

At baseline, maximal muscle CS and mitochondrial electron transport chain complex I–IV activities did not differ between elderly and young individuals (Figure 3A–E). Six weeks of aerobic training increased muscle CS activity by 31% in elderly individuals ($p < 0.05$), which was the same as that observed in the young individuals (45%) (Figure 3A). Eight weeks of deconditioning decreased CS activity in the elderly individuals by 18% ($p < 0.05$), while CS activity remained at post-training level in young individuals (Figure 3A). The training-induced increases in complex I (163% and 152%; Figure 3B), II (63% and 58%; Figure 3C), III (63% and 49%; Figure 3D), and IV (51% and 40%; Figure 3E) activities were similar in elderly and young individuals. In elderly individuals, 8 weeks of deconditioning decreased complex I (Figure 3B), II (Figure 3C), III (Figure 3D), and IV activities (Figure 3E) by 40%, 8%, 25%, and 26% ($p < 0.05$), respectively, whereas only complex I (26%; Figure 3B) and II (9%; Figure 3C) activities decreased in young individuals after 8 weeks of deconditioning ($p < 0.05$). Interestingly, the change in enzyme activity with deconditioning significantly correlated with change in endurance capacity for complex I ($r = 0.47$, $p < 0.05$) and tended to correlate for complex III ($r = 0.43$, $p = 0.05$) and CS ($r = 0.39$, $p = 0.09$), whereas the change in enzymatic activity for complex II and IV was not significantly correlated to the change in endurance capacity with deconditioning.

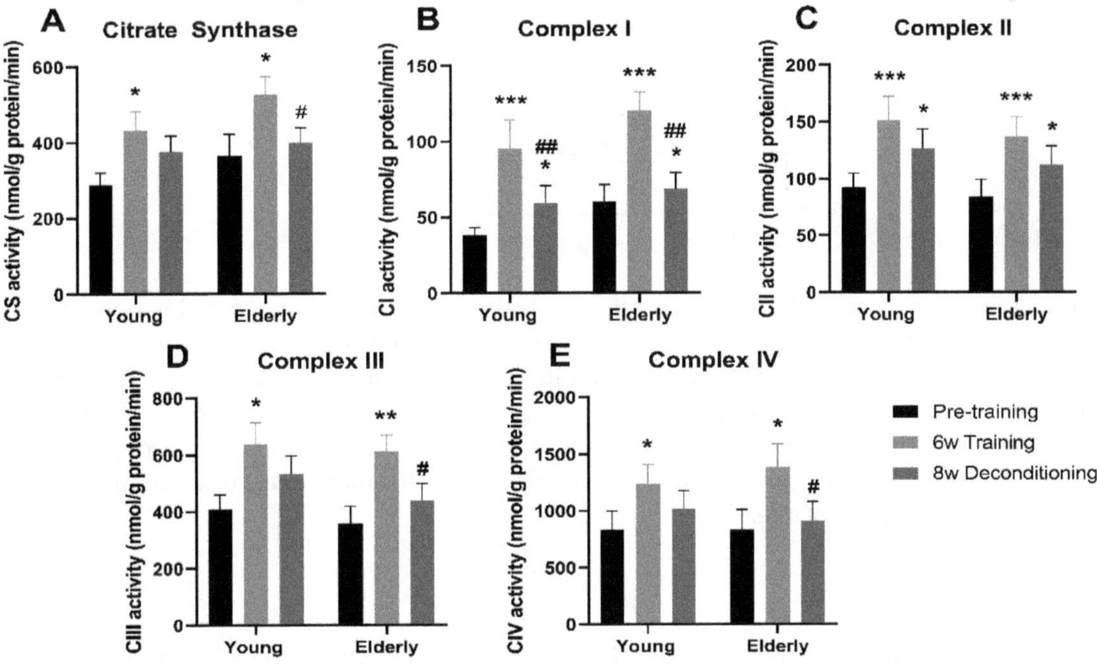

Figure 3. Mitochondrial enzyme activities. Maximal enzyme activity of citrate synthase (CS; **A**), and mitochondrial complex I (**B**), II (**C**), III (**D**), and IV (**E**) in skeletal muscle pre and post six weeks of aerobic exercise training and after subsequent 8 weeks of deconditioning in young and elderly individuals. $n = 10$ in young group and $n = 11$ in the elderly group. */**/*** $p < 0.05/0.01/0.001$, significantly different from pretraining within age group. #,## significantly different from 6 weeks of training within age group.

When correcting mitochondrial electron transport chain complex I–IV activities individually to CS activity, to take mitochondrial content into account, complex II (−26%) and III (−31%) activities were overall lower in the elderly compared with the young individuals pretraining and also after training and deconditioning ($p < 0.05$), whereas the CS-corrected complex I and IV activity was similar between young and elderly at all time points.

3.4. Apoptosis Markers: Cleaved Caspase 3 and Bcl2

There was no effect of aerobic training on cleaved caspase-3 protein content in either the elderly or the young individuals. Pretraining, elderly individuals had a 48% lower expression of cleaved caspase-3 protein content compared with young individuals ($p < 0.05$); however, after aerobic training and deconditioning, there was no longer any difference between the two groups (Figure 4A). Bcl2 protein expression decreased by 21% and 20% after aerobic training to a similar extent in the elderly and young individuals ($p < 0.05$), respectively; however, after 8 weeks of deconditioning, this was not different from pretraining levels in both groups (Figure 4B).

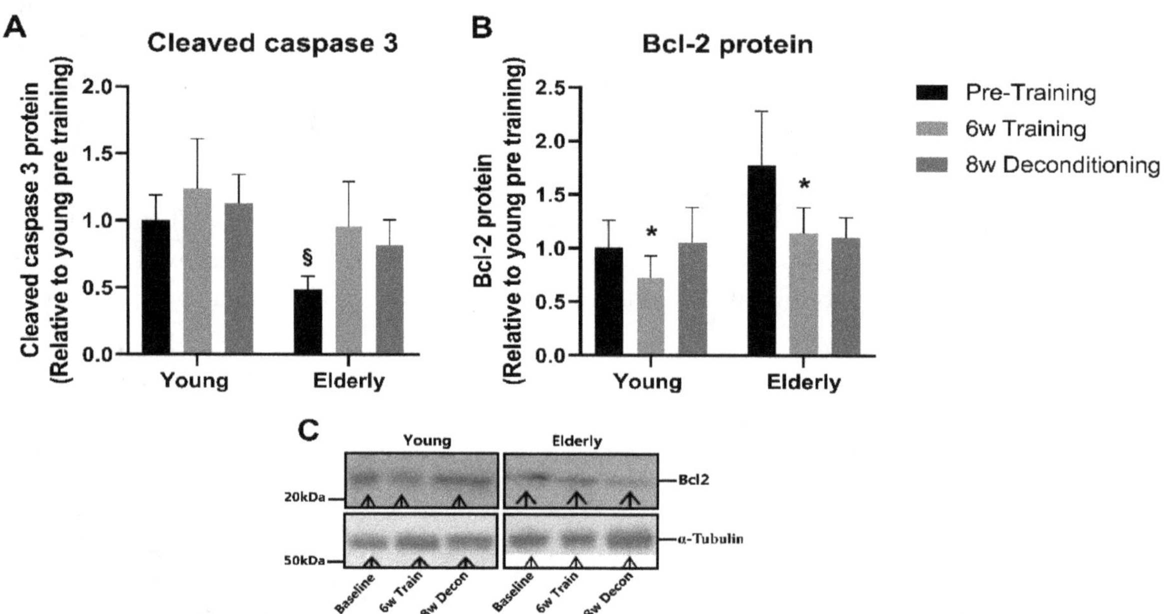

Figure 4. Apoptosis markers. Protein expression of cleaved caspase-3 (**A**) and B-cell lymphoma 2 (Bcl2) (**B**) in skeletal muscle pre and post 6 weeks of aerobic exercise training and after subsequent 8 weeks deconditioning period in young and elderly individuals. $n = 10$ in young group and $n = 11$ in the elderly group; however, due to lack of samples, only $n = 6$ in both groups in (**B**). (**C**) representative Western blots. Values are arbitrary units (means ± SE) and expressed relative to young group pretraining. § $p < 0.05$, young vs. elderly group within pretraining. * $p < 0.01$, main effect of training compared to pretraining independently of age.

4. Discussion

Age-related loss of muscle mass and function may be related to changes in mitochondrial function with age and an impaired response to adapt to the physical activity level. However, only a few studies investigated age-related changes in mitochondrial function in response to aerobic training and deconditioning. In the present study, we investigated age-related changes of aerobic capacity, mitochondrial function, and apoptotic signaling markers with aerobic training and deconditioning and found that (1) only 6 weeks of aerobic training efficiently improved maximal aerobic capacity and mitochondrial function in the elderly individuals, (2) the training effect on aerobic capacity, endurance, mitochondrial enzyme activities, and apoptosis signaling markers in the elderly individuals was similar to that found in the young individuals despite an age difference of more than 50 years, and (3) with deconditioning, the training-induced increases in endurance and mitochondrial enzyme activities decreased in a faster manner in elderly compared with young individuals.

It was suggested that differences in aerobic capacity in elderly versus young healthy humans, at least in part, may be a result of differences in the ability to gain and maintain VO_{2peak} with age [13,21,22]. However, in the present study, 6 weeks of intensive aerobic exercise training resulted in the same increase in VO_{2peak} in elderly individuals compared with that found in young, gender-matched, sedentary individuals, indicating a similar ability to increase oxidative capacity in elderly vs. young individuals. Although the training period was longer than in the present (8–16 weeks), the effect on aerobic capacity was overall the same as previously observed [12–17]. The increase in VO_{2peak} in the present study was found after only 6 weeks of aerobic training, suggesting that elderly individuals can increase oxidative capacity after a relatively short training period to the same extent as that seen in young healthy individuals.

Citrate synthase has been shown to be a strong marker of mitochondrial content. Thus, maximal CS activity strongly correlated with mitochondrial volume measured by electron microscopy in skeletal muscles of healthy, young men [41]. Moreover, maximal CS activity correlated with the improvement in mitochondrial volume after 6 weeks of aerobic training in skeletal muscle of young individuals [42]. In the literature, it has been debated whether there is an age-related decline in mitochondrial enzyme activities, since results from studies investigating this have been ambiguous. Several studies found decreased activity of CS and complex I–IV in muscle of elderly [15,43–47], indicating an age-related decline in mitochondrial content and function. Supporting this view, a study investigating the effect of age on mitochondrial content by transmission electron microscopy found a decrease in the content of mitochondria in elderly compared with young individuals [47]. In contrast, in the present study, CS and mitochondrial complex activities were similar at baseline between young and elderly, as we also recently showed between a similar cohort of young (~22 years) and elderly individuals (~82 years) [36] and in accordance with several other studies [13,48–50]. Interestingly, when mitochondrial complex activities were corrected relative to CS activity to take mitochondrial content into account, in the present study, complex II and III activities were lower in the elderly compared with the young individuals, implying a loss in the electron transport chain efficiency relative to mitochondrial content. It is possible that the mixed results from studies investigating the effect on age and mitochondrial function in part are related to differences in the pretraining level of physical activity in the investigated elderly individuals. Interestingly, in the present study, elderly individuals were able to increase CS activity (+31%) and mitochondrial complex activities (ranging between 61–163%) with training that matched that found in the healthy young individuals, which emphasizes that the ability to respond to an increase in demand in muscle enzymes in tricarboxylic acid (TCA) cycle and oxidative phosphorylation is preserved at least to the eighth decade of life. The few studies that investigated CS and/or mitochondrial complex activities in elderly of 60–80 years of age did not compare results to young but found a similar increase after 12–16 weeks of training [13,15,16,43], suggesting a similar ability of elderly of 60 and 80 years of age to respond to aerobic training. A recent study with only 6 weeks of high-intensity exercise training also showed improved CS activity and mitochondrial complex protein contents in "younger" elderly (63 years old) men and women [12], which, together with the intense protocol in the present study, underscores that mitochondria can adapt to even short-term training interventions in elderly of both 60 and 80 years of age, when the intensity and frequency of the training are high.

In addition to the exercise training intervention, we included a subsequent deconditioning period to evaluate mitochondrial dynamics in aged human skeletal muscle, which, to our knowledge, has not been studied previously in elderly healthy individuals. Deconditioning after exercise training was investigated in a few studies in healthy young individuals, and data implied that oxidative capacity, muscle mitochondrial protein content, and enzyme activities return to pretraining levels after 6–8 weeks in young individuals [23–27]. In the present study, mitochondrial content judged by CS and mitochondrial complex activities returned to pretraining levels after 8 weeks of deconditioning in the elderly, which was not seen in the young healthy individuals. Thus, enzyme activity of CS and complex I, III, and IV decreased in the elderly to a larger extent than in the young individuals. This indicates that the turnover rate of mitochondrial enzymes in the TCA cycle, as well as the oxidative phosphorylation, is fast and even more rapid in skeletal muscle of elderly. Thus, it seems as the ability to obtain oxidative capacity and increase mitochondrial volume with intensive aerobic training is preserved with age, but is lost faster in aged than in young muscle during subsequent deconditioning. A sedentary lifestyle in elderly individuals may, therefore, be even more deleterious to muscle health than in young individuals.

Endurance capacity is essential in order to maintain independence, reduce incidence of disability, and sustain a high quality of life in older people. In the present study, we found that 6 weeks of intensive aerobic exercise resulted in a remarkable increase in the time to exhaustion during an endurance test in the elderly individuals by 2.4-fold. Moreover, this training-induced increase in endurance was likely, at least in part, mediated by an improved exercise economy, reflecting the capacity to turn oxygen consumption into mechanical work and, hence, lower usage of VO_2 at the given power. This finding suggests a functional relevance of the training-induced increase in muscle mitochondrial respiratory enzyme activities, through an improved ability to sustain a high energy-production and also a more energy-efficient power production over a longer period of time. The present study is, to our knowledge, the first to demonstrate that the effect on aerobic capacity and muscle mitochondrial function and efficiency seemingly translates into functional improvement of endurance and exercise economy in elderly. In this line, it should be mechanistically studied in future investigations whether aerobic exercise training prevents sarcopenia by improving mitochondrial function and dynamics [51]. Interestingly, with deconditioning, a faster decrease in endurance capacity was observed among elderly compared with young individuals in accordance with similar decreases in CS and mitochondrial complex activities, indicating that, although elderly individuals improve endurance with training in the same manner as young individuals, aerobic endurance seems to be lost faster in elderly individuals, likely related to enhanced degradation of muscle mitochondrial enzymes. To support this notion, we found, despite the modest number of participants in the present study, that the loss of enzyme activity of CS and complex I and III in response to deconditioning tended to correlate to the reduction in endurance capacity. Of note, the faster decline in mitochondrial enzyme activity with deconditioning was in the present study observed in elderly of ~80 years of age, and it remains to be clarified whether 60–75-year-old individuals that are often investigated in the scientific literature would be more affected by deconditioning compared with young individuals. Importantly, a faster decline in endurance performance during deconditioning contrasts with the loss of strength performance after 6 weeks of resistance training, which we recently showed to be similar between young and elderly individuals (~82 years) after comparable 8 weeks of deconditioning [36].

Even though some studies in rodents indicated that apoptosis may play a role during muscle senescence [32], the involvement of age-related apoptosis of skeletal muscle and its regulation with training and deconditioning is poorly understood. Caspase-3 plays an important role in mediating cell death, and Bcl2 is thought to be an antiapoptotic driver. Interestingly, we found a lower muscle content of active caspase-3 (cleaved caspase-3) and a similar Bcl2 expression in the elderly compared with young individuals at baseline. This indicates, at least in healthy elderly individuals, that markers of the muscle intrinsic apoptotic pathway are not upregulated. These findings contrast with findings in rodents, in which increased apoptosis in old muscle of rodents was suggested on the basis of findings of an increased expression of proapoptotic marker cleaved caspase-3 protein [31] and a lower expression of the antiapoptotic Bcl2 protein [28–30]. Moreover, in the present study, caspase-3 activity remained similar in elderly and young skeletal muscle after 6 weeks of aerobic training, indicating that exercise training does not induce a higher apoptosis activity. In contrast, Bcl2 protein content decreased slightly in response to training to the same extent in young and elderly, implying either less antiapoptotic signaling after training independently of age or that Blc2 content is not directly coupled to apoptosis rate. To our knowledge, this study is the first to investigate apoptotic markers with training and deconditioning in human muscle of elderly compared with young individuals.

Although we only investigated a few markers of a complex signaling, the present results do not substantiate the hypothesis that increased apoptosis with time is the mediator of age-related muscle mass. The faster decline with deconditioning in endurance capacity and mitochondrial enzyme activity could relate to an age-related decline in mitochondrial fusion/fission regulation or an impaired matching of lysosomal mitophagy flux to the demand in aged muscle during deconditioning [51]. In support of the latter, we previously showed in young individuals that 3 weeks of one-legged aerobic training improved the capacity for autophagosomal formation [40], which is also found to occur in elderly [52], emphasizing the importance of physical activity to improve or maintain lysosomal mitophagic capacity. From studies in rodents [53–55] and humans [52], it is known that both muscle disuse and aging are associated with impaired mitophagy regulation, and it is, hence, likely that impaired mitophagy and mitochondrial function with deconditioning contribute to accelerated impairment in elderly, which should be addressed in future studies. Overall, accelerated decline in mitochondrial function and sarcopenia seems not to be driven by increased muscle apoptosis in human muscle, and further investigations are needed to elucidate the responsible molecular mechanisms driving sarcopenia and age-related inactivity-induced mitochondrial impairments.

The present study had some limitations that must be acknowledged. It was suggested that potential sex-specific adaptations to aerobic training exist [12]. We recognize that the present study included both men and women but that the number of participants was not optimal to detect an intervention × sex interaction; however, the present study was primarily designed to investigate the effects of training and deconditioning in elderly vs. young individuals. Studies with more subjects are warranted to evaluate potential sex-specific age-related adaptations to training and deconditioning.

5. Conclusions

In the present study, we found that 6 weeks of aerobic training efficiently improved maximal aerobic capacity and mitochondrial function in elderly individuals to the seemingly same extent as in young individuals despite an age difference of more than 50 years. This implies that aerobic exercise training is a potent tool to combat age-related loss of aerobic capacity and mitochondrial function. However, with deconditioning, we present the novel finding that the training-induced increases in performance and mitochondrial enzyme activities seemingly decreased in a faster manner in elderly compared with young individuals. This accelerated loss of mitochondrial function in the elderly with deconditioning could play a role in the development of mitochondrial dysfunction and sarcopenia during aging, and responsible mechanisms need to be investigated further in future studies.

Author Contributions: Conceptualization, S.P.A. and T.D.J.; methodology, S.P.A., F.D.T., T.K., and T.D.J.; investigation, A.M.F., S.P.A., K.A.N.Q., F.D.T., T.K., M.C.Ø., and T.D.J.; resources, T.K., J.V. and T.D.J.; data curation, A.M.F., S.P.A., K.A.N.Q., T.D.K.; writing—original draft preparation, A.M.F., K.A.N.Q., T.D.J.; writing—review and editing, A.M.F., S.P.A., K.A.N.Q., F.D.T., T.K., M.C.Ø., J.V. and T.D.J.; visualization, A.M.F.; supervision, T.K., J.V. and T.D.J.; project administration, S.P.A. and T.D.J.; funding acquisition, J.V. All authors have read and agreed to the published version of the manuscript.

Acknowledgments: We thank Tessa Munkeboe Hornsyld and Danuta Goralska-Olsen at the Copenhagen Neuromuscular Center, University of Copenhagen, Denmark for excellent technical assistance. Lastly, we would like to gratefully recognize the volunteers for participating in this invasive and demanding study.

References

1. Fuggle, N.; Shaw, S.; Dennison, E.; Cooper, C. Sarcopenia. *Best Pr. Res. Clin. Rheumatol.* **2017**, *31*, 218–242. [CrossRef] [PubMed]
2. Proctor, D.N.; Joyner, M.J. Skeletal muscle mass and the reduction of VO2 max in trained older subjects. *J. Appl. Physiol.* **1997**, *82*, 1411–1415. [CrossRef] [PubMed]
3. Myers, J.; Prakash, M.; Froelicher, V.; Do, D.; Partington, S.; Atwood, J.E. Dat Exercise Capacity and Mortality among Men Referred for Exercise Testing. *N. Engl. J. Med.* **2002**, *346*, 793–801. [CrossRef] [PubMed]

4. Blair, S.N.; Kohl, H.W., III; Paffenbarger, R.S., Jr.; Clark, D.G.; Cooper, K.H.; Gibbons, L.W. Physical fitness and all-cause mortality. A prospective study of healthy men and women. *JAMA* **1989**, *262*, 2395–2401. [CrossRef]
5. Posner, J.D.; McCully, K.K.; Landsberg, L.A.; Sands, L.; Tycenski, P.; Hofmann, M.T.; Wetterholt, K.L.; Shaw, C.E. Physical determinants of independence in mature women. *Arch. Phys. Med. Rehabil.* **1995**, *76*, 373–380. [CrossRef]
6. Peterson, C.M.; Johannsen, D.L.; Ravussin, E. Skeletal Muscle Mitochondria and Aging: A Review. *J. Aging Res.* **2012**, *2012*, 1–20. [CrossRef]
7. Johnson, M.L.; Robinson, M.M.; Nair, K.S. Skeletal muscle aging and the mitochondrion. *Trends Endocrinol. Metab.* **2013**, *24*, 247–256. [CrossRef]
8. Turner, D.L.; Hoppeler, H.; Claassen, H.; Vock, P.; Kayser, B.; Schena, F.; Ferretti, G. Effects of endurance training on oxidative capacity and structural composition of human arm and leg muscles. *Acta Physiol. Scand.* **1997**, *161*, 459–464. [CrossRef]
9. Hoppeler, H.; Howald, H.; Conley, K.; Lindstedt, S.L.; Claassen, H.; Vock, P.; Weibel, E.R. Endurance training in humans: Aerobic capacity and structure of skeletal muscle. *J. Appl. Physiol.* **1985**, *59*, 320–327. [CrossRef]
10. Holloszy, J.O. Biochemical adaptations in muscle. Effects of exercise on mitochondrial oxygen uptake and respiratory enzyme activity in skeletal muscle. *J. Boil. Chem.* **1967**, *242*, 2278–2282.
11. Tarnopolsky, M.A.; Rennie, C.D.; Robertshaw, H.A.; Fedak-Tarnopolsky, S.N.; Devries, M.C.; Hamadeh, M.J. Influence of endurance exercise training and sex on intramyocellular lipid and mitochondrial ultrastructure, substrate use, and mitochondrial enzyme activity. *Am. J. Physiol. Integr. Comp. Physiol.* **2007**, *292*, R1271–R1278. [CrossRef] [PubMed]
12. Chrøis, K.M.; Dohlmann, T.L.; Søgaard, D.; Hansen, C.V.; Dela, F.; Helge, J.W.; Larsen, S. Mitochondrial adaptations to high intensity interval training in older females and males. *Eur. J. Sport Sci.* **2019**, *20*, 135–145. [CrossRef] [PubMed]
13. Konopka, A.R.; Suer, M.K.; Wolff, C.A.; Harber, M.P. Markers of Human Skeletal Muscle Mitochondrial Biogenesis and Quality Control: Effects of Age and Aerobic Exercise Training. *J. Gerontol. Ser. A Boil. Sci. Med. Sci.* **2013**, *69*, 371–378. [CrossRef]
14. Menshikova, E.V.; Ritov, V.B.; Fairfull, L.; Ferrell, R.E.; Kelley, D.E.; Goodpaster, B.H. Effects of Exercise on Mitochondrial Content and Function in Aging Human Skeletal Muscle. *J. Gerontol. Ser. A Boil. Sci. Med. Sci.* **2006**, *61*, 534–540. [CrossRef]
15. Short, K.R.; Vittone, J.L.; Bigelow, M.L.; Proctor, D.N.; Rizza, R.A.; Coenen-Schimke, J.M.; Nair, K.S. Impact of aerobic exercise training on age-related changes in insulin sensitivity and muscle oxidative capacity. *Diabetes* **2003**, *52*, 1888–1896. [CrossRef] [PubMed]
16. Konopka, A.R.; Douglass, M.D.; Kaminsky, L.A.; Jemiolo, B.; Trappe, T.A.; Trappe, S.; Harber, M.P. Molecular Adaptations to Aerobic Exercise Training in Skeletal Muscle of Older Women. *J. Gerontol. Ser. A Boil. Sci. Med. Sci.* **2010**, *65*, 1201–1207. [CrossRef]
17. Broskey, N.T.; Greggio, C.; Boss, A.; Boutant, M.; Dwyer, A.; Schlueter, L.; Hans, D.; Gremion, G.; Kreis, R.; Boesch, C.; et al. Skeletal Muscle Mitochondria in the Elderly: Effects of Physical Fitness and Exercise Training. *J. Clin. Endocrinol. Metab.* **2014**, *99*, 1852–1861. [CrossRef]
18. Seals, D.R.; Hagberg, J.M.; Hurley, B.F.; Ehsani, A.A.; Holloszy, J.O. Endurance training in older men and women. I. Cardiovascular responses to exercise. *J. Appl. Physiol. Respir. Environ. Exerc. Physiol.* **1984**, *57*, 1024–1029. [CrossRef]
19. Seals, D.R.; Reiling, M.J. Effect of regular exercise on 24-hour arterial pressure in older hypertensive humans. *Hypertension* **1991**, *18*, 583–592. [CrossRef]
20. De Vito, G.; Bernardi, M.; Forte, R.; Pulejo, C.; Figura, F. Effects of a low-intensity conditioning programme on V˙O2max and maximal instantaneous peak power in elderly women. *Graefes Arch. Clin. Exp. Ophthalmol.* **1999**, *80*, 227–232. [CrossRef]
21. Wang, E.; Næss, M.S.; Hoff, J.; Albert, T.L.; Pham, Q.; Richardson, R.S.; Helgerud, J. Exercise-training-induced changes in metabolic capacity with age: The role of central cardiovascular plasticity. *AGE* **2013**, *36*, 665–676. [CrossRef] [PubMed]
22. Örlander, J.; Aniansson, A. Effects of physical training on skeletal muscle metabolism and ultrastructure in 70 to 75-year-old men. *Acta Physiol. Scand.* **1980**, *109*, 149–154. [CrossRef]

23. Fritzen, A.M.; Thøgersen, F.D.; Thybo, K.; Vissing, J.; Krag, T.O.B.; Ruiz-Ruiz, C.; Risom, L.; Wibrand, F.; Høeg, L.D.; Kiens, B.; et al. Adaptations in Mitochondrial Enzymatic Activity Occurs Independent of Genomic Dosage in Response to Aerobic Exercise Training and Deconditioning in Human Skeletal Muscle. *Cells* **2019**, *8*, 237. [CrossRef] [PubMed]
24. Coyle, E.F.; Martin, W.H.; Sinacore, D.R.; Joyner, M.J.; Hagberg, J.M.; Holloszy, J.O. Time course of loss of adaptations after stopping prolonged intense endurance training. *J. Appl. Physiol.* **1984**, *57*, 1857–1864. [CrossRef] [PubMed]
25. Coyle, E.F.; Martin, W.H.; Bloomfield, S.A.; Lowry, O.H.; Holloszy, J.O. Effects of detraining on responses to submaximal exercise. *J. Appl. Physiol.* **1985**, *59*, 853–859. [CrossRef]
26. Klausen, K.; Andersen, L.B.; Pelle, I. Adaptive changes in work capacity, skeletal muscle capillarization and enzyme levels during training and detraining. *Acta Physiol. Scand.* **1981**, *113*, 9–16. [CrossRef]
27. Jeppesen, T.D.; Schwartz, M.; Olsen, D.B.; Wibrand, F.; Krag, T.O.B.; Duno, M.; Hauerslev, S.; Vissing, J. Aerobic training is safe and improves exercise capacity in patients with mitochondrial myopathy. *Brain* **2006**, *129*, 3402–3412. [CrossRef]
28. Song, W.; Kwak, H.-B.; Lawler, J.M. Exercise Training Attenuates Age-Induced Changes in Apoptotic Signaling in Rat Skeletal Muscle. *Antioxid. Redox Signal.* **2006**, *8*, 517–528. [CrossRef]
29. Kwak, H.-B.; Song, W.; Lawler, J.M. Exercise training attenuates age-induced elevation in Bax/Bcl-2 ratio, apoptosis, and remodeling in the rat heart. *FASEB J.* **2006**, *20*, 791–793. [CrossRef]
30. Chung, L.; Ng, Y.-C. Age-related alterations in expression of apoptosis regulatory proteins and heat shock proteins in rat skeletal muscle. *Biochim. Biophys. Acta* **2006**, *1762*, 103–109. [CrossRef]
31. Dirks-Naylor, A.J.; Leeuwenburgh, C. Aging and lifelong calorie restriction result in adaptations of skeletal muscle apoptosis repressor, apoptosis-inducing factor, X-linked inhibitor of apoptosis, caspase-3, and caspase-12. *Free Radic. Boil. Med.* **2004**, *36*, 27–39. [CrossRef] [PubMed]
32. Leeuwenburgh, C. Role of Apoptosis in Sarcopenia. *J. Gerontol. Ser. A Boil. Sci. Med. Sci.* **2003**, *58*, M999–M1001. [CrossRef] [PubMed]
33. Dordevic, A.L.; Bonham, M.P.; Ghasem-Zadeh, A.; Evans, A.; Barber, E.M.; Day, K.; Kwok, A.; Truby, H. Reliability of Compartmental Body Composition Measures in Weight-Stable Adults Using GE iDXA: Implications for Research and Practice. *Nutrients* **2018**, *10*, 1484. [CrossRef] [PubMed]
34. Swain, D.P. Energy cost calculations for exercise prescription: An update. *Sports Med.* **2000**, *30*, 17–22. [CrossRef]
35. Bergstrom, J. Percutaneous needle biopsy of skeletal muscle in physiological and clinical research. *Scand. J. Clin. Lab. Invest.* **1975**, *35*, 609–616. [CrossRef] [PubMed]
36. Fritzen, A.M.; Thøgersen, F.D.; Qadri, K.A.N.; Krag, T.; Sveen, M.-L.; Vissing, J.; Jeppesen, T.D. Preserved Capacity for Adaptations in Strength and Muscle Regulatory Factors in Elderly in Response to Resistance Exercise Training and Deconditioning. *J. Clin. Med.* **2020**, *9*, 2188. [CrossRef]
37. Wibrand, F.; Jeppesen, T.D.; Frederiksen, A.L.; Olsen, D.B.; Duno, M.; Schwartz, M.; Vissing, J. Limited diagnostic value of enzyme analysis in patients with mitochondrial tRNA mutations. *Muscle Nerve* **2009**, *41*, 607–613. [CrossRef]
38. Birchmachin, M.; Briggs, H.; Saborido, A.; Bindoff, L.A.; Turnbull, D. An Evaluation of the Measurement of the Activities of Complexes I-IV in the Respiratory Chain of Human Skeletal Muscle Mitochondria. *Biochem. Med. Metab. Boil.* **1994**, *51*, 35–42. [CrossRef]
39. Krähenbühl, S.; Talos, C.; Wiesmann, U.; Hoppel, C.L. Development and evaluation of a spectrophotometric assay for complex III in isolated mitochondria, tissues and fibroblasts from rats and humans. *Clin. Chim. Acta* **1994**, *230*, 177–187. [CrossRef]
40. Fritzen, A.M.; Madsen, A.B.; Kleinert, M.; Treebak, J.T.; Lundsgaard, A.-M.; Jensen, T.E.; Richter, E.A.; Wojtaszewski, J.F.; Kiens, B.; Frøsig, C. Regulation of autophagy in human skeletal muscle: Effects of exercise, exercise training and insulin stimulation. *J. Physiol.* **2016**, *594*, 745–761. [CrossRef]
41. Larsen, S.; Nielsen, J.; Hansen, C.N.; Nielsen, L.B.; Wibrand, F.; Stride, N.; Schrøder, H.D.; Boushel, R.; Helge, J.W.; Dela, F.; et al. Biomarkers of mitochondrial content in skeletal muscle of healthy young human subjects. *J. Physiol.* **2012**, *590*, 3349–3360. [CrossRef] [PubMed]
42. Lundby, A.-K.M.; Jacobs, R.A.; Gehrig, S.; De Leur, J.; Hauser, M.; Bonne, T.C.; Flück, D.; Dandanell, S.; Kirk, N.; Kaech, A.; et al. Exercise training increases skeletal muscle mitochondrial volume density by enlargement of existing mitochondria and not de novo biogenesis. *Acta Physiol.* **2017**, *222*, e12905. [CrossRef]

43. Ghosh, S.; Lertwattanarak, R.; Lefort, N.; Molina-Carrion, M.; Joya-Galeana, J.; Bowen, B.P.; Garduño-García, J.J.; Abdul-Ghani, M.; Richardson, A.; DeFronzo, R.A.; et al. Reduction in Reactive Oxygen Species Production by Mitochondria From Elderly Subjects With Normal and Impaired Glucose Tolerance. *Diabetes* **2011**, *60*, 2051–2060. [CrossRef]
44. Boffoli, D.; Scacco, S.; Vergari, R.; Solarino, G.; Santacroce, G.; Papa, S. Decline with age of the respiratory chain activity in human skeletal muscle. *Biochim. Biophys. Acta* **1994**, *1226*, 73–82. [CrossRef]
45. Rooyackers, O.E.; Adey, D.B.; Ades, P.A.; Nair, K.S. Effect of age on in vivo rates of mitochondrial protein synthesis in human skeletal muscle. *Proc. Natl. Acad. Sci. USA* **1996**, *93*, 15364–15369. [CrossRef] [PubMed]
46. Tonkonogi, M.; Fernström, M.; Walsh, B.; Ji, L.L.; Rooyackers, O.; Hammarqvist, F.; Wernerman, J.; Sahlin, K. Reduced oxidative power but unchanged antioxidative capacity in skeletal muscle from aged humans. *Pflügers Arch.* **2003**, *446*, 261–269. [CrossRef]
47. Crane, J.D.; Devries, M.C.; Safdar, A.; Hamadeh, M.J.; Tarnopolsky, M.A. The Effect of Aging on Human Skeletal Muscle Mitochondrial and Intramyocellular Lipid Ultrastructure. *J. Gerontol. Ser. A Boil. Sci. Med. Sci.* **2009**, *65*, 119–128. [CrossRef]
48. Brierley, E.; Johnson, M.; James, O.; Turnbull, D. Effects of physical activity and age on mitochondrial function. *QJM Int. J. Med.* **1996**, *89*, 251–258. [CrossRef]
49. Barrientos, A.; Casademont, J.; Rötig, A.; Miro, O.; Urbano-Márquez, Á.; Rustin, P.; Cardellach, F. Absence of Relationship between the Level of Electron Transport Chain Activities and Aging in Human Skeletal Muscle. *Biochem. Biophys. Res. Commun.* **1996**, *229*, 536–539. [CrossRef]
50. Gouspillou, G.; Sgarioto, N.; Kapchinsky, S.; Purves-Smith, F.; Norris, B.; Pion, C.H.; Barbat-Artigas, S.; Lemieux, F.; Taivassalo, T.; Morais, J.A.; et al. Increased sensitivity to mitochondrial permeability transition and myonuclear translocation of endonuclease G in atrophied muscle of physically active older humans. *FASEB J.* **2013**, *28*, 1621–1633. [CrossRef]
51. Casuso, R.A.; Huertas, J.R. The emerging role of skeletal muscle mitochondrial dynamics in exercise and ageing. *Ageing Res. Rev.* **2020**, *58*, 101025. [CrossRef] [PubMed]
52. Arribat, Y.; Broskey, N.T.; Greggio, C.; Boutant, M.; Alonso, S.C.; Kulkarni, S.S.; Lagarrigue, S.; Carnero, E.A.; Besson, C.; Canto, C.; et al. Distinct patterns of skeletal muscle mitochondria fusion, fission and mitophagy upon duration of exercise training. *Acta Physiol.* **2018**, *225*, e13179. [CrossRef] [PubMed]
53. Kang, C.; Yeo, D.-W.; Ji, L.L. Muscle immobilization activates mitophagy and disrupts mitochondrial dynamics in mice. *Acta Physiol.* **2016**, *218*, 188–197. [CrossRef] [PubMed]
54. Vainshtein, A.; Tryon, L.D.; Pauly, M.; Hood, D.A. Role of PGC-1α during acute exercise-induced autophagy and mitophagy in skeletal muscle. *Am. J. Physiol. Physiol.* **2015**, *308*, C710–C719. [CrossRef]
55. Carter, H.N.; Kim, Y.; Erlich, A.T.; Zarrin-Khat, D.; Hood, D.A.; Erlich, A.T. Autophagy and mitophagy flux in young and aged skeletal muscle following chronic contractile activity. *J. Physiol.* **2018**, *596*, 3567–3584. [CrossRef]

15

Diagnosis, Treatment and Prevention of Sarcopenia in Hip Fractured Patients: Where we are and where we are Going

Gianluca Testa [1,*], Andrea Vescio [1], Danilo Zuccalà [1], Vincenzo Petrantoni [1], Mirko Amico [1], Giorgio Ivan Russo [2], Giuseppe Sessa [1] and Vito Pavone [1]

1 Department of General Surgery and Medical Surgical Specialties, Section of Orthopaedics and Traumatology, University Hospital Policlinico-San Marco, University of Catania, 95124 Catania, Italy; andreavescio88@gmail.com (A.V.); danilozuccala90@gmail.com (D.Z.); vpetrantoni1@gmail.com (V.P.); amico_mirko87@hotmail.com (M.A.); giusessa@unict.it (G.S.); vitopavone@hotmail.com (V.P.)

2 Department of General Surgery and Medical Surgical Specialties, Urology Section, University Hospital Policlinico-San Marco, University of Catania, 95124 Catania, Italy; giorgioivan.russo@unict.it

* Correspondence: gianpavel@hotmail.com

Abstract: Background: Sarcopenia is defined as a progressive loss of muscle mass and muscle strength associated to increased adverse events, such as falls and hip fractures. The aim of this systematic review is to analyse diagnosis methods of sarcopenia in patients with hip fracture and evaluate prevention and treatment strategies described in literature. Methods: Three independent authors performed a systematic review of two electronic medical databases using the following inclusion criteria: Sarcopenia, hip fractures, diagnosis, treatment, and prevention with a minimum average of 6-months follow-up. Any evidence-level studies reporting clinical data and dealing with sarcopenia diagnosis, or the treatment and prevention in hip fracture-affected patients, were considered. Results: A total of 32 articles were found. After the first screening, we selected 19 articles eligible for full-text reading. Ultimately, following full-text reading, and checking of the reference list, seven articles were included. Conclusions: Sarcopenia diagnosis is challenging, as no standardized diagnostic and therapeutic protocols are present. The development of medical management programs is mandatory for good prevention. To ensure adequate resource provision, care models should be reviewed, and new welfare policies should be adopted in the future.

Keywords: sarcopenia; hip fracture; diagnosis; treatment; prevention; dual-energy X-ray absorptiometry; bisphosphonate; β-hydroxy-β-methylbutyrate; exercise intervention

---

1. Introduction

Sarcopenia-related falls and fractures play an important role in our society due to the increased average age of the population [1]. Hip fractures are becoming an evolving and more current problem, as well as one of the most serious medical and social concerns. Hip fractures result in enhanced mortality, perpetual physical morbidity and reduced activities of daily living (ADL) [2,3], with a decrease of the quality of life for caregivers and an increased economic impact on society and government spending [4–6]. Nowadays, the prevention of hip fractures is considered crucial for preserving an acceptable quality of life in older patients. For these reasons, the role of the muscles trophism and function is crucial to prevent traumas in older patients [1]. Ageing is inversely related to the mass and strength of skeletal muscles, and their loss accelerates after 65 years of age, leading to an increased risk of adverse outcomes [7]. For the last 30 years, a considerable effort has been made to understand the condition of sarcopenia, and several definitions have been proposed. Sarcopenia was first defined by

Rosenberg as an age-associated loss of skeletal muscle mass [8], but recently, it has been identified as a disease, and is included in the ICD-10 code (M62.84) [9]. Several disease descriptions were suggested during the last 20 years, but substantial operative variances are present concerning definitions, including nomenclature, the technique of assessment of lean mass, the technique of standardization of lean mass to body size, cut-points for weakness and cut-points for slowness [10]. One of the most accepted was described by the EWGSOP (European Working Group on Sarcopenia in Older Persons), updated in 2018 (EWGSOP2), considering sarcopenia as a "progressive loss of muscle mass and muscle strength, associated to an increased likelihood of adverse events, such as falls, fractures, physical disability and death" [7]. Several authors investigated the differences in sarcopenia cases, agreeing with EWGSOP1 and EWGSOP2 and noting substantial discordance and limited overlap of the definitions [11,12]. Nevertheless, the EWGSOP2 is crucial suggestion to evaluate a possible condition of sarcopenia by measuring the muscle strength, muscle mass and physical performance [13]. Aging is related to variations in body structure and uncontrolled weight loss. The progressive loss of skeletal muscle mass (SMM) and strength promotes functional and physical disability, leading to poor quality of life [7]. The body composition changes were reported in several studies [7,14,15]. Cruz-Jentoft et al. [7] showed a loss of muscle strength in older patients through measurement grip strength with a dynamometer. Hida et al. [14] demonstrated a greater sarcopenia prevalence and more diminished leg muscle mass in subjects following a hip fracture than uninjured subjects with the same age. The most efficient technique to date, dual energy X-ray absorptiometry (DXA), assesses lean mass [16]. Bioelectrical impedance analysis (BIA), CT, and MRI can be used in selected cases [16]. DXA has several advantages, including low cost, low irradiation exposure and easy availability and usability. However, the difficulty of performing this examination in patients with hip fracture or in subjects undergoing recent orthopaedic surgery, due to post-surgical pain and immobility, the use of machines with non-uniform calibrations between them and the lack of universally shared protocols, makes DXA not always reliable in the quantification of MM and in the instrumental diagnosis of sarcopenia [11,17]. No specific drugs have been approved for the treatment of sarcopenia and the literature lacks evidence [16]. Research activity is focused on developing new drugs for sarcopenia, although progress has not been straightforward. Initial interest in selective androgen receptor modulators is related to small phase I and II trials [18,19]. For these reasons, the interest in sarcopenia is rising in orthopaedic surgery, due to the high prevalence of older patients, especially those suffering for hip fractures [20], and sarcopenia could be considered as a hip fracture risk factor.

The aim of this systematic review was to analyse diagnosis methods of sarcopenia in patients with hip fracture and evaluate prevention and treatment strategies described in literature.

2. Experimental Section

2.1. Study Selection

From their date of inception to 19th March 2020, two independent authors (AV and GT) systematically reviewed the main web-based databases, Science Direct and PubMed, agreeing to the Preferred Reporting Items for systematic Reviews and Meta-Analyses (PRISMA) recommendations [19]. The research string used was "sarcopenia AND (diagnosis OR treatment OR prevention) AND (femoral neck fracture OR hip fracture)". In order to extract the number of patients, mean age at treatment, sex, type of treatment, follow-up, and year of the study a standard data entry form was used for each included original manuscript. Three independent reviewers (MA, PV and DZ) performed the quality evaluation of the studies. Discussing conflicts about data were resolved by consultation with a senior surgeon (VP).

2.2. Inclusion and Exclusion Criteria

Eligible studies for the present systematic review included sarcopenia diagnosis, treatment and prevention in hip-fractured patients. The original titles and abstracts examination were selected using the following inclusion criteria: Sarcopenia, hip fractures, diagnosis and treatment and prevention with a minimum average of 6-months follow-up in last 20 years. The exclusion criteria were: Patients' cohort with no sarcopenia diseases, less than 6 months of symptoms and no human trials. Each residual duplicate, articles related on other issues or with inadequate technical methodology and available abstract were ruled out.

2.3. Risk of Bias Assessment

According to the ROBINS-I tool for nonrandomized studies [21], a three-stage assessment of the studies included risk of bias assessment was performed. The first step involved the design of the systematic review, the next phase was the assessment of the ordinary bias discovered in these manuscripts and the final was about the total risk of bias. "Low risk" and "Moderate risk" studies were considered acceptable for the review. The assessment was separately performed by three authors (MA, PV and DZ). Any discrepancy was discussed with the senior investigator (VP) for the final decision. All the authors agreed on the result of every stage of the assessment.

3. Results

3.1. Included Studies

Thirty-two manuscripts were recovered. Twenty-four articles were chosen, following the exclusion of duplicates. At the end of the first screening, according to the selection criteria previously described, nine articles were chosen as eligible for full-text reading. Metanalysis or systematic reviews were eliminated from the study. Finally, after reading the complete articles and examining the reference list, we chose seven manuscripts comprised of randomized controlled human trials (hRCT), prospective and retrospective cohort or series studies, according to previously described criteria. A selection and screening method PRISMA [22] flowchart is provided in Figure 1.

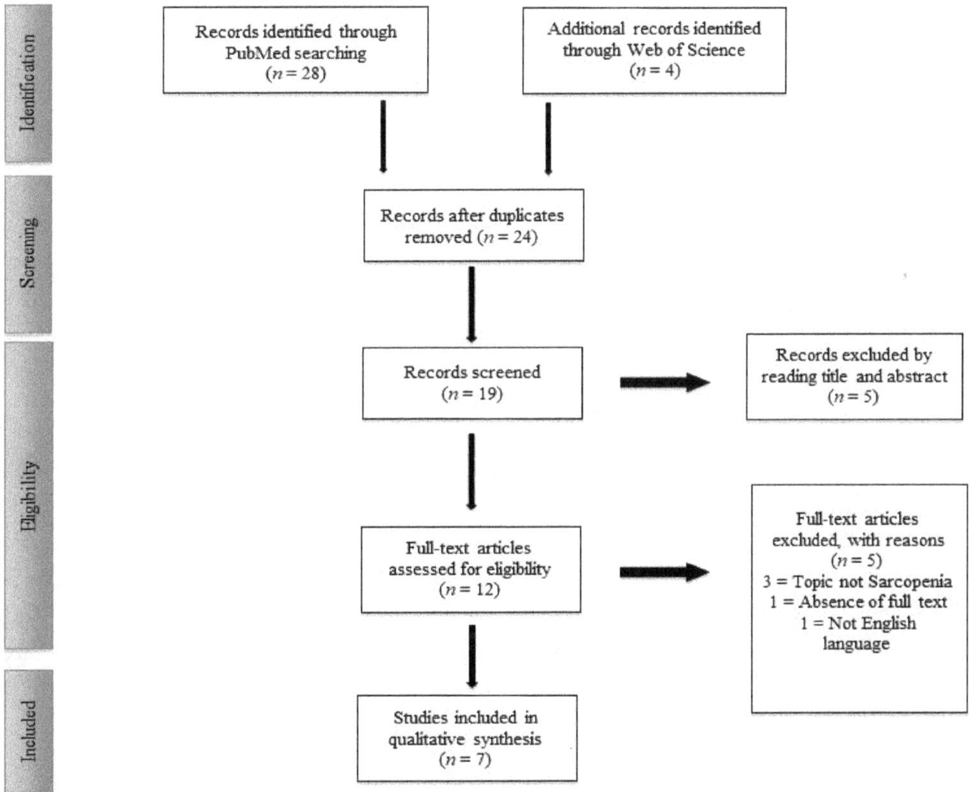

Figure 1. PRISMA (Preferred Reporting Items for Systematic Reviews and Meta-Analysis) flowchart.

3.2. The Diagnosis of Sarcopenia in Patients Affected by Hip Fracture

Kramer et al. [23] performed biopsies of vastus lateralis to assess the muscle changes. The sample was divided in to three groups: Healthy young women (HYW) (18–25 years), healthy older women (HEW) (>65 years) and older women (>65 years) affected by traumatic hip fracture (FEW). FEW Type 2 fibers (2.609 ± 185 μm^2) were noted significantly smaller compared to HEW (3.723 ± 322 μm^2; $p = 0.03$) and HYW (4.755 ± 335 μm^2; $p < 0.001$).

Hansen et al. [16] compared the Computed Tomography (CT) and dual-energy X-ray absorptiometry (DXA) efficiency in the assessment of midthigh muscle mass (SMM) and midthigh cross-sectional area (CSA) respectively, after a hip fracture with 12 months follow-up. The two measures were significantly linked to baseline ($r = 0.86$, $p < 0.001$). Ratios of midthigh fat to lean mass were comparably related (interclass correlation coefficient = 0.87, $p < 0.001$). Data of the change from baseline to follow-up showed a low correlation (interclass correlation coefficient = 0.87, $p = 0.019$). The assessment of muscle mass by DXA-derived midthigh slice has been shown to be reasonably accurate in comparison to a single-slice CT technique in this sample of frail older patients.

Villani et al. [24] evaluated the agreement degree between DXA and bioelectrical impedance spectroscopy (BIS) associated to corrected arm muscle area (CAMA). No significant changes ($p = 0.78$) were found when comparing fat-free mass (FFM) with BIS (FFMBIS) to FFM with DXA (FFMDXA) mean bias. Nevertheless, when included as an independent covariate, gender demonstrated an influence on variation in the mean bias over time ($p = 0.007$). The influence of BMI had no effect on change in the mean bias ($p = 0.19$). Similarly, no significant changes in the mean bias were observed between SMMDXA and SMMCAMA across each assessment time point ($p = 0.18$). At each assessment follow-up, both the techniques were observed overestimated SMM and FFM.

3.3. Treatment of Sarcopenia in Patients Affected by Hip Fracture

Flodin et al. [25] evaluated the efficacy of nutritional supplementation on body composition (BC), handgrip strength (HGS) and health-related quality of life (HRQoL) in 79 hip-fractured patients (mean age 79 ± 9 years). Patients were divided into a protein and bisphosphonate group (PB) group, bisphosphonate-only group (BO) and a control group (CG) with 12 months follow-up. All groups included the CG, received calcium and Vitamin D supplementation. No significant differences in changes of FFM Index, HGS and HRQoL were detected during the follow-up period between the groups.

Invernizzi et al. [26] assessed the essential amino acid supplementation (AAS) in hip-fractured patients. Thirty-two patients (sarcopenia-affected = 71.9%) underwent to a 2-month rehabilitative protocol combined with dietetic counselling. The AA group (16 subjects) had an AAS, while the NAA group did not receive AAS. According to Janssen criteria, both groups were divided in subgroups: Sarcopenic (Sac) and non-sarcopenic (No-Sac) patients. At 2 months follow-up, the Sac AA group ($n = 10$) obtained better significant results in the Iowa Level of Assistance scale (ILOA) and all the primary outcomes ($p < 0.017$) compared to Sac NAA cohort ($n = 13$). The No-Sac groups had similar results.

Malafarina et al. [27] investigated the effectiveness of β-hydroxy-β-methylbutyrate (HMB) oral NS on muscle mass and nutritional markers (BMI, proteins) in patients >65 years with hip fracture. Fifty-five patients (IG) received standard diet plus HMB NS and 52 patients (CG) received standard diet only. The authors used the EWGSOP criteria to diagnose sarcopenia and its prevalence among the entire population was 72%. The sarcopenia diagnostic markers were gait speed (GS), HGS and BC (assessed with BIA). Positive results were recorded in IG for grip work index ($p = 0.188$), muscle mass (MM) ($p = 0.031$) and appendicular lean mass (aLM) ($p = 0.020$). GS analysis did not show a significant difference ($p = 0.367$).

3.4. Prevention of Sarcopenia in Patients Affected by Hip Fracture

In a study by Ding-Cheng Chan et al. [28], 110 patients over 50 years of age with high-risk fracture underwent 3-month exercise interventions. According to different modalities of the exercise, the cohort were randomly divided into integrated care (IC) group and machine-based low extremities exercise (LEE) group. The authors observed a gain in limb mass in the entire cohort (1.13%, $p < 0.05$) with a significant change in the LEE group (1.13%, $p < 0.01$). Both groups obtained significant improvement in muscle strength measured with curl, press and leg extension, grip strength, gait speed, chair stand test and time up and go test. Improvements were seen in leg curl in the LEE group (29.78%, $p = 0.001$).

The most important results of the included articles were summarized (Table 1).

Table 1. Included studies summary. Dual-energy X-ray absorptiometry (DEXA); healthy young women (HYW); healthy elderly women (HEW); elderly women with a hip fracture (FEW); Dual-energy X-ray absorptiometry (DEXA); BIS (bioletrical impedance spectroscopy); corrected arm muscle area (CAMA); Fat-free mass (FFM) with BIS (FFMBIS); FFM with DXA (FFMDXA); handgrip strength (HGS) and health-related quality of life (HRQoL); Timed Up and Go test (TUG); Iowa Level of Assistance scale (ILOA); Mini Nutritional Assessment–Short Form (MNA-SF); Barthel index (BI); Functional Ambulation Categories (FAC).

Author	Sample	Intervention	Outcome Measures	Results	Limits of the Study
Kramer et al., 2017	15 HYW (age: 20.3 ± 0.4 years), 15 HEW (age: 78.8 ± 1.7 years), and 15 FEW (age: 82.3 ± 1.5 years)	Muscle biopsies and immunohistochemistry	Muscle fibre type distribution, myonuclear and satellite cell content	FEW resulted in atrophy of muscle fibres Type I and II, associated to a general deterioration in muscle fibres Type II size. Atrophy of Type II muscle fibre in these subjects is associated to a decrease in myonuclear content of Type II muscle fibre.	No measures of muscle mass and/or strength. No data about men
Hansen et al., 2007	30 patients over 60 years old with hip fractures affected in community living patients (not nursing houses, no dementia, no terminally ill)	DEXA-derived midthigh slice has been found to be reasonably accurate in comparison with a single-slice CT technique	Muscle mass and composition	Superior accessibility and simplicity of DEXA utilize. DEXA errors inherent suggest that it should be used to studying groups of patients rather than individuals and in longitudinal trials.	Patients with non-traumatic neck hip fracture
Villani et al., 2012	79 Patients with hip fracture, free in the community.	BIS; DEXA	FFM and SMM, and CAMA	BIS demonstrated sufficient agreement against DXA.	Predictive power and Repeatability
Flodin et al., 2015	79 patients divided in 3 groups: Group N (26 patients); Group B (28 patients); Group C (25 patients)	Group N: 40 g of protein and 600 kcal combined with risedronate and calcium 1 g and vit D 800 IE; Group B: Same of Group N + bisphosphonates alone once weekly for 12 months; Group C: Control. All groups received conventional rehabilitation	Body composition; HGS; HRQoL at 0, 6 and 12 months postoperatively	No considerable variation in baseline attributes was observed between the groups. There was a positive correlation between FFMI and aLMI, $r = 0.92$, $p < 0.01$.	Small number of study subjects. The use of different devices of DXA measurements inflict uncertainties on the validity of the results

Table 1. *Cont.*

Author	Sample	Intervention	Outcome Measures	Results	Limits of the Study
Invernizzi et al., 2018	32 patients over 65 years old divided in two groups: Sarcopenic and non-sarcopenic.	Physical exercise rehabilitative programme and received a dietetic counselling. One group was supplemented with two sachets of 4 g/day of essential amino acids.	HGS, TUG, ILOA, Nutritional assessment, HRQoL baseline (T0) and after 2 months of treatment (T1)	At T1 follow-up, statistically significant differences in all the outcomes ($p < 0.017$) in sarcopenic patient who received AA supplementation.	Small size, the use of BIA to calculate the SMI.
Malafarina et al., 2017	107 patients: Group control (CG), Group intervention (IG)	CG: standard diet (1500 kcal); IG: CG+oral nutritional supplementation (CaHMB 0.7 g/100 mL, 25(OH)D 227 IU/100 mL and 227 mg/100 mL of calcium). All patients received Physical therapy	Body composition, HGS, MNA-SF, BI, FAC	BMI and lean mass were constant in IG patients, while reduced in the CG. The vitamin D and proteins and concentration had improved more in the IG than in the CG. ADL recovery of was more frequent in the IG (68%) than in the CG (59%) ($p = 0.261$)	Patients received physiotherapy 5 days por week. No follow-up after discharge. Diagnostic criteria for sarcopenia.
Chan et al., 2018	110 participants divided in Integrated group (IG) and Low extremity group (LEG)	IC: 15 min warm-up + Resistance training (30 min) + Balance training (10 min) at least once a week for 12 weeks. LEG: 12-week machine based lower extremity resistance exercise twice per week (30 min each). All participants had received a lecture on prevention of osteoporosis, sarcopenia and fall-related injury	Body composition; Gait speed (m/s), chair stand test and timed up-and-go test. Hip and L-spine BMD.	Decrease in weight ($p < 0.01$) and limb fat ($p < 0.001$) were noted in IC group. Im LLE group, Significant variations were detected in limb mass ($p < 0.01$). No variation in the cohorts regarding change on body composition. Significant enhancement in muscle strength in both the cohorts. After 3 months, significant improvement for leg strength but higher gain in LEE on leg curl performance ($p = 0.001$). BMD of L-spine improved but similar after 3 months.	BMD tests were not strictly performed on all participants.

4. Discussion

4.1. General Considerations and Key Findings

According to the review findings the diagnosis is still a challenge. The lack of an optimal instrumental tool for diagnosis in hip-fractured patients demonstrates the crucial role of physicians in these cases. The diagnosis is not instrumental data but the correct analysis of the clinical examination and patients' physical status evaluation in association with the results of the tool. At the same time, the nutritional supplementation and hip fracture prevention exercise program are mandatory to avoid the variances in body composition after midlife. Therefore, body composition evaluation is a crucial element for measuring health status in older adults.

The higher incidence of fractures, especially in the spinal column and femoral neck, is attributable to the condition of osteopenia or osteoporosis. Several authors have debated the correlation of bone mineral density (BMD) to muscle mass (MM). However, this association is controversial. Gillette-Guyonnet et al. [29] and Walsh et al. [30] claimed there was no muscle–bone relationship. On the other hand, Locquet et al. exhaustively explored the correlation between muscle and identified a subpopulation affected by the reduction in bone and muscle mass [31]. Moreover, Hirschfeld et al. suggested considering the two condition as a new pathologic disorder, where the subjects affected should be defined as "osteosarcopenic patients" [32]. The controversial findings should be explained by the different diagnosis protocols used. In fact, the sarcopenia diagnosis is often challenging, and there is not an instrumental method or standard algorithm commonly accepted for the evaluation. EWGSOP2 suggests combining clinical tests and instrumental investigations to evaluate the muscle strength, physical performance and muscle mass [11].

4.2. Sarcopenia Diagnosis in Hip-Fractured Patients

Determining grip strength is easy, inexpensive and routine in clinical practice. The evaluation requires calibrated handheld dynamometer use under well-definite exam circumstances with interpretive data from appropriate reference populations [11,33]. On the other hand, the technique measurements can be influenced by the examiner [33]. Similarly, the chair stand test (also called the chair rise test), aims to assess the quantity of time that the patient needs to rise five times from a seated position without using their arms [30]. The Gait Speed test is helpful in the evaluation of physical performance. The principles are the Short Physical Performance Battery (SPPB), and the Timed-Up and Go test (TUG), but the results can be influenced by patient compliance. The Gait Speed test is a rapid, secure and reliable test to assess sarcopenia by EWGSOP2 [11]. The patient walks for 4 m while the clinical staff records the walking speed using an electronic device or manually with a stopwatch. A Gait Speed of ≤0.8 m/s is a severe sarcopenia marker [34–36]. The SPPB is a complex test aimed to analyse gait speed using a balance test and a chair stand test. The highest score is 12 points, and a score of ≤8 points suggests inadequate physical performance. The TUG test assesses the taken time to rise from a standard chair, walk 3 m away, turn around, walk back and sit down again. A score of >20 s is indicative of poor physical performance [37].

Due to the reduced mobility in the hip-fractured patients, and consecutively, to the impossibility in performing the main tests used to assess the disease, the instrumental tools are important part of diagnosis, even if they can replace the clinical evaluation.

DXA is a more widely accessible tool to establish MM [38], and can be defined as total body SMM, as ASM or as muscle cross-sectional area of specific muscle groups [16]. New methods have been studied, including midthigh muscle measurement by CT or MRI, BIS, psoas muscle measurement with CT, the detection of specific biomarkers and other tests [16,24,25]. CT and MRI allow for a precise and detailed study of soft tissues and they offer reliable and universally shared data. On the other hand, these methods have a high cost and it is difficult to find institutes where it is possible to quickly perform them. Moreover, CT exposes patients to a high rate of irradiation [16,34]. Hansen et al. [16] compared SMM estimated by DXA to midthigh muscle CSA, determined by CT, in a group of older patients with hip fracture, observing a positive correlation between CT-determined midthigh muscle CSA and DXA-derived midthigh SMM. The assessment of MM and body composition by DXA-derived midthigh slice has been shown to be reasonably accurate in comparison to a single-slice CT technique in this sample of frail older patients [16].

BIS is another technique used to estimate SMM. The measurement is not a direct evaluation of MM, but an estimation on the whole-body electrical conductivity, through conversion equations [37]. BIS needs highly trained personnel, and the institutes where it can be performed are very difficult to find. Villani et al. [24] compared BIS associated to CAMA and DXA, noting BIS were reliable, but the difficulties in carrying out the examination and in the use of conversion equations led to DXA as the preferred reference technique. Muscle mass evaluation is not the only parameter that can be associated to sarcopenia. A low muscle quality is considered as one of the diagnosis criteria by EWGSOP [11]. Muscle quality is one of the main determinants of muscle function, depending on different factors (fibre composition, architecture, metabolism, intermuscular adipose tissue, fibrosis, motor unit activation) [39]. In particular, the decline of type II muscle fibres (II-MF) is responsible for muscle mass reduction [40].

Kramer et al. [22] performed vastus lateralis biopsies in different groups, confirming a significant II-MF atrophy in older women with hip fractures when compared to healthy older or young women. Since muscle atrophy is associated to loss of function, the author suggested that II-MF atrophy could lead to a higher risk of falls and consequent fractures. This study has some limits. There was no measure of strength and the sample was exclusively female, but the findings could be relevant to treat sarcopenia and to understand the II-MF atrophy causes. The histological diagnosis of sarcopenia could be a valuable way to understand physiopathology of sarcopenia in patients with hip fractures, even if it is not obviously suitable for routine diagnosis.

4.3. Sarcopenia Treatment in Hip-Fractured Patients

The treatment of sarcopenia in patients affected by hip fractures is a multidisciplinary challenge and, according to our findings, great attention should be given to nutritional status. Malnutrition is a highly prevalent condition in the geriatric population affected by this fracture [27]. Therefore, oral nutritional supplementation (ONS), in addition to rehabilitation programs, has become the subject of debate between different authors. Flodin et al. [25] investigated the effects of protein-rich supplementation and bisphosphonate on body composition, handgrip strength and quality of life in patients with hip fracture at 12-months follow-up. In a group, the combination of bisphosphonates and protein supplementation had no significant effects on handgrip strength (HGS), body composition and health-related quality of life (HRQoL). In another group, a positive effect of protein-rich supplementation and bisphosphonates on HGS and HRQoL was demonstrated.

Malafarina et al. [27] showed good results using oral nutritional supplementation with β-hydroxy-β-methylbutyrate (HMB). This approach improves MM, function and general nutritional status in hip-fractured patients [27]. HMB, a metabolite of leucine, has beneficial effect on MM and function in older people [41], but considering the lack of evidence focused on hip-fractured people, more investigations are needed in the treatment of sarcopenia with HMB in these patients. On the other hand, the role of a nutritional intervention without exercise for the treatment of sarcopenia is debated [41]. Although many studies have described good results in increasing protein intake in the older population [42,43], the timing and distribution is unclear [44].

4.4. Sarcopenia Prevention in Hip-Fractured Patients

Despite the few studies focused on sarcopenia prevention in our study, it could be considered the major area of research for future clinical activity and observational epidemiological trials [39] in order to identify and modify the sarcopenia risk factors. A midlife lifestyle approach could be more proper to limit the sarcopenia incidence [45].

Physical activity programs have been suggested as a relevant technique in reducing the risk of hip fracture in older patients [46,47]. In the study by Piastra et al. [47], data showed a significant improvement in MM, muscle mass index, and handgrip strength in muscle reinforcement training group, demonstrating that a muscle reinforcement program moved participants from a condition of moderate sarcopenia at baseline to a condition of normality. Ding-Cheng Chan et al. [28] evaluated effects of programs in community-dwelling older adults with high risk of fractures (> or =3% for hip fracture). The exercise authors clarified the lack of differences in the types of exercise to improve sarcopenia when compared an integrated care model to a lower extremity exercise model. However, several authors promoted rehabilitation protocols for hip-fractured patients, consisting of oral nutritional supplementation with proteins and amino acids and exercise programs [46,47]. Singh et al. [47] proposed a new rehabilitation protocol in the older with hip fracture after orthopaedic surgery. The 12-month rehabilitation program was characterized by a high-intensity progressive resistance training and a targeted treatment of balance, osteoporosis, nutrition, vitamin D and calcium, depression, home safety and social support. The authors showed a statistically significant reduction in mortality, nursing home hospitalization and disability, especially in those subjects with a systematic good health status.

A life course approach to prevention is paramount and offers chance to intervention when lifestyle changes, inspiring the increase of physical activity with immediate to lifelong advantages for skeletal muscle health [16].

4.5. Limits of the Study

The limits of the study are represented by the heterogenicity of the definition of sarcopenia and by the tools considered to assess the patient functional outcome. We extensively searched and identified all relevant last 20 years sarcopenia diagnosis-, treatment- and prevention-related articles. Therefore, risk of bias assessment showed moderate overall risk, which could influence our analysis. Moreover, in the diagnosis section, only instrumental tool evaluations without clinical assessment were detected.

5. Conclusions

Sarcopenia is a physiological condition and contributes to the increased risk of falls and hip fractures in the older population. However, the diagnosis of sarcopenia is challenging, especially in hip-fractured patients, and there are currently no standardised diagnostic and therapeutic protocols. The development of medical management programs is mandatory for good prevention. To ensure adequate resource provision, care models should be reviewed, and new welfare policies should be adopted in the future.

Author Contributions: Conceptualization, G.T., A.V. and V.P. (Vito Pavone); methodology, A.V.; software, M.A.; validation, G.T., V.P. (Vincenzo Petrantoni) and G.I.R.; formal analysis, A.V.; investigation, M.A., V.P. (Vincenzo Petrantoni) and D.Z.; resources, A.V.; data curation, G.T.; writing—original draft preparation, D.Z.; writing—review and editing, G.T. and A.V.; visualization, G.I.R.; supervision, G.S.; project administration, V.P. (Vito Pavone); funding acquisition, V.P. (Vito Pavone). All authors have read and agreed to the published version of the manuscript.

References

1. Auais, M.; Morin, S.; Nadeau, L.; Finch, L.; Mayo, N. Changes in frailty-related characteristics of the hip fracture population and their implications for healthcare services: Evidence from Quebec, Canada. *Osteoporos. Int.* **2013**, *24*, 2713–2724. [CrossRef]
2. Kitamura, S.; Hasegawa, Y.; Suzuki, S.; Sasaki, R.; Iwata, H.; Wingstrand, H.; Thorngren, K.G. Functional outcome after hip fracture in Japan. *Clin. Orthop. Relat. Res.* **1998**, *348*, 29–36. [CrossRef]

3. Cummings, S.R.; Melton, L.J. Epidemiology and outcomes of osteoporotic fractures. *Lancet* **2002**, *359*, 1761–1767. [CrossRef]
4. Marottoli, R.A.; Berkman, L.F.; Leo-Summers, L.; Cooney, L.M., Jr. Predictors of mortality and institutionalization after hip fracture: The New Haven EPESE cohort. Established Populations for Epidemiologic Studies of the Elderly. *Am. J. Public Health* **1994**, *84*, 1807–1812. [CrossRef]
5. Saltz, C.; Zimmerman, S.; Tompkins, C.; Harrington, D.; Magaziner, J. Stress among caregivers of hip fracture patients. *J. Gerontol. Soc. Work* **1998**, *30*, 167–181. [CrossRef]
6. Duclos, A.; Couray-Targe, S.; Randrianasolo, M.; Hedoux, S.; Couris, C.M.; Colin, C.; Schott, A.M. Burden of hip fracture on inpatient care: A before and after population-based study. *Osteoporos. Int.* **2009**, *21*, 1493–1501. [CrossRef] [PubMed]
7. Cruz-Jentoft, A.J.; Baeyens, J.P.; Bauer, J.M.; Boirie, Y.; Cederholm, T.; Landi, F.; Martin, F.C.; Michel, J.P.; Rolland, Y.; Schneider, S.M.; et al. Sarcopenia: European consensus on definition and diagnosis: Report of the European Working Group on sarcopenia in older people. *Age Ageing* **2010**, *39*, 412–423. [CrossRef] [PubMed]
8. Rosenberg, I.H. Sarcopenia: Origins and clinical relevance. *Clin. Geriatr. Med.* **2011**, *27*, 337–339. [CrossRef]
9. International Classification of Diseases 11th Revision (Version 04/2019). Foundation Id. Available online: http://id.who.int/icd/entity/1254324785 (accessed on 23 December 2019).
10. Cawthon, P.M. Recent progress in sarcopenia research: A focus on operationalizing a definition of sarcopenia. *Curr. Osteoporos. Rep.* **2018**, *16*, 730–737. [CrossRef]
11. Reiss, J.; Iglseder, B.; Alzner, R.; Mayr-Pirker, B.; Pirich, C.; Kässmann, H.; Kreutzer, M.; Dovjak, P.; Reiter, R. Consequences of applying the new EWGSOP2 guideline instead of the former EWGSOP guideline for sarcopenia case finding in older patients. *Age Ageing* **2019**, *48*, 719–724. [CrossRef]
12. Villani, A.; McClure, R.; Barrett, M.; Scott, D. Diagnostic differences and agreement between the original and revised European Working Group (EWGSOP) consensus definition for sarcopenia in community-dwelling older adults with type 2 diabetes mellitus. *Arch. Gerontol. Geriatr.* **2020**, *89*, 104081. [CrossRef]
13. Bruyère, O.; Beaudart, C.; Reginster, J.Y.; Buckinx, F.; Schoene, D.; Hirani, V.; Cooper, C.; Kanis, J.A.; Rizzoli, R.; Cederholm, T.; et al. Assessment of muscle mass, muscle strength and physical performance in clinical practice: An international survey. *Eur. Geriatr. Med.* **2016**, *7*, 243–246. [CrossRef]
14. Hida, T.; Ishiguro, N.; Shimokata, H.; Sakai, Y.; Matsui, Y.; Takemura, M.; Terabe, Y.; Harada, A. High prevalence of sarcopenia and reduced leg muscle mass in Japanese patients immediately after a hip fracture. *Geriatr. Gerontol. Int.* **2013**, *13*, 413–420. [CrossRef]
15. Gentil, P.; Lima, R.M.; Jacó de Oliveira, R.; Pereira, R.W.; Reis, V.M. Association between femoral neck bone density and lower limb fat-free mass in postmenopausal women. *J. Clin. Densitom.* **2007**, *10*, 174–178. [CrossRef] [PubMed]
16. Cruz-Jentoft, A.J.; Sayer, A.A. Sarcopenia. *Lancet* **2019**, *393*, 2636–2646. [CrossRef]
17. Hansen, R.D.; Williamson, D.A.; Finnegan, T.P.; Lloyd, B.D.; Grady, J.N.; Diamond, T.H.; Smith, E.U.; Stavrinos, T.M.; Thompson, M.W.; Gwinn, T.H.; et al. Estimation of thigh muscle cross-sectional area by dual-energy X-ray absorptiometry in frail elderly patients. *Am. J. Clin. Nutr.* **2007**, *86*, 952–958. [CrossRef]
18. Dalton, J.T.; Barnette, K.G.; Bohl, C.E.; Hancock, M.L.; Rodriguez, D.; Dodson, S.T.; Morton, R.A.; Steiner, M.S. The selective androgen receptor modulator GTx-024 (enobosarm) improves lean body mass and physical function in healthy elderly men and postmenopausal women: Results of a double-blind, placebo-controlled phase II trial. *J. Cachexia Sarcopenia Muscle* **2011**, *2*, 153–161. [CrossRef]
19. Papanicolaou, D.A.; Ather, S.N.; Zhu, H.; Zhou, Y.; Lutkiewicz, J.; Scott, B.B.; Chandler, J. A phase IIA randomized, placebo-controlled clinical trial to study the efficacy and safety of the selective androgen receptor modulator (SARM), MK-0773 in female participants with sarcopenia. *J. Nutr. Health Aging* **2013**, *17*, 533–543. [CrossRef]
20. Hong, W.; Cheng, Q.; Zhu, X.; Zhu, H.; Li, H.; Zhang, X.; Zheng, S.; Du, Y.; Tang, W.; Xue, S.; et al. Prevalence of Sarcopenia and Its Relationship with Sites of Fragility Fractures in Elderly Chinese Men and Women. *PLoS ONE* **2015**, *10*, e0138102. [CrossRef]
21. Moher, D.; Liberati, A.; Tetzlaff, J.; Altman, D.G.; PRISMA Group. Preferred reporting items for systematic reviews and meta-analyses: The PRISMA statement. *PLoS Med.* **2009**, *6*, e1000097. [CrossRef]

22. Sterne, J.A.; Hernán, M.A.; Reeves, B.C.; Savović, J.; Berkman, N.D.; Viswanathan, M.; Henry, D.; Altman, D.G.; Ansari, M.T.; Boutron, I.; et al. ROBINS-I: A tool for assessing risk of bias in non-randomised studies of interventions. *BMJ* **2016**, *355*, 4919. [CrossRef] [PubMed]
23. Kramer, I.F.; Snijders, T.; Smeets, J.; Leenders, M.; van Kranenburg, J.; den Hoed, M.; Verdijk, L.B.; Poeze, M.; van Loon, L. Extensive Type II Muscle Fiber Atrophy in Elderly Female Hip Fracture Patients. *J. Gerontol. A Biol. Sci. Med. Sci.* **2017**, *72*, 1369–1375. [CrossRef] [PubMed]
24. Villani, A.M.; Miller, M.; Cameron, I.D.; Kurrle, S.; Whitehead, C.; Crotty, M. Body composition in older community-dwelling adults with hip fracture: Portable field methods validated by dual-energy X-ray absorptiometry. *Br. J. Nutr.* **2013**, *109*, 1219–1229. [CrossRef]
25. Flodin, L.; Cederholm, T.; Sääf, M.; Samnegård, E.; Ekström, W.; Al-Ani, A.N.; Hedström, M. Effects of protein-rich nutritional supplementation and bisphosphonates on body composition, handgrip strength and health-related quality of life after hip fracture: A 12-month randomized controlled study. *BMC Geriatr.* **2015**, *15*, 149. [CrossRef]
26. Invernizzi, M.; de Sire, A.; D'Andrea, F.; Carrera, D.; Renò, F.; Migliaccio, S.; Iolascon, G.; Cisari, C. Effects of essential amino acid supplementation and rehabilitation on functioning in hip fracture patients: A pilot randomized controlled trial. *Aging Clin. Exp. Res.* **2019**, *31*, 1517–1524. [CrossRef]
27. Malafarina, V.; Uriz-Otano, F.; Malafarina, C.; Martinez, J.A.; Zulet, M.A. Effectiveness of nutritional supplementation on sarcopenia and recovery in hip fracture patients. A multi-centre randomized trial. *Maturitas* **2017**, *101*, 42–50. [CrossRef]
28. Chan, D.C.; Chang, C.B.; Han, D.S.; Hong, C.H.; Hwang, J.S.; Tsai, K.S.; Yang, R.S. Effects of exercise improves muscle strength and fat mass in patients with high fracture risk: A randomized control trial. *J. Formos. Med. Assoc.* **2018**, *117*, 572–582. [CrossRef]
29. Gillette-Guyonnet, S.; Nourhashemi, F.; Lauque, S.; Grandjean, H.; Vellas, B. Body composition and osteoporosis in elderly women. *Gerontology* **2000**, *46*, 189–193. [CrossRef]
30. Walsh, M.C.; Hunter, G.R.; Livingstone, M.B. Sarcopenia in premenopausal and postmenopausal women with osteopenia, osteoporosis and normal bone mineral density. *Osteoporos. Int.* **2006**, *17*, 61–67. [CrossRef]
31. Locquet, M.; Beaudart, C.; Bruyère, O.; Kanis, J.A.; Delandsheere, L.; Reginster, J.Y. Bone health assessment in older people with or without muscle health impairment. *Osteoporos. Int.* **2018**, *29*, 1057–1067. [CrossRef]
32. Hirschfeld, H.P.; Kinsella, R.; Duque, G. Osteosarcopenia: Where bone, muscle, and fat collide. *Osteoporos. Int.* **2018**, *28*, 2781–2790. [CrossRef]
33. Roberts, H.C.; Denison, H.J.; Martin, H.J.; Patel, H.P.; Syddall, H.; Cooper, C.; Sayer, A.A. A review of the measurement of grip strength in clinical and epidemiological studies: Towards a standardised approach. *Age Ageing* **2011**, *40*, 423–429. [CrossRef]
34. Beaudart, C.; McCloskey, E.; Bruyère, O.; Cesari, M.; Rolland, Y.; Rizzoli, R.; Araujo de Carvalho, I.; Amuthavalli Thiyagarajan, J.; Bautmans, I.; Bertière, M.C.; et al. Sarcopenia in daily practice: Assessment and management. *BMC Geriatr.* **2016**, *16*, 170. [CrossRef] [PubMed]
35. Maggio, M.; Ceda, G.P.; Ticinesi, A.; De Vita, F.; Gelmini, G.; Costantino, C.; Meschi, T.; Kressig, R.W.; Cesari, M.; Fabi, M.; et al. Instrumental and non-instrumental evaluation of 4-meter walking speed in older individuals. *PLoS ONE* **2016**, *11*, e0153583. [CrossRef] [PubMed]
36. Rydwik, E.; Bergland, A.; Forsén, L.; Frändin, K. Investigation into the reliability and validity of the measurement of elderly people's clinical walking speed: A systematic review. *Physiother. Theory Pract.* **2012**, *28*, 238–256. [CrossRef]
37. Podsiadlo, D.; Richardson, S. The timed 'Up & Go': A test of basic functional mobility for frail elderly persons. *J. Am. Geriatr. Soc.* **1991**, *39*, 142–148.
38. Treviño-Aguirre, E.; López-Teros, T.; Gutiérrez-Robledo, L.; Vandewoude, M.; Pérez-Zepeda, M. Availability and use of dual energy X-ray absorptiometry (DXA) and bio-impedance analysis (BIA) for the evaluation of sarcopenia by Belgian and Latin American geriatricians. *J. Cachexia Sarcopenia Muscle* **2014**, *5*, 79–81. [CrossRef]
39. McGregor, R.A.; Cameron-Smith, D.; Poppitt, S.D. It is not just muscle mass: A review of muscle quality, composition and metabolism during ageing as determinants of muscle function and mobility in later life. *Longev. Healthspan* **2014**, *3*, 9. [CrossRef]

40. Nilwik, R.; Snijders, T.; Leenders, M.; Groen, B.B.; van Kranenburg, J.; Verdijk, L.B.; van Loon, L.J. The decline in skeletal muscle mass with aging is mainly attributed to a reduction in type II muscle fiber size. *Exp. Gerontol.* **2013**, *48*, 492–498. [CrossRef]
41. Malafarina, V.; Reginster, J.Y.; Cabrerizo, S.; Bruyère, O.; Kanis, J.A.; Martinez, J.A.; Zulet, M.A. Nutritional Status and Nutritional Treatment Are Related to Outcomes and Mortality in Older Adults with Hip Fracture. *Nutrients* **2018**, *10*, 555. [CrossRef]
42. Bauer, J.; Biolo, G.; Cederholm, T.; Cesari, M.; Cruz-Jentoft, A.J.; Morley, J.E.; Phillips, S.; Sieber, C.; Stehle, P.; Teta, D.; et al. Evidence-based recommendations for optimal dietary protein intake in older people: A position paper from the PROT-AGE Study Group. *J. Am. Med. Dir. Assoc.* **2013**, *14*, 542–559. [CrossRef] [PubMed]
43. Deer, R.R.; Volpi, E. Protein intake and muscle function in older adults. *Curr. Opin. Clin. Nutr. Metab. Care* **2015**, *18*, 248–253. [CrossRef] [PubMed]
44. Dodds, R.; Kuh, D.; Aihie Sayer, A.; Cooper, R. Physical activity levels across adult life and grip strength in early old age: Updating findings from a British birth cohort. *Age Ageing* **2013**, *42*, 794–798. [CrossRef]
45. Landi, F.; Calvani, R.; Picca, A.; Marzetti, E. Beta-hydroxy-beta-methylbutyrate and sarcopenia: From biological plausibility to clinical evidence. *Curr. Opin. Clin. Nutr. Metab. Care* **2019**, *22*, 37–43. [CrossRef]
46. Piastra, G.; Perasso, L.; Lucarini, S.; Monacelli, F.; Bisio, A.; Ferrando, V.; Gallamini, M.; Faelli, E.; Ruggeri, P. Effects of Two Types of 9-Month Adapted Physical Activity Program on Muscle Mass, Muscle Strength, and Balance in Moderate Sarcopenic Older Women. *Biomed. Res. Int.* **2018**, *2018*, 5095673. [CrossRef]
47. Singh, N.A.; Quine, S.; Clemson, L.M.; Williams, E.J.; Williamson, D.A.; Stavrinos, T.M.; Grady, J.N.; Perry, T.J.; Lloyd, B.D.; Smith, E.U.; et al. Effects of High-Intensity Progressive Resistance Training and Targeted Multidisciplinary Treatment of Frailty on Mortality and Nursing Home Admissions After Hip Fracture: A Randomized Controlled Trial. *J. Am. Med. Dir. Assoc.* **2012**, *13*, 24–30. [CrossRef] [PubMed]

Permissions

All chapters in this book were first published by MDPI; hereby published with permission under the Creative Commons Attribution License or equivalent. Every chapter published in this book has been scrutinized by our experts. Their significance has been extensively debated. The topics covered herein carry significant findings which will fuel the growth of the discipline. They may even be implemented as practical applications or may be referred to as a beginning point for another development.

The contributors of this book come from diverse backgrounds, making this book a truly international effort. This book will bring forth new frontiers with its revolutionizing research information and detailed analysis of the nascent developments around the world.

We would like to thank all the contributing authors for lending their expertise to make the book truly unique. They have played a crucial role in the development of this book. Without their invaluable contributions this book wouldn't have been possible. They have made vital efforts to compile up to date information on the varied aspects of this subject to make this book a valuable addition to the collection of many professionals and students.

This book was conceptualized with the vision of imparting up-to-date information and advanced data in this field. To ensure the same, a matchless editorial board was set up. Every individual on the board went through rigorous rounds of assessment to prove their worth. After which they invested a large part of their time researching and compiling the most relevant data for our readers.

The editorial board has been involved in producing this book since its inception. They have spent rigorous hours researching and exploring the diverse topics which have resulted in the successful publishing of this book. They have passed on their knowledge of decades through this book. To expedite this challenging task, the publisher supported the team at every step. A small team of assistant editors was also appointed to further simplify the editing procedure and attain best results for the readers.

Apart from the editorial board, the designing team has also invested a significant amount of their time in understanding the subject and creating the most relevant covers. They scrutinized every image to scout for the most suitable representation of the subject and create an appropriate cover for the book.

The publishing team has been an ardent support to the editorial, designing and production team. Their endless efforts to recruit the best for this project, has resulted in the accomplishment of this book. They are a veteran in the field of academics and their pool of knowledge is as vast as their experience in printing. Their expertise and guidance has proved useful at every step. Their uncompromising quality standards have made this book an exceptional effort. Their encouragement from time to time has been an inspiration for everyone.

The publisher and the editorial board hope that this book will prove to be a valuable piece of knowledge for researchers, students, practitioners and scholars across the globe.

List of Contributors

Ana Coto-Montes
Department of Morphology and Cellular Biology, Medicine Faculty, University of Oviedo, Julian Claveria, s/n, Oviedo 33006, Spain
Department of Cellular and Structural Biology, UTHSCSA, San Antonio, TX 78229, USA

Dun X. Tan and Russel J. Reiter
Department of Cellular and Structural Biology, UTHSCSA, San Antonio, TX 78229, USA

Jose A. Boga
Department of Cellular and Structural Biology, UTHSCSA, San Antonio, TX 78229, USA
Service of Microbiology, Hospital Universitario Central de Asturias, Avenida de Roma, s/n, Oviedo 33011, Spain

Carlotta Roncaglione and Paolo Rossi
Geriatric Unit, Fondazione IRCCS Ca' Granda Ospedale Maggiore Policlinico, 20122 Milan, Italy

Sarah Damanti and Domenico Azzolino
Geriatric Unit, Fondazione IRCCS Ca' Granda Ospedale Maggiore Policlinico, 20122 Milan, Italy
Phd Course in Nutritional Sciences, University of Milan, 20122 Milan, Italy

Beatrice Arosio and Matteo Cesari
Geriatric Unit, Fondazione IRCCS Ca' Granda Ospedale Maggiore Policlinico, 20122 Milan, Italy
Department of Clinical Sciences and Community Health, University of Milan, 20122 Milan, Italy

Maria L. Petroni, Maria T. Caletti and Giulio Marchesini
Unit of Metabolic Diseases and Clinical Dietetics, Sant'Orsola-Malpighi Hospital, "Alma Mater" University, via G. Massarenti 9, 40138 Bologna, Italy

Riccardo Dalle Grave
Department of Eating and Weight Disorders, Villa Garda Hospital, via Monte Baldo 89, 37016 Garda (VR), Italy

Alberto Bazzocchi
Diagnostic and Interventional Radiology, IRCCS Istituto Ortopedico Rizzoli, via G.C. Pupilli 1, 40136 Bologna, Italy

Maria P. Aparisi Gómez
Department of Radiology, Auckland City Hospital, Park Road, Grafton, 1023 Auckland, New Zealand

Anne-Julie Tessier
School of Human Nutrition, McGill University, 21111 Lakeshore Rd, Ste-Anne-de-Bellevue, QC H9X 3V9, Canada
Research Institute of the McGill University Health Centre, 1001 Décarie Blvd, Montreal, QC H4A 3J1, Canada

Stéphanie Chevalier
School of Human Nutrition, McGill University, 21111 Lakeshore Rd, Ste-Anne-de-Bellevue, QC H9X 3V9, Canada
Research Institute of the McGill University Health Centre, 1001 Décarie Blvd, Montreal, QC H4A 3J1, Canada
Department of Medicine, McGill University, 845 Sherbrooke St. W, Montreal, QC H3A 0G4, Canada

Máximo Bernabeu-Wittel, Álvaro González-Molina and Manuel Ollero-Baturone
Internal Medicine Department, Hospital Universitario Virgen del Rocío, 41013 Sevilla, Spain

Raquel Gómez-Díaz
General and Multiple Use Laboratory, Instituto de Biomedicina de Sevilla, 41013 Sevilla, Spain

Sofía Vidal-Serrano
Internal Medicine Department, Hospital San Juan de Dios del Aljarafe, 41930 Sevilla, Spain

Jesús Díez-Manglano
Internal Medicine Department, Hospital Royo Villanova, 50015 Zaragoza, Spain

Fernando Salgado
Internal Medicine Department, Hospital Regional, 29010 Málaga, Spain

María Soto-Martín
Internal Medicine Department, Hospital Juan Ramón Jiménez, 21005 Huelva, Spain

Ilse J. M. Hagedoorn, Milou M. Oosterwijk and Gozewijn D. Laverman
Division of Nephrology, Department of Internal Medicine, Ziekenhuisgroep Twente, 7609 PP Almelo, The Netherlands

Bert-Jan F. van Beijnum
Faculty of Electrical Engineering, Mathematics and Computer Science, University of Twente, 7522 NB Enschede, The Netherlands

Niala den Braber and Miriam M. R. Vollenbroek-Hutten
Division of Nephrology, Department of Internal Medicine, Ziekenhuisgroep Twente, 7609 PP Almelo, The Netherlands
Faculty of Electrical Engineering, Mathematics and Computer Science, University of Twente, 7522 NB Enschede, The Netherlands

Gerjan Navis and Stephan J. L. Bakker
Division of Nephrology, Department of Internal Medicine, University of Groningen, University Medical Center Groningen, 9713 GZ Groningen, The Netherlands

Christina M. Gant
Division of Nephrology, Department of Internal Medicine, University of Groningen, University Medical Center Groningen, 9713 GZ Groningen, The Netherlands
Department of Internal Medicine, Meander Medisch Centrum, 3813 TZ Amersfoort, The Netherlands

Mariana Cevei and Felicia Cioara
Psychoneuro Sciences and Rehabilitation Department, Faculty of Medicine & Pharmacy, University of Oradea, 410087 Oradea, Romania

Roxana Ramona Onofrei
Department of Rehabilitation, Physical Medicine and Rheumatology, "Victor Babeş" University of Medicine and Pharmacy Timişoara, 300041 Timişoara, Romania

Dorina Stoicanescu
Microscopic Morphology Department, "Victor Babeş" University of Medicine and Pharmacy Timişoara, 300041 Timişoara, Romania

Jacobo Á. Rubio-Arias
LFE Research Group, Department of Health and Human Performance, Faculty of Physical Activity and Sport Science-INEF, Universidad Politécnica de Madrid, 28040 Madrid, Spain

Raquel Rodríguez-Fernández
Department of Methodology of Behavioral Sciences, Faculty of Psychology, Universidad Nacional de Educación a Distancia (UNED), 28040 Madrid, Spain

Luis Andreu
International Chair of Sports Medicine, Universidad Católica San Antonio de Murcia (UCAM), 30107 Murcia, Spain
Faculty of Sports, Universidad Católica San Antonio de Murcia (UCAM), 30107 Murcia, Spain

Domingo J. Ramos-Campo
Faculty of Sports, Universidad Católica San Antonio de Murcia (UCAM), 30107 Murcia, Spain

Luis M. Martínez-Aranda
Faculty of Sports, Universidad Católica San Antonio de Murcia (UCAM), 30107 Murcia, Spain
Neuroscience of Human Movement Research Group (Neuromove), Universidad Católica San Antonio de Murcia (UCAM), 30107 Murcia, Spain

Alejandro Martínez-Rodriguez
Department of Analytical Chemistry, Nutrition and Food Science, Faculty of Science, Alicante University, 03690 Alicante, Spain

Frank D. Thøgersen, Khaled Abdul Nasser Qadri, Thomas Krag, John Vissing and Tina D. Jeppesen
Department of Neurology, Copenhagen Neuromuscular Center, Rigshospitalet, DK-2100 Copenhagen, Denmark

Andreas Mæchel Fritzen
Department of Neurology, Copenhagen Neuromuscular Center, Rigshospitalet, DK-2100 Copenhagen, Denmark
Molecular Physiology Group, Department of Nutrition, Exercise, and Sports, Faculty of Science, University of Copenhagen, DK-2100 Copenhagen, Denmark

Marie-Louise Sveen
Department of Neurology, Copenhagen Neuromuscular Center, Rigshospitalet, DK-2100 Copenhagen, Denmark
Novo Nordisk A/S, DK-2860 Søborg, Denmark

Nejc Šarabon
Faculty of Health Sciences, University of Primorska, Polje 42, SI-6310 Izola, Slovenia
InnoRenew CoE, Human Health Department, Livade 6, SI6310 Izola, Slovenia
S2P, Science to practice, Ltd., Laboratory for Motor Control and Motor Behavior, Tehnološki Park 19, SI-1000 Ljubljana, Slovenia

Žiga Kozinc
Faculty of Health Sciences, University of Primorska, Polje 42, SI-6310 Izola, Slovenia
Andrej Maruši˘c Institute, University of Primorska, Muzejski Trg 2, SI-6000 Koper, Slovenia

Stefan Löfler
Physiko- & Rheumatherapie, Institute for Physical Medicine and Rehabilitation, 3100 St. Pölten, Austria
Centre of Active Ageing—Competence Centre for Health, Prevention and Active Ageing, 3100 St. Pölten, Austria

Christian Hofer
Ludwig Boltzmann Institute for Rehabilitation Research, 3100 St. Pölten, Austria

Raquel Fábrega-Cuadros, Agustín Aibar-Almazán, Antonio Martínez-Amat and Fidel Hita-Contreras
Department of Health Sciences, Faculty of Health Sciences, University of Jaén, 23071 Jaén, Spain

Francisco Miguel Martínez-Arnau
Department of Physiotherapy, University of Valencia, 46010 Valencia, Spain
Frailty and Cognitive Impairment Research Group (FROG), University of Valencia, 46010 Valencia, Spain

Cristina Buigues, Rosa Fonfría-Vivas and Omar Cauli
Frailty and Cognitive Impairment Research Group (FROG), University of Valencia, 46010 Valencia, Spain
Department of Nursing, University of Valencia, 46010 Valencia, Spain

Marianna Avola, Giulia Rita Agata Mangano and Michele Vecchio
Department of Biomedical and Biotechnological Sciences, Section of Pharmacology, University Hospital Policlinico-San Marco University of Catania, 95123 Catania, Italy

Sebastiano Mangano
Department of General Surgery and Medical Surgical Specialties, Section of Orthopaedics and Traumatology, University Hospital Policlinico-San Marco, University of Catania, 95123 Catania, Italy

Gianluca Testa, Andrea Vescio and Vito Pavone
Department of General Surgery and Medical Surgical Specialties, Section of Orthopaedics and Traumatology, University Hospital Policlinico-San Marco, University of Catania, 95123 Catania, Italy
Department of General Surgery and Medical Surgical Specialties, Section of Orthopaedics and Traumatology, University Hospital Policlinico-San Marco, University of Catania, 95124 Catania, Italy

Søren Peter Andersen and Mette C. Ørngreen
Department of Neurology, Copenhagen Neuromuscular Center, Rigshospitalet, DK-2100 Copenhagen, Denmark

Danilo Zuccalà, Vincenzo Petrantoni, Mirko Amico and Giuseppe Sessa
Department of General Surgery and Medical Surgical Specialties, Section of Orthopaedics and Traumatology, University Hospital Policlinico-San Marco, University of Catania, 95124 Catania, Italy

Giorgio Ivan Russo
Department of General Surgery and Medical Surgical Specialties, Urology Section, University Hospital Policlinico-San Marco, University of Catania, 95124 Catania, Italy

Index

Printed in the USA
CPSIA information can be obtained
at www.ICGtesting.com
JSHW051406091023
49903JS00006B/301